WOMAN'S HOUR
BOOK
of
HEALTH

By women,
for women,
about women

Dr Ann McPherson and Nancy Durham

For Gill + Richard
love
Nancy.

BBC BOOKS

Published by BBC Books, an imprint of BBC Worldwide Ltd,
Woodlands, 80 Wood Lane, London W12 OTT

First published in 1998

ISBN 0 563 37028 9

Art Directed by Jane Coney
Design styling by Town Group Creative
Designed by Ann Burnham
Graphs by Ben Cracknell
Charts by Ann Burnham
Illustrations by Alan Burton

Printed and bound in Great Britain by Butler & Tanner Ltd, Frome and London
Cover printed by Belmont Press Ltd, Northampton

Contents

The Authors

Dr Ann McPherson is a family doctor in Oxford and is not only highly experienced in helping others, but also, having recently had breast cancer herself, has had to take 'a dose of her own medicine' as a patient. This experience was partially responsible for her wanting to write the present book using women's own experiences. As a leading expert on the health of women she has already created the definitive book on women's health for GPs, *Women's Problems in General Practice*, first published in 1984. This continues to be the bestseller in the Oxford University General Practice series and is now in its 4th edition. Her experiences as a doctor, writer and mother also led her to co-author, with Aidan Macfarlane, a series of books for teenagers including *Diary of a Teenage Health Freak*, which has been made into two successful TV series and sold more than half a million copies as well as being available in twenty-two other languages. She is also the BBC Thames Valley Radio Doctor, doing a monthly phone-in on all matters of health. She is married to Klim McPherson who is Professor of Epidemiology at the London School of Hygiene and Tropical Medicine. They have three children, aged twenty-eight, twenty-six and twenty-two. She is a fellow of Green College and the Royal College of General Practitioners.

Nancy Durham is a journalist renowned for her coverage of war and politics from a human perspective. Since moving to Britain from Canada in 1984 she has reported from thirty-one countries for the BBC and CBC TV and Radio. Nancy is one of the new TV pioneers: reporter, producer, and camera operator in one, gathering material on her own whether in Britain, Bosnia, Rwanda, or in the cockpit of a MiG 29 jet fighter where she filmed the Hungarian Air Force at work. Her vivid portrayals of the lives of women around the world have been featured on *Woman's Hour* since 1985. Nancy has covered women's stories of survival in war in Mozambique, Malawi and throughout the Balkans. During the Balkan war she travelled in a hay wagon with Serb refugee mothers fleeing their homes. She has documented the Albanian women's fight for equality, and the trouble with sex, contraception and abortion in both China and Romania. During the unrest in Kosovo, Yugoslavia, in March 1998, she filmed in the operating rooms of the Albanians' illegally run hospitals. Nancy Durham has also lectured on journalism in the former Czechoslovakia, Romania, China, and at London's Westminster University.

Acknowledgements

This book is a collaboration between ourselves and many others: the many women who talked candidly to us about their most intimate physical and mental health experiences; the dozens of women who told their stories to *Woman's Hour*; and a few men who shared with us their views of the opposite sex. We thank them for sharing their thoughts and experiences.

BBC Radio 4's *Woman's Hour* (WH) is the creation of a talented team, and every member of it is a contributor to our book. Karen Deco's WH report on grief and Claire Jenkins's feature on sex therapy were especially helpful to us. We thank presenter Jenni Murray for always asking great questions. We salute former WH editor Sally Feldman who, with support from Angie Nehring, conceived the idea for this book. Nadine Grieve, Managing Editor of Topical Features, joined the project in its final year – she was always encouraging and made many helpful suggestions. WH Editor, Emma Selby, acting editor Hazel Castell and health producer Jayne Egerton helped bring the book home in the last months. Salley Rear, our loyal liaison at WH for four years, supplied us with endless show tapes thus keeping us up to date with the latest in WH medical news.

Dr Alison Bigrigg and Dr Mollie McBride both acted as consultants on this book, and we appreciate their careful reading of the manuscript and their perceptive comments.

We acknowledge the many other experts who were generous with their time and advice: Dr Joan Austoker on screening, Professor David Barlow on infertility, Professor Michael Baum on breasts, Dr Joan Bassey on bone mineral density, Toni Bellafield on contraception, Dr William Bird on exercise and calories, Professor Colin Blakemore on the mind, Ophthalmologist Professor Anthony Bron on cataracts, Jane Hanna and Alison Campbell for advice on health service complaints, Psychotherapist Frances Campbell, Epidemiologist Eileen Clarke, Professor Christopher Conlan on HIV, Dr Angela Coulter on who gets referred to hospital, Dr Rodney Dawber on skin, Professor John Guillebaud and Dr Elizabeth Greenhall on contraception, Dr Gillian Lockwood on infertility, Alison Macfarlane of the National Perinatal Epidemiology Unit, Dr William C. Orr on sleep, Dr Simon Plint on hypertension, Professor Richard Peto on smoking and health, Dr Margaret Rees on the menopause and periods, Dermatologist Professor Terence Ryan, Halina St James, Tracey Berry and Kevin Martin on alternative medicine, Dermatologist Vanessa Venning, Kaye Wellings on sex, and Gynaecologist Janice Willet on screening.

The researchers at the BBC News and Information Library in Broadcasting House were fast and fantastic. We thank Claire Panter and Penny Young of BBC Broadcasting Research for their work on the *Woman's Hour* survey as well as all the women who participated in the study.

Several organizations and government agencies gave us background briefings, diagrams and statistics. We thank The British Heart Foundation; The British Pregnancy Advisory Service; The Department for Education and Employment; Ann Barker, Laurence Knight and Chris Warburton at the Department of Health; Effective Health Care Bulletins; Euromonitor; The Family Planning Association and its Contraceptive Education Service; Sean Larkins and Catherine Evans at the Health Education Authority; The Human Fertilisation and Embryology Authority; The National Sports Medicine Institute of the UK; The NHS Centre for Reviews and Dissemination; The National Childbirth Trust; The National Osteoporosis Society; The Nuffield Institute for Health; David Marder, Rebecca Wood and Alison Wright at the Office for National Statistics; The Office of Population and Census Surveys; Jennifer Guy at the Ontario Medical Association; Simon Barber at the Public Health Laboratory Service; Quit; The Sports Council; Marie Stopes International; The University of Leeds; The University of York; Noorece Ahmed at The Wellcome Trust.

Our data on miscarriage comes from research by Dr Christopher Everett writing in the *British Medical Journal* Volume 315, 5 July 1997. Statistics on types of birth delivery come from the House of Commons Health Committee replies written to Questions 1995–6. We are also indebted to the authors of the *National Survey of Sexual Attitudes and Lifestyles* and all of the authors of *Women's Health in General Practice* edited by Ann McPherson and Deborah Waller.

Michele Wates, author of *Disabled Parents: Dispelling the Myths*, published by NCT and the Radcliffe Medical Press, advised us on women and disability. We are grateful to Joy Archibald for allowing us to quote from her late daughter's diary. Jeannette Matthey died of breast cancer in October 1993, aged 37. We also thank Rebecca Armstrong, Charly Smith, Jennifer Chevalier and Margaret Corrigan for their help with research and fact-checking.

We thank Heather Holden-Brown, formerly of BBC Books, for commissioning the book. Nicola Copeland inherited it and treated it as if it were her own. Our copy-editor, Susan Martineau, was enthusiastic and thorough. We also thank Melissa Lombardelli and all the members of the publicity and marketing team for their enthusiasm in promoting this book. And it has been a delight to work day to day with our project editor, Lara Speicher, who gave the manuscript her critical eye while providing us with constant encouragement.

We are in debt to many unnamed friends, relatives and colleagues who cheerfully allowed us to interrogate them. This was often informal but nevertheless invaluable to us.

Ann would like to give special thanks to Klim McPherson for his advice on matters epidemiological; and her three children Sam, Tess and Beth who along with Klim tolerated her distracted state during the writing of the book – together with James and Jane they especially helped with the final details. Rachel Miller, Deborah Waller, Aidan Macfarlane, Jacky Maxmin and Lyz Minton all helped in their individual ways to see this book through to completion. They provided chat, laughter, meals and cups of tea as well as encouragement and critical comment, especially when the going got tough.

Nancy thanks her husband Bill Newton-Smith for his infinite cheer as well as his philosophical comments on the manuscript. She thanks all her family for their encouragement, but especially her parents Bess and Warren whose pursuit of long and healthy lives is a constant inspiration. Her two WSDs Apple and Rain are an inspiration to her for everything, but especially the health and hopes of young women. She is especially indebted to nine outstanding women (who know who they are). They brought this book to life for her, and spirited her through the writing of it.

Dr Ann McPherson and Nancy Durham
Oxford, 1998

Introduction

This health book is unique. Even before we began we had riches. Our resource base is a BBC Radio Four programme which has been informing women for over half a century. We have drawn from hundreds of interviews and feature reports broadcast on *Woman's Hour*. The *Woman's Hour* voice is often but not exclusively a woman's voice; some are famous but most are not. They come from all walks of British life and sometimes from abroad. All of these voices are represented here: Dusty Springfield reveals how she felt upon discovering her breast cancer and Lesley talks about what it is like to be dying from it; Julie Andrews muses on the power of her ageing voice; Linda describes the thrill of a revived sex life; Honor Blackman says her beauty is probably in her genes; Mandy talks about the grief of losing her husband at the age of thirty-seven.

We did not rely exclusively on *Woman's Hour*. We conducted about seventy interviews over three years with women of all ages and in all stages of life. Most of the interviews were carried out in the UK, but we also talked to several North American women, including medical experts, to compare notes and health concerns over our two continents. We asked them questions on all matters of health: periods, menopause, sex, beauty, anxiety and ageing. We returned to several of our 'subjects' on many occasions to ask further questions. Some women have been identified – these are usually the experts and the famous – others we refer to by their first names, and in a few cases, with the use of a pseudonym. Women's ages were not always available. Women talked to us in a remarkably candid way revealing the most intimate details of their private lives. Their stories tell of triumph over illness, and are always loaded with the lessons of experience and experiment. Their stories are inspirational and informative, although their views are their own and other people may not always agree with them.

Throughout the writing of this book, we also monitored the news for developments on the women's health front. Such is the pace of discovery in medicine that there is something new practically every day, casting doubt on old beliefs, shedding light on new ones. We also include the results of a women's health survey especially commissioned for our book (see Chapter 1). Everyone's health is obviously of great importance to them and to those close to them. Women, however, for all the years of liberation, are still the major carers both for children and the elderly. Women have to be healthy and are doing well. Female life expectancy at birth is now eighty years whilst for men it is seventy-five. One hundred and fifty years ago the figures were forty-two years for women, forty for men. Tuberculosis and infections associated with childbirth were the main causes of death for women in the 1800s with TB accounting for 26 per cent of deaths in women under forty-five as recently as 1930. Today, heart disease and cancer are the major killers of women.

At the beginning of the century, free health care for women was limited to those who had jobs outside the home, however, all pregnant women were cared for by their local health authorities. In 1939 the Women's Health Enquiry Committee found women's main complaints were anaemia, headaches, constipation, rheumatism, gynaecological trouble, dental problems, varicose veins and ulcerated legs. Today headaches and gynaecological problems are the number one complaints of women, while the other ailments from the above list written on the eve of the Second World War are unchanged. But there has been a revolution in the way reproduction is handled – the birth control pill changed women's lives forever and brought new problems with it. Now a new pill, Hormone Replacement Therapy, is revolutionizing middle age.

The modern woman has more contact with doctors than ever before, especially when it comes to contraception, pregnancy and infant checks. Women are dominant in the health professions where they work as nurses, physiotherapists and midwives, and women now make up over 50 per cent of new medical students. The National Health Service, formed in 1948, gave all women – for the first time – access to universal free health care in the UK. Today the NHS is fighting to continue to deliver arguably the best free health care on earth.

Poverty continues to be the main threat to women's health. Poorer women are more likely to have baby deaths, more illness and to die earlier. Professional women live longer and enjoy a healthier life. Overall, though, women do have a better quality of life now than in the past. Women know how to live well and how to get the help they need from the health services. When the modern woman sees doctors and other health professionals, she meets them on a much more level playing field than her grandmother could have imagined. There is so much health information available, through the media and the internet, that it can be difficult to sift through, to decide what to believe and whom to trust. We offer this book as a reliable guide to help women make decisions based on the best scientific evidence available. Sometimes there will be no obvious right or wrong treatment. Dealing with uncertainty makes choices even more difficult, but decisions about health and treatment are best made in partnership with carers and loved ones. There will be times when an exhausted or anxious patient may want others to take decisions but such moments should be chosen, not forced.

Like *Woman's Hour* itself we hope to inform and offer a diversity of opinion – as well as entertain. We look at the key areas of women's health, and this book can be read from start to finish or dipped into. We have not included every single disease and certainly not many which are common to men too. It is a sort of recipe book for health, and we hope readers will compare methods and remedies and learn what works best. This book belongs to all of the women who told their stories and to all of the women who see themselves through them.

introduction

women's health concerns

Kelly, 21: Breast cancer scares me. It's not like I expect to get it tomorrow. I just think it's really frightening how risky it is … and how little people know about it.

Jennifer, 44: *As women we really sort of analyse our bodies and what's wrong with them ... this part's too flabby and this part's too this and too that.*

Marge, 24: *You have to go to the doctor regularly to deal with birth control. That sums up the problem of being a woman. But you're far more in tune with your body than a man is with his. Men don't have a clue what goes on inside them.*

Our bodies are a constant source of wonder and worry. In 1994 BBC Broadcasting research commissioned a special survey for *Woman's Hour* called What Women Think About Their Health. We wanted to know how well women are and how well women think they are. We wanted to know what women think they should do in order to stay healthy, and whether they act on this. We wanted to discover what worries us and what does not, and we wanted to find out how women feel about their doctors. National Opinion Poll (NOP) conducted face-to-face interviews with 531 women throughout Great Britain aged sixteen and up. Each woman also completed a questionnaire. The women in the survey were representative of women across the country, with NOP taking age and region, working status and social class into consideration.

Highlights from the Survey

- Only one in ten women say their health is excellent but nearly half say it's very good.
- One in ten women do not feel in control of their lives.
- Headaches are women's most common health complaint.
- Younger women complain more about their health than older women do.
- Women worry more about getting breast cancer than any other disease.
- More than half of the women interviewed consider themselves overweight.
- Two-thirds of women feel they could do more to stay healthy.
- Two-thirds of women see male doctors and do not mind.
- Only 2 per cent of women see complementary medicine as better than conventional medicine but nearly half see it as a good addition to conventional medicine.

women's health concerns

Which Health Issues Do Women Worry About?

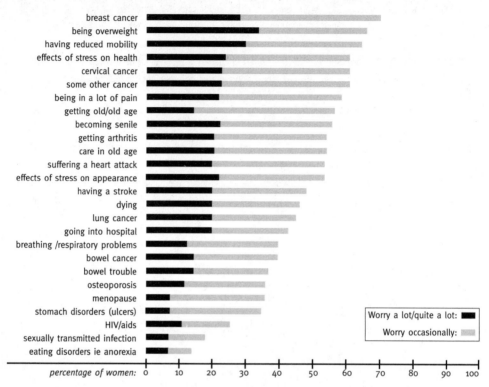

The survey found that our various worries do not always match the health risk in reality. Most women worry about illnesses they do not have now and are never likely to have. For instance, women worry about getting breast cancer more than any other disease, with younger women doing most of the worrying even though they are least at risk. Older women are much more likely to develop breast cancer yet 80 per cent of sixteen to forty-four year olds worry about the possibility (see Chapter 10 for more on breast cancer).

Breast cancer *is* something to worry about. It remains a great mystery and more research must be done to crack it. But we studied figures provided by the National Statistics Office to see just how much of a danger it really is. Breast cancer comes number four on the list of causes of death in women in England and Wales. These figures are for women of all ages so they can look misleading. Younger women are more likely to die in an accident, older women of pneumonia. The six most common causes of death in women (in order) are as follows:

1 Heart disease	4 Breast cancer
2 Stroke	5 Lung cancer
3 Pneumonia	6 Bronchitis

Unlike breast cancer, the number one killer, heart disease, is no mystery. We know something about what causes it and what can be done to help prevent it. Few women are fully aware of the seriousness of the risk of heart disease. In Chapter 13 we explain what you can do to reduce your risk.

Most Common Cancer Deaths, Men and Women, UK 1995

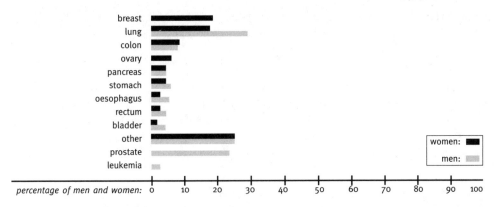

Causes of Death in Women under 75, UK 1995

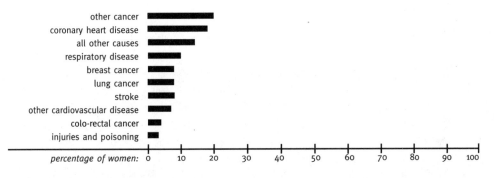

In women and men under the age of thirty-five the most common cause of death is car accidents. In 1996, 336 women died in this way and 1238 men. After that, suicide and cancer were the main causes of death in this age group.

women's health concerns

Worries About Weight

The big demon for so many of us is our weight and our survey found that we worry about it more than anything else. Over half of the women interviewed – and particularly middle-aged women – said they were overweight, although four out of five women still considered their health to be good.

> **Linda, 50:** *I'd like to be thin. But I can't. I can't diet. I just can't do it so I don't. I used to be thin but I'm not and I've accepted that I'm not ... I am what I am. Like it or lump it. I don't like it but I shut my eyes to it.*

> **Margaret, 58:** *I could lose a stone and a half and I would look alright then I think. I eat to comfort myself if I'm feeling a bit depressed.*

Although at least 60 per cent of women have been on a diet at some point in their lives and one in five women are dieting right now, only a small number of women who consider themselves to be overweight are in fact seriously overweight. Yet we still struggle with dieting even though it is generally accepted that taking more exercise and eating a healthy diet are better for your health than any crash diet could ever be.

> **Linda, 41:** *I would like to have a little card, when I die, that says I leave my fat arse to Michelle Pfeiffer and now you live with it! I could donate my thighs to Liz Hurley.*

Is That Me in a Few Years' Time?

The survey found – not surprisingly – that women's concerns about their health vary with age. Younger women complain more about health problems than older women do and they worry more about dying (68 per cent of sixteen to twenty-four year olds) than older women do (35 per cent of over sixty-fives). This suggests that the longer you live the more accepting you become of the inevitable. The big worry of older women is loss of mobility.

> **Marion:** *You do find as you get older that you can't do as much as you thought you could ten years ago. When you see somebody ... who can't move or maybe has a stroke, reduced to a wheelchair, forced to rely on what help is available ... you think 'Is that me in a few years' time?'*

How Worries Vary by Age (percentage of women who worry)

Ages 16–24	%	Ages 45–64	%
Breast cancer	82	Having reduced mobility	76
Cervical cancer	77	Senility	68
Effects of stress on appearance	73	Breast cancer	67
Being overweight	69	Being overweight	65
Being in a lot of pain	69	Other cancer	61
Dying	68	Stroke	60
Other cancer	67	Effects of stress on health	60
HIV/AIDS	64	How will be looked after in old age	58
Effects of stress on health	61	Heart attack	58
Lung cancer	59	Cervical cancer	54
		Arthritis	54
Ages 25–44			
Breast cancer	78	**Age 65+**	
Effects of stress on health	75	Having reduced mobility	72
Cervical cancer	74	Arthritis	65
Being overweight	72	Senility	64
Other cancer	68	How will be looked after in old age	62
Getting old	63	Being in a lot of pain	56
Having reduced mobility	62	Stroke	51
Being in a lot of pain	59	Getting old	49
Effects of stress on appearance	57	Being overweight	47
Arthritis	55	Other cancer	40
		Heart attack	39
		Going into hospital	39
		Bowel trouble	39

The older we get the more likely we are to suffer from muscular aches and pains, and arthritis. Three-quarters of women over sixty-five have muscular problems. More than two-thirds of women over sixty-five suffer from arthritis.

> **Bess, 74:** *I began to get worse and worse and I eventually couldn't straighten out my legs. I couldn't extend my arm out to turn the lamp on ... I couldn't bend to go to the toilet. It is awful recalling that now. I couldn't get into the tub. I did eventually have someone help me getting into the tub so I could have a shower but I couldn't bend my knees and get up into the shower. I was just devastated because I was used to being such an active person.*

Loss of mobility not only means loss of independence, it can also mean you are cut off from friends. This is a common concern of women as we age.

> **Rose, 53:** *I worry about being old and being alone and not having the contact with people one has now. Old people get quite solitary.*

What Do Women Suffer From?

Women's most common complaint, according to our survey, is the headache. Stress, anxiety, illness, and tiredness can all give you a headache. Most of them get better on their own or with just a little help from aspirin or paracetamol. But migraines are something quite different. They are more common in women. They can be triggered by food such as chocolate and red wine and some women find they have a cyclical connection with their periods. If migraines do not settle with non-prescription drugs ask your doctor about prescription drugs, such as sumatriptine, which is effective. Marina gets migraines:

> **Marina, 49:** *They railroad what you want to do, they set you off course. Describing pain's really difficult ... the pain ... overtakes you, you can't do anything else. You just have to lie there and wait for it to stop ... the pain moves around. It is insistent throbbing pain ... it can go quite quickly. Or the pain can last two days ... I think they're stress-related certainly.*

Coughs and colds run a close second to the headache. Period pains are the main complaint of younger women – 75 per cent of sixteen to twenty-four year olds and 69 per cent of twenty-five to forty-four year olds have problems with their periods – and period pain is one of the major reasons girls miss school. (See Chapter 2 for more about period problems.)

Incontinence

Although incontinence was not a worry that featured in the survey, from our interviews with women it is clear that this concerns them. Our bodies produce two to three pints of urine per day. How often we need to pee varies from woman to woman. Some lucky women sleep through the night without needing to urinate, while others of us are up again and again. How frequently we pee may depend upon how much we have had to drink, what time of the month it is (with some women having to pee more frequently just before a period), whether we have given birth or had gynaecological surgery. If we are very overweight we may have to pee more frequently under the pressure of extra weight.

Whatever the cause, women often complain of having to pee too frequently and incontinence (uncontrollable peeing) is a common women's problem. (We discuss what you can do about it on pages 335–6.) Incontinence can be a problem whether you are in good shape or bad shape, able-bodied or disabled, but when we are disabled incontinence may be an even bigger challenge to manage:

> **Wendy, 46, has Multiple Sclerosis which has damaged her muscle control:**
> *I remember saying to myself I think I could cope with anything but being incontinent, but the fact is you can cope with that just as well ... When you actually decide to use a wheelchair it's a liberation because you can do things you couldn't do ... in terms of your social life and everything ... I have a friend who uses a catheter and she says I feel so proud about having this secret skill.*

What Do Women Suffer From?

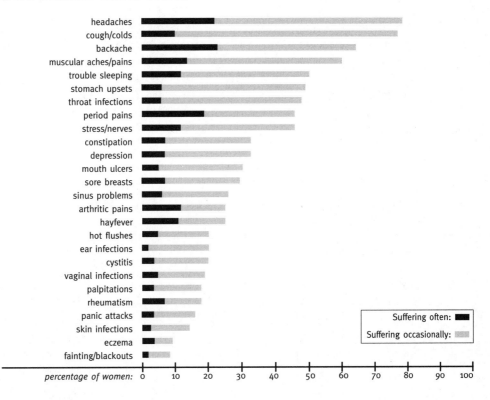

How Does Suffering Vary by Age?

Ages 16–24	%	Ages 45–64	%
Headaches	89	Cough/colds	77
Cough/colds	82	Headaches	74
Period pains	75	Backache	64
Stomach upsets	59	Muscular aches/pains	64
Throat infections	56	Trouble sleeping	53
Backache	55	Stress/nerves	52
Muscular aches/pains	52	Throat infections	45
Trouble sleeping	49	Stomach upsets	44
Stress/nerves	47	Arthritis	37
Depression	36	Hot flushes	34
Ages 25–44		**Age 65+**	
Headaches	89	Muscular aches/pains	74
Cough/colds	80	Cough/colds	70
Period pains	69	Backache	70
Backache	66	Arthritis	68
Muscular aches/pains	54	Headaches	56
Throat infections	53	Trouble sleeping	54
Stress/nerves	52	Rheumatism	47
Stomach upsets	51	Stomach upsets	38
Sore breasts	46	Constipation	35
Trouble sleeping	45	Depression	31

What's Important to Keep Healthy?

The survey asked women what they thought was important to do – or not do – to stay healthy. Here are their top five answers:

- Cut down or stop smoking.
- Reduce stress.
- Get a good night's sleep.
- Be in control of one's life.
- Cut down on fatty foods.

Women also said they consider it important to watch their weight, relax as much as possible, eat regular meals, get regular check-ups, take exercise and watch their alcohol intake.

Smoking and Health

Cathy, 41: *I listened to my kids tell me not to smoke ... I told myself that the day was coming ... I went to see my doctor and told him I needed his help ... he was so supportive and positive ... He suggested the strongest patch for me to begin with. I would need to apply it for approximately four weeks before we would consider going to the next lower strength.*

The effects of smoking on our health have been scrupulously studied. Smoking causes lung cancer, heart disease and is a major factor in a host of other diseases. Smoking is one of the things women mention most frequently as something to avoid in order to stay healthy. Yet the survey's findings on women and smoking are discouraging. One in four women smokes and those most likely to pick up the habit are girls and young women. Forty per cent of sixteen to twenty-four year olds smoke compared with 16 per cent of women over

What's Important to Keep Healthy?

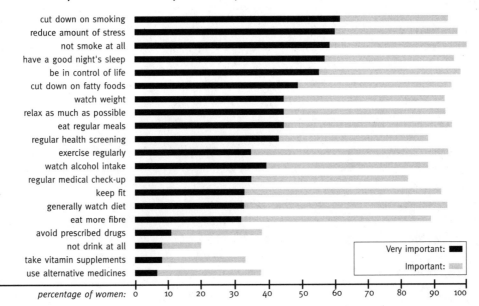

percentage of women:

Legend:
Very important: ■
Important: ▨

sixty-five. One-quarter of women are ex-smokers. Professor Richard Peto of the Imperial Cancer Research Fund, Oxford, says: 'If women smoke like men, they will die like men.' And so we *are* dying like men.

There is a time lag before the effects of smoking seriously harm your health. In the UK women started smoking heavily during the Second World War and we are now seeing the damage. In Scotland, where women have smoked more heavily, more women die from lung cancer than breast cancer.

It is assumed that everyone knows about the risk of smoking. But most people do not realize just how dangerous it is. Women who start to smoke young and keep on smoking have a fifty-fifty chance of being killed by it. Compare deaths from smoking with deaths from cervical cancer: in the UK there are under 2000 deaths a year from the latter and up to 50,000 deaths in women from smoking-related illnesses. It has been estimated that half the women killed by tobacco in the European Union are in the UK. Women are smoking less than they used to but the decline has been slower than in men. Women in unskilled jobs are three times more likely to smoke than those in professional jobs. One in three girls smokes by the age of sixteen, even though they know smoking is deadly. Young women say they smoke because they like it and because their friends do it. Sometimes it is linked to looks. Girls claim it helps them stay thin, distracting them from food, keeping them from bingeing. There is no evidence at all for this. Older women may smoke because they feel it helps them cope with their lives. They say they know about heart disease and lung cancer but after a hard day at work and with the children in bed, they long for a cigarette.

Cathy, 41: *Sunday night will be it. The last night of smoking. I feel excited, I feel scared, I feel sad – I'm going to give up an old friend ... an old enemy! ... drive those grieving thoughts away! Replace them with the thoughts of no more daily worrying about cancer. No more having to save my money for smokes. No more smelly clothes. Happy children. The list goes on.*

Nicotine is highly addictive. Ask anyone who is addicted to cigarettes and they will tell you the addiction is so strong that it is quite impossible to imagine life without them. The physical addiction is a big part of it. But so is a person's social life. Smoking is associated with before-dinner drinks, with after-dinner coffees, visits to certain friends, and evenings at the pub.

Women smokers, like men, die prematurely from lung cancer, heart disease and emphysema (a condition where the lung tissue is damaged, making breathing difficult). There are also some conditions specific to women. Smokers are more likely to have irregular periods and the menopause occurs two to three years earlier in women who smoke. Smokers are also

women's health concerns

more likely to develop osteoporosis (see pages 323–7) and they are up to four times more likely to develop cervical cancer (see pages 374–9). The risk of having a heart attack or a stroke whilst on the oral contraceptive pill is increased tenfold if you smoke. Smoking can impair your fertility and in pregnant women it can cause miscarriage, stillbirth, and low birthweight. There is no doubt that not smoking prevents disease.

Tips for Stopping

- Do it with a friend – if you have someone you trust who also wants to quit you could support one another by being available to talk each other out of cravings, since they will probably occur at different times for each of you.
- Try not telling anyone at all – this way you will not be bothered by well-meaning but irritating questions about your progress.
- Set a date to stop – and stick to it.
- Try not to think of forever – go without for a day. Make a decision about the following day when it arrives, and so on. Tell yourself you can have one tomorrow if you *really* want one.
- Quit on holiday – it may sound odd but quitting in a new environment can help because you will be in a place where you have no smoking habits, such as smoking in a favourite chair, or room, or place outdoors. Cigarettes and hot beaches clash, and they are not great on heavy-duty walking holidays either.
- Quit when you are ill – when you have a wretched cold or flu you sometimes feel less like smoking (although the ability of even the most ill people to smoke is remarkable!). If you are able to quit during an illness you may ease the initial withdrawal period. By the time you really want to smoke again you will have been through the worst few days.
- Do some manual work. Get your hands busy. Knit, paint, clean something.
- Initially avoid situations where you would always smoke.
- Use nicotine patches or gum – they really do work.

Detox Diary – What Happens When You Stop Smoking?

If you have been a typical one pack a day smoker (20–25 cigarettes), this is what happens after you stop smoking:

- 20 minutes – blood pressure and pulse rate return to normal.
- 8 hours – nicotine and carbon monoxide levels in the blood reduce by half, oxygen levels return to normal.
- 24 hours – carbon monoxide will be eliminated from the body. Lungs start to clear out mucus and other smoking debris.
- 48 hours – there is no nicotine left in the body. Ability to taste and smell is greatly improved.

women's health concerns

- 72 hours – breathing becomes easier. Bronchial tubes begin to relax and energy levels increase.
- 2–12 weeks – circulation improves.
- 3–9 months – coughs, wheezing and breathing problems improve as lung function is increased by up to 10 per cent.
- 5 years – risk of heart attack falls to about half that of a smoker.
- 10 years – risk of lung cancer falls to half that of a smoker. Risk of heart attack falls to the same as someone who has never smoked.

> **Cathy, 41:** *I awaken Monday morning and apply my patch. I'm a non-smoker. I can do it. I want a cigarette. I'm not going to have one ... I get busy. The next few days are different without cigarettes. I turn for one often and have to remember that I don't smoke ... every bit of me wants one ... the moments pass, the days pass. There are times when I need to be alone, to curl up and feel bad for myself ... the weeks go by ... when Dr M. was sure my cravings were becoming more infrequent, more bearable, he put me on a slightly weaker patch ... he was very careful not to rush it. We talked a lot about how I felt ... I couldn't have done it without his patient approach and my submission to it.*

Patches are no longer available on the National Health Service, but the cost of a patch kit is cheaper than maintaining a smoking habit. Patches work by feeding you small amounts of nicotine which is intended to reduce your craving for a cigarette until the amount is so low you can give up the patch and the cigarettes altogether.

Pregnancy is sometimes a strong incentive to give up with one in four women quitting at that time and 40 per cent cutting down prior to or during the pregnancy. Forty per cent of the quitters restart three months after the baby is born.

> **Cathy:** *Two years and three months tonight at midnight since I last inhaled or had anything to do with a smoke! It has gone so quickly. I just keep telling myself that the moment will pass and it does.*

Passive Smoking

There is now no doubt that passive smoke (the smoke non-smokers inhale from smokers) is harmful and cancer deaths linked to passive smoke inhalation are well documented. Obviously the smokier the atmosphere is, the greater the potential danger but exactly how much smoke is necessary to harm you is not known. A 1997 review of the world literature on passive smoking found that non-smoking members in a family where someone does smoke have about a 25 per cent increased risk of lung cancer and heart disease, compared with being in a family where no one smokes. If you do smoke be considerate of others who may not have the nerve to say no to you even when you offer not to smoke.

> **Honor Blackman, Actress, 70:** *I don't smoke, I hate smoking now, I must say, and smoky atmospheres are really rotten for my chest.*

Alcohol and Health

More recently alcohol has come under scientific scrutiny and it has come in for praise. Red wine in particular has been singled out for its benevolent qualities. A glass a day is thought to help reduce cholesterol in our blood (see page 332). The same glass has also been praised for its help in managing stress, thus lowering the risk of heart attack. There is even some evidence that women who never drink may have an increased risk of heart disease.

> **Ann, 50:** *I find drinking very relaxing and particularly after a very, very fraught day that first sip just signals that you can wind down. It's probably not the alcohol as much as just stopping for a moment and thinking, 'Oh I've actually got some time to stop and relax'.*

According to our survey it appears that most women are reasonably careful about drinking, although it is known that respondents in surveys tend to underestimate how much alcohol they drink.

The recommended intake of alcohol is no more than 2–3 glasses of wine a day which equals 14–21 units per week. One unit is a small glass of wine, a half pint of beer, or one short measure of spirits. Remember, these are guidelines. Some women may drink a little more than this and still be considered moderate drinkers. But if you find yourself feeling

How Often Do Women Drink?

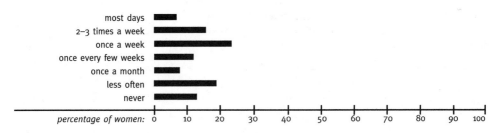

unwell the day after drinking, and notice that drinking interferes with your work or home life you probably need to consider cutting down. Remember, too, that a pub measure is small. Some wine glasses hold enough to count for several measures.

Women drink less than men. Figures from the 1994 Health Survey for England show that although women drink more now than in the past, 12 per cent of women reported they had not had a drink in twelve months, compared to 7 per cent of men. Fifty-eight per cent drank fewer than 8 units per week and only 2 per cent drank excessively at over 35 units per week. One in five women said they had been at least slightly drunk in the past three months. Women and men drink different types of drink. Whereas beer tends to be a man's drink whatever his age, usually only young women are beer drinkers with the majority of middle-aged women preferring wine, and older women spirits. For women, the higher your social class, the more you drink.

Although some alcohol is good for our health and protects against heart disease, stroke and even some types of gallstones, too much alcohol is not. There is an array of medical problems associated with long-term heavy drinking including high blood pressure, liver cirrhosis, cancers of the liver, mouth and oesophagus, mental illness and brain damage. Heavy drinking in pregnancy can damage the developing baby but there is no evidence that one or two glasses of wine a week causes problems. For more on alcohol see Chapter 5.

Keeping Control of Your Life

The *Woman's Hour* survey found that women think staying in control of their lives is as important as getting a good night's sleep.

Nine in ten women felt they were in control of their lives. The one in ten who did not were much more likely to suffer illness and depression (see Chapter 5 for more on depression and anxiety). Two-thirds of women thought they could do more to stay healthy and they believed reducing stress is an important part of that.

How in Control of Your Life Do You Feel?

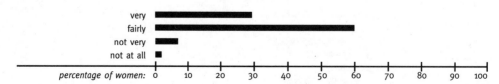

Reducing Stress

Stress is difficult to measure. What is stressful for one person might not be for the next. But life's inevitable upsets and changes are generally considered stressful for most people: the death of a loved one, separation and divorce, losing a job, changing jobs, job demotion and job promotion, having an accident, an illness, a major operation, and moving house. Our lives are full of day-to-day stresses that result from the struggle for survival at work and home. We hurry to make deadlines, catch trains, race to the shops before closing, rush to be home in time for the children. We stay late at work to stay on top.

There is no way to avoid stress altogether but what seems to be most important of all is whether or not we have control over the stress in our lives. In studies, men (women are often not considered in medical research) who felt in control of the stress in their lives had fewer heart attacks. So we simply do not know the long-term effect of stress on a young mother who bravely makes her way through the trenches of domesticity when her children are young.

> **Henrietta:** *How I see myself is as a very tired, worn-out person ... my children in my buggy are getting heavier and bigger every day. I'm getting weaker. My day is endlessly washing and cleaning and ironing that nobody on the street outside would know that I've done ... It's not a thankless job having children but ... I'm completely out of control of my own life ... These jobs have to be done but nobody's actually going to know if my children are wearing clean clothes or not. As soon as I've done it, it's going to have to be done again and this whole lifestyle is incredibly stressful day after day after day.*

Women who do feel in control of their lives take time to maintain that control.

> **Celia, 41:** *I don't do anything obvious like go and have a massage or anything. It's more sorting myself out. Just getting my life straight. Getting my room sorted out. My desk cleared, my bills written, find a new bit of make-up to try. Quite small-scale things can be very therapeutic.*

Some of us are natural-born managers of stress and strain.

> **Margaret Thatcher:** *Most able women I know, women who climbed to the top ... got there through merit ... We're pretty independent people and if there is a difference, let me say this: it's often women who are left to cope and that's what makes us very practical and very able.*

Good health, less stress, and more exercise are clearly important to women. Fifty-six per cent of the women in the survey said keeping fit is important to maintaining their health.

> **Jennifer, 44:** *I've always [exercised] for mental reasons rather than physical reasons ... I'm not trying to have a flatter stomach. I'm not trying to have smaller hips ... for the last twelve years I have used it as a way of getting rid of stress. I actually don't know how people don't do it because if I didn't do it I think I'd go bonkers. Then the side benefit is that I think I am physically fit.*

Women and Their Doctors

> **Ann, 50:** *I have a fabulous female doctor who is always very busy but always makes time to listen to my problems and gives excellent advice.*

Thirty-eight per cent of the women surveyed had been to the doctor in the last month. Nine out of ten women in the survey had seen their doctor in the past year. Doctors are ranked way ahead of pharmacists, friends, books and the media in terms of importance as a source of health information, according to our survey. However, we get most of our information from friends and the media. Eighty-two per cent of women agree their doctors are overworked with 42 per cent saying they would like more time with their doctor. Two-thirds of women see a male doctor and are reasonably satisfied with this, although they do prefer to see women doctors when it comes to discussing certain matters.

> **Joanna:** *One time when I had thrush I just plucked up the courage to go. And then when I came face-to-face with the GP I just didn't know what to say to him. And then he asked me all these questions. I suppose they have to. But questions like, 'Does it hurt when you make love, have you been itching, is there a discharge?' Obviously they are questions they have to ask but you just feel so terrible about it.*

Our survey showed that older women are much less shy with their doctors and are more comfortable talking about sex in the surgery than younger women are. Once again, age brings confidence and experience that makes it easier to discuss private matters. If your worries are interfering with life's enjoyment it is a good idea to see your doctor.

The Worries Never Stop

Just when we think we have got it all sorted, just when we think we have control, new worries come along. Many women stop worrying about themselves and turn all their anxiety towards the children!

Linda, 50: *You worry about your children when they're grown up, very much so. And my husband's children. Everybody's children! Then you worry about grandchildren.*

Vera, 66: *I think children are the biggest worry. If you've got children they are always at the back of your mind. Are they going to turn out well? What sort of a world are they going to grow up in because the world is altered from when we were young.*

chapter 2

periods

Katie, 13: A month ago I had my first period. I was very relieved because all of my friends had theirs. I was also relieved to find everything was working properly in my body ... Unbelievably I am actually looking forward to when I get my next one because it makes me feel like a proper adult!

Most of us have about thirty years to get to know our periods. It is a long, intimate exploration. It is a special relationship and an expensive one. Assuming we spend three pounds a month on tampons, towels for light days and towels for heavy ones, at today's prices that would be a total of £1080 for a lifetime's supply. That is a lot of money but we can be grateful for what it buys us nowadays:

> **Jennifer, 44:** *When I look back I can't believe what we had to wear when we were little girls. Those belts with the little metal hooks and they'd get caught in your pubic hair and then you had this great big wad between your legs and you're a little stick of a thing! When I think of it I can't believe we had to wear it but that's what you wore.*

Of course, most of us nowadays know what to expect when it arrives, but until relatively recently many young women were not even told about their periods.

> **Bess, 74:** *My first period. I just found this blood on my pants and nobody had said anything to me about what was going to happen about a period and I just called my mother and ... said Mum, look. She just said one thing and that was stay away from boys. Can you imagine? That's all she told me ... I probably didn't even know what the significance of that was.*

The mystery of menstruation and fascination with menstrual blood is as old as woman herself. In some cultures periods are called 'moon' and some women actually believe periods are regulated by the moon. Although the menstrual interval can be approximately equal to the lunar month there is no evidence to link the two. Menstrual blood has been thought to cure epilepsy, gout, malaria and boils. It was supposed to make iron rust and copper turn green. In some cultures, even to talk about menstruation is taboo. The word taboo itself comes from the Polynesian *tabu* which means 'menstruation' as well as 'unclean' and 'sacred'. According to some religions, or simply to tradition, during menstruation women may be forbidden to have sex or to have any contact with men. They may not be allowed to bathe, wash their hair, or even prepare food. Tradition has it that women are thought to be unclean when they menstruate. Sometimes it is superstition, sometimes strict belief. Just think of the names used to describe our periods: the curse, the devil's gateway – words that not only reflect superstition but also the nuisance our periods can be.

> **May, 71:** *You didn't have a bath. You didn't wash your feet. You never wet anything when you had your period. You didn't dare. Always be something wrong if you did. You'd really have a bloody good scrub after!*

In this chapter we look at how our periods work and what to do when they go wrong. This is your guide, through from your first period to your last. The way we manage our periods is constantly changing. We have more control over them now than ever before. We can alter our periods, starting and stopping for convenience, to help us become pregnant, to avoid pregnancy altogether or simply to take a break from them for a special occasion. What has not changed is the intricate monthly interactive process between our brains and our ovaries which produces a period.

The Normal Hormonal Changes with Periods

We have two sets of hormones which govern our menstrual cycles. Every month their levels go up and down, sending negative and positive feedback messages to different parts of the body and brain. Our ovaries produce the hormones oestrogen and progesterone. The pituitary gland, a small gland in the brain, produces two more hormones: LH – luteinizing hormone, and FSH – follicular stimulating hormone.

The diagram opposite shows how oestrogen levels go up and then come down during the first half of the cycle. In the second half, once the egg has been released from the ovary, the oestrogen levels go up again this time along with progesterone. The first half of the monthly cycle is called the follicular phase – this is when the egg is maturing in the ovary. The luteal phase is when the egg pops out of the ovary leaving behind the *corpus luteum* which produces the oestrogen and progesterone for the second half of the cycle.

Meanwhile the LH and FSH hormone levels are also going up and down. The levels of these hormones are interdependent. The FSH is affected by the level of oestrogen. If there is too much oestrogen the pituitary gland stops producing FSH. This is called 'negative' feedback. When the oestrogen level gets high enough it stimulates the pituitary to produce a twenty-four-hour surge of the other hormone, LH. The LH surge triggers the egg to be released from the ovary. This is called ovulation. Some women know when they ovulate just by the change in mucus discharge. It varies through the month, becoming more slippery at the time of ovulation. Some women feel a short sharp pain which is caused by the release of the egg. There are kits available from chemists to test your urine if you want to know when you ovulate (see Chapters 8 and 12).

Changes during the Menstrual Cycle

Pituitary hormones

LH
FSH

Growth and   *Ovulation*   *Growth and degeneration of*
maturation of follicle   *corpus luteum*

Changes in the ovary

Ovarian hormones

Oestrogen

DAY I

Progesterone

Infertile ◄——— *Fertile* ———► *Infertile*

**Cervix
and
mucus**

Menses   *Thick mucus*   *Thinner*   *Watery peak*   *Thicker*   *Thick*
                            changing   *mucus*   *mucus*

Following ovulation the FSH and LH levels drop and the oestrogen and progesterone levels rise. If you do not get pregnant, the oestrogen and progesterone levels drop again at the end of the cycle and you have a period. Individual variations in the ups and downs of these hormones help to explain why periods are long or short and whether your periods are close together or far apart. Measurement of these hormones (see page 42) can help to explain some period problems and may also help to find out why you might not be getting pregnant.

These hormones are also involved in changing the make-up of the lining of the uterus and it is this lining which falls away every time you have a period. Yet more hormones called prostaglandins make tiny curly blood vessels open and close appropriately whilst you have your period to prevent too much bleeding. Prostaglandin hormone levels are often too high in women who have extremely heavy or painful periods. The drugs sometimes prescribed to alleviate this block the action of prostaglandins (see page 37).

periods

The 'Normal' Period

What is normal for one woman may be considered abnormal by another. Women commonly consider their periods to be too heavy, too light, too messy, too frequent, too infrequent, too late, too early, too painful, too long, too short. It seems there is no perfect period.

> **Kate, 21:** *It wasn't very heavy the first time. It only lasted two or three days and it didn't settle down until about three months after my first one ... At the beginning they weren't heavy and they were completely painless ... but when I was about fifteen or sixteen I started getting pains. I still do get them but not very bad. My periods are fairly regular and I normally get quite bad period pain on my first day and then they're fine. They're short, five days at the most.*
>
> **Celia, 41:** *They used to be quite heavy and quite frequent and now they're much more normal. Two to three days every twenty-eight days, so pretty standard. But for about fifteen years they were embarrassingly heavy – a packet of tampons a day, maybe for two days. Real flooding. But it's just sort of settled down, maybe it was a bit better after I had my children.*
>
> **Jennifer, 44:** *They get shorter as I've been getting older. I can remember when I was younger it was every thirty-two days, then it somehow switched to thirty. Now it's bouncing all over the place but it's about every twenty-six days ... I think my shortest period was nineteen days in between.*

There is so much variation that it is impossible to say what is normal. The important thing about periods is what is normal for you. You might have what you consider to be long-lasting periods or short – and if they are fairly consistent and not outrageously heavy or painful this is probably 'normal' for you. Your periods may vary with your age, weight, stress levels and the pills you take. Twenty-eight-day cycles have wrongly become synonymous with being normal and healthy as there is a wide range of normal. Twelve-year-old girls usually have their periods every thirty-five days, compared with twenty-seven days at forty-three years of age and fifty-two days by the time you are fifty-five if you are still menstruating. Fifty per cent of women have periods lasting five to six days, but 20 per cent bleed for more than seven days and 1 per cent more than twelve days.

Many women notice their cycles match those of their closest friends. It is a fascinating fact, that women who live or work together do tend to have cycles which converge. This is thought to be mediated by chemicals which we secrete called pheromones, which are also involved in sexual attraction.

How Much Blood is in a Period?

Again, the range of 'normal' is quite wide. But we do have an idea of what the 'average' blood loss is, thanks to a group of women who volunteered to send off their sanitary towels and tampons to a research laboratory for analysis. The results showed the average blood loss per period to be about six to eight teaspoonfuls, or 35 millilitres. About 90 per cent of the blood is lost in the first three days. Blood is only one component in the monthly discharge. What makes it seem much heavier are the additional cells from the lining of the uterus and mucus from the cervix. The discharge can be light red or dark red, thick or thin. Women use anything from ten to fifty tampons during one period. How many tampons or sanitary towels you use depends on how long your period is, how often you change the tampons, which size and absorbency you use and, of course, how heavy your discharge is. If you think you are losing too much blood then you should consult your doctor.

What Can Go Wrong with Periods

Every woman experiences about 400 menstruations in her life. A 1990 UK Mori poll found 31 per cent of women reported they had heavy periods; nearly 40 per cent said their periods were painful; 5–10 per cent had sought help from a doctor for period problems. Periods are in the top ten reasons for going to the doctor. If you decide to see your doctor for period problems you will be asked for all the details of your cycle – how long your periods are and how regular. So it helps to keep a diary like the one shown below. Make a copy and shade in the days when you have your period.

Ninety-five per cent of girls start their periods between the ages of eleven and fifteen. If you have not had a period by the age of sixteen it is a good idea to see your doctor. It is usually just a variation of the norm, but can be caused by a problem in the development of the uterus, due to an abnormality in the chromosomes called Turners syndrome, or because there is something wrong in the ovary or pituitary glands.

DAY/MONTH	1	2	3	4	5	6	7	8	9	10	11	12	13	14	15	16	17	18	19	20	21	22	23	24	25	26	27	28	29	30	31	TOTAL

When Your Periods Are too Heavy

Clots, flooding and forever having to change pads and tampons mean your periods are too heavy. Doctors write more than three-quarters of a million prescriptions for this condition each year in England and Wales. Menorrhagia – the medical term for heavy periods – is the reason for a third of all referrals to a gynaecologist. It is also the most common reason for having a hysterectomy or removal of the womb. Each year in the UK, 40,000 hysterectomies are performed for heavy periods. Heavy periods can be an indication that something is wrong or they can be part of the 'normal variation' of your cycle. If you think your periods are too heavy or if they have become much heavier, see your doctor. The doctor should discuss the pattern of your periods with you and do a vaginal examination to check your womb and ovaries. A more general medical history and examination may also help sort out the problem. A cervical smear test (see pages 373–9) should also be carried out if you have not had one in the past three years.

Heavy periods sometimes cause anaemia – because you lose more iron in the period blood than your body can replace – so a blood test may be arranged to check for this and iron tablets may be prescribed. Anaemia often results if heavy periods persist for several months. The symptoms of anaemia usually come on gradually making you feel more and more tired and/or dizzy. If you are under forty it is unlikely you will need further tests unless treatment with iron pills does not work. In about half the cases of women having heavy periods no obvious physical cause is actually found. Doctors call it 'unexplained' and put it down to 'hormones'. When there *is* a physical explanation one of the most common causes is fibroids which grow inside the uterus (see pages 36–7). Other common causes are polyps or endometriosis (which can also cause very painful periods – see pages 37, 38–40) and recently it has been found that they can sometimes be linked to a clotting disorder of the blood. Only very rarely is cancer found to be the cause. Occasionally there is something more generally wrong, such as an under-active thyroid gland. If you use an intrauterine device (IUD) as your method of contraception this may also cause heavy periods (see pages 208–9).

Many women with heavy periods decide just to put up with them. Exercising, eating properly and keeping fit may help you cope better but there is no evidence that this actually helps 'cure' heavy periods. Whether or not a cause is found, there is almost always something you can do to make heavy periods lighter.

Drug Treatment for Heavy Periods
There are several over-the-counter or prescription drug treatments which may help with heavy periods if the cause of them is not a physical problem such as a fibroid.

Synthetic Non-hormone Drugs These include ibuprofen (Nurofen) which can be bought over the counter, or prescription medicines like mefenamic acid (Ponstan), tranexamic acid and ethamsylate. The good thing about these tablets is that they only need to be taken during the heavy periods. They have few side effects and reduce bleeding in 80 per cent of women. Ibuprofen and mefenamic acid both reduce bleeding and pain. Tranexamic acid and ethamsylate reduce bleeding but do not alleviate pain. Always check pill bottle labels for warnings, carefully read the instructions, and talk to your pharmacist. Some painkillers, especially aspirin and ibuprofen, should not be taken if you have stomach problems or suffer from asthma.

Each of these drugs works in a different way so if one does not help, try another. Tranexamic acid is said to reduce bleeding by 50 per cent and mefenamic acid by 25 per cent. Tranexamic acid is not prescribed very often but you can ask for it. However, occasionally you may experience side effects when taking these medicines. Nausea, dizziness, stomach upsets, or lightheadedness are symptoms. If this happens to you, ask your doctor about trying an alternative.

Hormone Treatment The most commonly used hormone treatment for heavy periods is the combined oral contraceptive pill, a good option whether or not contraception is also needed. Once again if one brand does not work, ask your doctor to prescribe another. The other hormone treatments used include progestogens (e.g. norethisterone) which are especially useful to stop a sudden torrential bleed but they are not good for helping with regular heavy periods.

Less Commonly Used Hormonal Drugs Danazol can stop periods altogether. The downside is that you may experience unpleasant side effects such as weight gain, acne and headaches. Gestrinone can also help as can LH RH agonists (see page 37), although these produce a pseudo-menopause and can only be used short term. These drugs are usually only prescribed by specialists. Recently it has been found that some types of HRT (hormone replacement therapy – see pages 60–71) may help women whose periods have become heavier as they approach the menopause.

periods

'Coil Treatment' or Intrauterine System (IUS)

Though most contraceptive coils actually make your periods heavier, a newer type of coil called Mirena, which slowly releases a very small amount of the hormone progestogen directly into the womb, makes periods lighter or stops them altogether. It also helps to alleviate pain but is of no use if the bleeding is related to fibroids. It works by thinning the lining of the uterus. Every woman should be offered this as an option, if drugs do not solve the problem, before surgery for heavy bleeding is considered. In Norway where it has been widely used, far fewer women need to have hysterectomies to cure their heavy periods. However, this coil is expensive and some doctors therefore do not offer it as an option, even though it is far cheaper than a hysterectomy. But do ask for it! The bonus is that it also acts as a contraceptive and can stay in place for at least three years.

Surgical Treatments and Tests

If your doctor cannot find a cause for the heavy periods and especially if you are over forty, you may be referred to hospital for further tests and to check for other conditions such as fibroids, polyps or possibly cancer developing in the uterus. For women under the age of forty, cancer is very rare. One study has shown that 4000 investigations had to be done to find one cancer. Even if you are over forty, cancer is not common, just a bit more likely. Hospital tests might include an ultrasound scan which can help see fibroids, a hysteroscopy to see if there is a polyp, or a type of D and C (dilatation and curettage) called an aspiration curettage. A small tube is inserted into the cervix and samples of the uterine lining are removed for testing. All of these tests are usually done as outpatient procedures often without the need for a general anaesthetic. (See also Chapter 15 for more information on all of these tests.) In the unlikely case that menorrhagia is due to a cancer in the uterus, hysterectomy is usually the treatment of choice often with radiotherapy treatment and chemotherapy, and/or hormone therapy in more advanced cases. Cancer of the uterus, if caught early, can be cured in at least 85 per cent of cases. If it has spread to other parts of the body the cure rate is only 10 per cent.

Fibroids

> **Francesca, 42:** *I found a doctor who made me feel very comfortable ... he removed the fibroids which helped to make my periods ... more normal and also gives me the possibility of having children, plus the fact that I now have a flatter stomach and I'm probably almost a size down as a result.*

Fibroids are round lumps of fibrous tissue that grow in the wall of the uterus. They can also occur on the outside of the uterus or protrude into the cavity of the uterus. We have no idea what causes them but they are very common. Nearly one-quarter of women over thirty-five have them. Often when fibroids are discovered it is to the woman's surprise. As they do not always cause a problem and do not usually do any harm other than sometimes causing heavy periods, you can remain unaware of them for a long time. In some women they are related to fertility problems (see Chapter 12). Only extremely rarely do they change into a cancer. Fibroids are more common in Afro-Caribbean women, but appear to cause fewer problems.

You can have one fibroid or lots of them. They can grow to the size of a grapefruit but are usually smaller. A doctor can sometimes feel them during a vaginal examination and they can be seen on an ultrasound scan. If they get very large you might even be able to feel a lump yourself if you press on the lower part of your abdomen. If they are small and not causing any problems there is no need to have anything done about them except to get them checked every year or so.

If the fibroids are very large, causing heavy periods or other trouble – like making you pee a lot by causing pressure on your bladder – you may need treatment. Hysterectomy used to be the usual treatment (see pages 359–61). However, if you are young and especially if you have not had children or completed your family, you will want to minimize surgery and certainly avoid hysterectomy if at all possible.

> **Margaret, 58:** *I had fibroids ... I used to have very, very heavy periods that went on for about ten days and I literally used to haemorrhage and the doctor said I should have [a hysterectomy] otherwise I'd be taken in as an emergency one day, I just wouldn't stop bleeding. So I went in and had it done.*

New ways of treating fibroids have been developed which involve only a small operation using a laparoscope (see page 364) or a hysteroscope (see pages 358–9). Another option is a myomectomy, a procedure which shells out the fibroid from the muscle of the uterus, leaving the uterus intact. The new progestogen coil (see page 36) sometimes helps shrink fibroids. There are also new drugs available which can shrink the fibroids called GnRH agonists. Unfortunately these drugs are not always successfu. If you are nearing the menopause you may not need an operation as fibroids tend to shrink after the menopause. However, if you take HRT (see pages 60–71) it can make fibroids grow bigger, or stop them from shrinking.

Polyps
Polyps are like little lumps of skin. They can occasionally grow quite large but they are not cancerous. They may develop on the surface of the cervix where they can cause bleeding between periods. Those in the lining of the womb can cause heavy periods or bleeding between periods. Sometimes a doctor can see one on the cervix, usually when a smear is taken. If a polyp is present on the cervix, your GP can simply twist it off. A hospital visit is necessary for the removal of polyps inside the uterus.

Painful Periods

This problem is known as dysmenorrhoea, a Greek name, meaning difficult monthly flow. The majority of women have discomfort with their periods at some time in their lives. Some get painful periods very soon after they start to menstruate. For others it becomes a problem in their mid-thirties or later. In the past women who complained of painful periods were unfairly labelled as neurotic. However, now we know that women who have painful periods have a uterus which contracts more during periods and the muscle of the uterus itself is more tense. Some of their hormone levels are also higher than in women who do not get painful periods.

Anecdotal accounts suggest that having an orgasm alleviates menstrual pain, because it is supposed to make blood rush from the area. Whether or not it does is not proven but some women do find it helps them, although we recognize that this may not suit you, or may not be acceptable in your culture or religion.

Over the counter drugs like ibuprofen (Nurofen) or mefenamic acid (Ponstan) on prescription solve the problem for 80–90 per cent of women with painful periods. Alternatively the combined oral contraceptive pill will often help and can be used whether or not contraception is needed as well. In a small number of women, however, there are other underlying causes for the pain. There can be something wrong in the uterus like a fibroid (see pages 36–7), endometriosis (see below), a polyp in the uterus (see page 37) or it can be related to the coil (IUD) used for contraception. Then the treatment will be for the underlying cause.

Endometriosis

The endometrium is the lining of cells inside the womb or uterus. But pieces of endometrium can sometimes be found *outside* the womb where they should not be: on the ovaries, fallopian tubes, intestines, and even on the lungs. When bits of endometrium are located in these sites the condition is called endometriosis. These wayward cells behave in the same way as the lining of the womb, that is, bleeding just like a period, once a month, but the blood has nowhere to go. This can result in cysts and sometimes scarring on the ovaries, fallopian tubes and uterus which if serious may result in infertility. Scarring is caused by the endometrial mass sticking to the walls of these organs. It can then – very painfully – tear away leaving scar tissue.

> **Sandra, 42:** *I must have had it for ten years before it was diagnosed. Twice I was rushed to hospital in excruciating pain. Each time the episode began during intercourse. And both times – a few years apart, and with different partners – the doctors thought I had appendicitis.*

Gemma: *Be persistent and if necessary ask to be referred for a second opinion but don't give up because I think if you're quite good at listening to your own body your body is telling you there is something not right.*

Theories and myths about the cause of endometriosis abound but there is little hard data. Patients and doctors alike find this very frustrating. There are claims that more than 1.5 million women in Great Britain suffer from it. The Endometriosis Society (see Useful Addresses on page 390) says the average time taken to make the diagnosis is seven years.

If you have mild endometriosis which does not cause any symptoms, you may not even know that you have it. There are no easy diagnostic tests available. Since the cause is not understood, trying to prevent and treat endometriosis is very difficult.

Annie: *My GP ... treated me initially for irritable bowel syndrome and when that didn't seem to help I was then sent to a gastroenterologist and had extensive tests – all of which showed that I was normal and then I was sent to a rheumatologist ... (finally) ... a junior doctor ... said, 'I think you may have endometriosis'.*

Endometriosis can cause many different symptoms and they can vary in severity: backache, diarrhoea, pain during intercourse, painful periods, puffy abdomen, pain during bowel movements, and pelvic pain can all be linked to the condition. If endometriosis is left this will not necessarily cause you problems, or the condition may worsen and become more damaging leading to infertility. It may be possible for your doctor to diagnose this disease on the history of your symptoms but a laparoscopy is the only way to make a certain diagnosis (see page 364).

Sandra, 42: *... the surgeon made three tiny holes. One below my navel and one over each side, just about where I think my ovaries are. It was great not to have a big painful scar but I was very sore and felt depressed after the anaesthetic. At the end of it all, I was told there was no chance of having children. I believed it without much difficulty because by then I had had so many investigations and heard so much explanation that I really could picture the situation. I was a mess inside.*

In the past endometriosis was thought to be something women in their thirties and forties developed. It is now being discovered in younger women, even in teenagers. It is difficult to know if this is due to greater awareness and increasing use of laparoscopes or whether it is genuinely becoming more common. Although some women with infertility are found to have endometriosis many women with it still get pregnant, especially if it is mild. Endometriosis sounds like – and can be – a miserable condition. But very many women with it live entirely normal lives without being bothered by it.

Treating Endometriosis Hormonal drug treatment can alter the balance of hormones. It works by suppressing hormones produced by our ovaries. The treatment should shrink the endometrial tissue. The most commonly used drug is a high-level progestogen oral contraceptive pill. Another way of treating it is by suppressing oestrogen using drugs such as danazol and GnRH agonists. However, they often have unpleasant side effects including hot flushes, weight gain and headaches (see page 50).

There are also surgical options when medical treatments fail or cannot be tolerated and the symptoms are severe. These include laser treatment to zap the cysts, or surgery to remove individual cysts. Unfortunately, once drug treatments stop and even after surgery, the condition often reappears. Removing the uterus and ovaries is only necessary if the endometriosis is extremely severe and all else fails. Treating endometriosis is not always easy. You may need to try different approaches before finding something which helps.

When Your Periods Seem Too Light

If your periods are very light, even as little as half a teaspoonful (2 ml) a month, this is nothing to worry about. Many women with light periods are only too grateful. For others a good flow is considered to be important.

No Periods

It is worrying when periods stop or one is missed for no apparent reason. We complain about our periods, but most women want to menstruate regularly, or at least to know there is nothing wrong if they do not. We usually associate having no periods with being pregnant, whether we want to be or not. We also connect loss of periods with loss of femininity or we worry that something else might be wrong.

If you normally have regular periods and they suddenly stop, first consider pregnancy. If there is no possible risk of this, or a pregnancy test is negative, there could be several other reasons for the interruption. The most likely one depends on your age and what is happening in your life. Some women just seem to skip a period every so often for no apparent reason and usually it is nothing to worry about. Sometimes there will be a specific reason why. These include stopping the contraceptive pill, excessive weight loss or exercise, stress and anxiety, the menopause, and travel across time zones.

Combined Oral Contraceptive Pill (COC)

After stopping the COC pill, it can take many months before you start ovulating and menstruating. This is more likely if your periods were irregular before you started on the pill. The best thing to do in these circumstances is just wait until your periods start again but if you are trying to get pregnant you might want to take a fertility drug (see page 303) to kickstart your ovaries back into action. If you do *not* want to get pregnant, remember that just because you are not having periods it does not always mean you are not ovulating, as you ovulate before your period comes. So you should still use contraception.

> **Ann, 40:** *I missed my periods for about four years when I stopped taking the pill. I went to see a specialist who did a bunch of tests. He said I was suffering from long-term effects of the pill and somehow it had stopped me ovulating. He put me on hormone pills and after about two months I became pregnant with my first child. Once I had the baby everything returned to normal. I had two more children after that.*

Weight Loss and Exercise

Over-dieting and anorexia (see page 142) are common reasons for periods stopping or, indeed, never starting in young women. If this is the cause your periods will only restart if you gain weight. Too much exercise can also interrupt periods. This is not new. Two thousand years ago the Greek doctor Soranus noticed that women who took too much exercise stopped having periods. This can happen to women joggers, athletes, and long-distance runners who overdo it. Sometimes the exercise itself interferes with periods, and sometimes the trouble is caused by weight loss due to over-exercise.

Studies have shown that excessive exercise and weight loss have an effect on the hypothalamus gland in the brain. The normal feedback pathways between the hypothalamus and pituitary in the brain and the ovaries are disrupted and normal periods stop. Periods usually return after several months once a normal diet and exercise routine are resumed.

Stress and Anxiety

This can also affect the hypothalamus making your periods stop for several months. This is very common at exam time, when you start a new job or when a relationship breaks up. The interruption in your periods is nothing to worry about.

Menopause

If you are between the ages of forty-five and fifty-five (although it can be much earlier or much later) when your periods stop, it is probably due to the menopause. Some women do have a premature menopause in their thirties and, very rarely, even earlier.

Jane, 50: *I was sad to hear I had passed through the menopause. I didn't even know, I didn't know much about it, I just didn't get my period any more. The doctor finally sent me for an ultrasound to confirm years after ... when I was about 40 but in fact I went through the menopause about age 35.*

It is rare for a woman's ovaries to stop functioning when she is in her twenties. Pregnancy in this case is difficult, though not impossible, with modern fertility treatments (see Chapter 12). If your periods stop and you think you are having an early menopause you will probably have other signs as well: hot flushes, night sweats and vaginal dryness (see Chapter 3). You should see your doctor for tests if you are worried about this.

When to Act When Your Periods Stop

This depends on many things like your age, whether it has happened before, and how worried you are. If your periods stop, do not return after six months, and you are definitely not pregnant, see your doctor, who may suggest a simple blood test to find out more about the way your hormones may be affecting your cycle. Your blood may show a hormonal imbalance, that you are not ovulating, or that you are in fact entering the menopause. Depending on your blood results you may need further investigations with ultrasound scans, or a laparoscopy (see page 364).

What the Blood Tests Look for

- FSH (Follicular stimulating hormone) – high at time of menopause.
- Oestrogen – low at menopause and if not ovulating.
- LH (luteinizing hormone) – high at time of menopause and during ovulation.
- Prolactin – raised in stress, with some drugs (including some antidepressants and the oral contraceptive pill) and, more *rarely*, when there are tumours on the pituitary gland.
- Testosterone – high if you have polycystic ovarian syndrome (see page 43).

Some doctors may also suggest a progestogen challenge test. This is where a low dose of progestogen such as medroxy-progesterone is taken once a day for seven days, following which a period should start. If you do not have a period after this, you should see your doctor.

Irregular Periods

Women often worry that something is wrong if their periods become irregular. But irregularities are usually normal, especially if they occur in your teens soon after starting your periods, or when you are approaching the menopause. Sometimes periods take time to settle down after you have given birth. During breast-feeding some women start to menstruate irregularly whilst others do not restart until they stop breast-feeding. If your periods become heavy as well as irregular or you bleed between periods or after sex, it is wise to get them checked to make sure there is nothing wrong.

PCOS

One reason for irregular periods is polycystic ovarian syndrome, PCOS. Typically PCOS is linked with infrequent or no periods, being overweight, having acne and rather a lot of hair on the face. If PCOS is suspected, blood tests are taken. High levels of luteinizing hormone (LH) and testosterone would suggest PCOS. Your ovaries also need to be checked to confirm the diagnosis – they will be full of cysts if it really is PCOS. But there is a problem in that not all women with these cysts have PCOS. If you examined the ovaries of all women, 20 per cent would have cysts but in only a small percentage would the cysts be a problem. Most women with PCOS do not ovulate regularly and may therefore have trouble getting pregnant without treatment. They are also slightly more likely to miscarry, possibly because of the high level of the hormone LH which interferes with the embryo developing in the wall of the uterus.

Treating PCOS is sometimes difficult. It is not always necessary unless you want to get pregnant or are bothered by the acne and/or hairiness. Losing weight by dieting can help and may improve many of the problems associated with PCOS. If the hairiness is a problem, the oral contraceptive pill, Dianette, containing a special anti-androgen (anti-male) hormone may help. If you are trying to get pregnant you may need to take fertility drugs to help stimulate your ovaries to ovulate. Or you may decide to do nothing, in which case be reassured there is no link with the cysts in PCOS and ovarian cancer though there is a very small increased risk of cancer of the uterus.

Bleeding Between Periods

You should always get this checked. If you are under forty it is rarely anything to worry about. The bleeding may be caused by a problem on the cervix such as a polyp or an ectropion. A polyp is like a flap of skin on the cervix which can easily be removed (by twisting it off) by the GP or at the hospital as an outpatient. You will feel a sharp, short pain. An ectropion or erosion is a raw area on the cervix which occurs in about 10 per cent of women and makes the cervix appear redder than usual, because the cells inside the cervix have grown out on to the surface of the cervix. These cells are more fragile than those usually on the outer part of the cervix and can sometimes become inflamed or bleed, especially if knocked during sex. It is thought that the cervical cells are influenced by hormones because erosions are more common during pregnancy and in women on the contraceptive pill. Erosions usually cause no problems, but if they cause bleeding or a lot of vaginal discharge they can be treated by cauterization usually by freezing or by applying a chemical such as silver nitrate. Cauterization should not hurt but it is uncomfortable.

periods

Some women bleed regularly in the middle of their cycle between periods – around the time of ovulation – because of hormonal changes. Sometimes women on the contraceptive pill or HRT, bleed between periods because of variations in hormonal levels and all you need to do is change the brand of pill or HRT.

If you are over forty it is more likely that your doctor will suggest further tests such as a hysteroscopy (see pages 358–9) or an aspiration curettage (see page 357–8). This is to check that there is no polyp or cancer in the lining of the womb causing the bleeding. Whatever your age very often no cause is found at all and the problem is rather vaguely put down to 'hormones'.

How to Postpone a Period

> **Alice:** *We had planned to get married on 12 June. I'd even planned it so that it was not when I had a period, not that it was going to be some big deal wedding night – that was long ago, but I just thought it would be nicer somehow. Then in April my period came ten days early just like that so the whole planning was messed up. No way did I want my period then. What if it leaked all over my dress as I walked down the aisle? My doctor gave me some pills to stop my period coming.*

There are ways to postpone a period if it is due to come at the wrong time. You can ask your doctor to prescribe a progestogen hormone such as norethisterone. Start taking it three days before the anticipated period and continue until you want to have a period. You can start on the combined oral contraceptive pill, but you need to do this at least one month in advance. If you are already on the pill and your pill-free week occurs when you do not want to have a bleed, you can prevent it by running two packs together without leaving a gap. Postponing a period in this way over several months is not at all harmful.

Sex and Periods

Like periods themselves there is enormous variation in our views about what is normal and what is not. For religious reasons some couples avoid intercourse at this time. But if you are comfortable with the idea of making love during your period there is no medical reason why you should not.

Kate, 21: *I don't normally have sex when I'm having a period and that's the only time I get sort of cross about having my period. I think it's the mess – I don't think it's embarrassment. I suppose I never really feel like it that much.*

Marge, 24: *I was off the pill for nearly a year and I used to look forward to having my periods because it meant I wasn't pregnant and I could have carefree sex. And then my doctor told me that wasn't strictly true so she kind of ruined the fun.*

It would be virtually impossible to become pregnant during your period if you have a regular cycle. However, if your cycle is not regular there is still a risk and there is also still the risk of getting a sexually transmitted infection if you do not use a condom.

Brenda, 50: *Years ago when no one was worried about Aids or anything else I had sex with someone I thought I knew fairly well. He wanted to use a condom and I didn't because I was on my period and wasn't worried about getting pregnant. What I got instead was herpes.*

Sex and periods are not just to do with how you feel about the mess. It is just as much about your sexual drive.

Sue, 42: *Immediately after my period I do desperately want sex. I feel refreshed and clean and ready to go again. For me it's the horniest time of the month, within a day or two of it stopping. But I certainly have no inclination just before my period.*

Premenstrual Syndrome (PMS)

Marge, 24: *Since I've been on the mini–pill I still get very bloated. But it's not as bad as it used to be. My bras still feel too small but my breasts no longer feel like they've got rocks in them and now I can run to catch the bus. For three days before I get a period I'm constantly hungry. I eat all day but then for three days after it's over I'm not at all hungry.*

Francesca, 42: *In my twenties I didn't think twice about my periods. They came and went. My mother used to complain about her periods and I always dismissed her complaints. She'd say I'm very hungry before my periods or I'm very moody and I always thought that she was making it up or being melodramatic ... I can say that in my late thirties and early forties I am very conscious of my monthly periods. My moods are much more extreme. I have more pain. I have many more symptoms. Nausea. Irritability. Bloated feeling. I find my periods much more hard to cope with now than I did.*

There has long been debate about periods and mood changes. But it is now widely accepted that premenstrual syndrome (PMS) is real and affects many women in different ways. Up to 90 per cent of women notice changes in their emotional and physical feelings which relate to their menstrual cycle. For most women this is not a big problem. But for a minority, about one in ten women, PMS can be serious. It used to be called premenstrual tension or PMT and was a frequent subject of jokes. The new name, where 'syndrome' replaces 'tension', is more accurate since the symptoms do not always include tension. Over 150 symptoms have been documented.

The table opposite shows some of the features of premenstrual syndrome. The most common symptoms are breast tenderness, bloatedness, anxiety, irritability and depression. But these symptoms are only due to PMS if you can show that they happen regularly most months, that they start one to fourteen days before menstruation begins and that all the symptoms disappear by the time your period has finished. If you get these symptoms throughout your cycle, or for most of it, this is *not* PMS. Although PMS is generally seen as a negative experience, studies have shown that 5–15 per cent of women actually feel better just before their periods. They say they have more energy, are more active and feel better overall. Women's reactions are very variable but most of us feel the lift right after our period starts.

Sue, 42: *I have quite typical PMS. I get aggravated easily. I feel very tired. I get headaches and I know I'm going to be ratty and I can't stop myself from being ratty. I just know it. That stops the second I actually get it.*

The Causes of PMS

There are many theories about what causes PMS. They include abnormal responses to normal levels of ovarian hormones, and abnormalities of the chemicals serotonin and B endorphin which are produced in the brain. There are also nutritional theories including deficiencies of vitamin B6 and essential fatty acids, low blood sugar and low magnesium

Symptoms of PMS

Physical symptoms	Psychological changes
• Breast tenderness	• Depression or feeling low
• Bloated feeling, possibly with swollen face, abdomen, or fingers	• Feeling upset
	• Tiredness, lethargy, or fatigue
• Headaches	• Tension or unease
• Appetite changes	• Anxiety
• Carbohydrate cravings	• Irritability
• Acne or skin rashes	• Clumsiness or poor co-ordination
• Constipation or diarrhoea	• Difficulty in concentrating
• Palpitations	• Changes in sexual interest
• Changes in sleep patterns	• Anger
• Muscular aches and stiffness	• Low self-esteem
• Abdominal pains or cramps	• Feeling unattractive
• Backache	• Jealousy
• Exacerbation of epilepsy, migraines, asthma, rhinitis, urticaria	• Insecurity

and calcium levels. Cultural, psychological and social theories have also been suggested. We do not know what causes it but it probably results from a mixture of all these factors interacting with life events. There is some evidence that women who smoke have more trouble with PMS.

How PMS Affects Work

Women who suffer badly from PMS, and even those with less severe symptoms, often worry that it is going to affect their performance at work. But studies rarely show this to be the case. It may be that women are so aware of the possibility that they over–compensate, or that they falsely perceive they are not doing well at work.

How PMS Affects Sex

It can affect and influence women's sexuality as well as the associated mood changes which interact with sexual feelings. In extreme cases PMS can be very damaging to relationships. Severe tiredness and breast tenderness may well interfere with sex. Some women feel much more sexy in the few days before a period. Other women feel sexier straight after.

Am I Neurotic if I Have PMS?

No you are not. But some researchers think you are. A debate over the existence of PMS was rekindled in 1997 when Australian scientists at Swinburne University of Technology in Victoria revealed their claim that PMS does not exist, but that women expect to have it and therefore they use the label to explain whatever symptoms they have around the time of their periods.

Treating PMS

There are many competing therapies which all claim to be the best treatment for PMS. Drugs, hormones, psychological remedies, acupuncture or homoeopathy are all on offer. Few treatments have been properly evaluated to see if they work. Where they have been studied most of them have been found wanting.

The Coping with PMS Plan

- Keep a chart or diary to find out what is actually happening. Carry on keeping it when you try different activities and treatments so that you can monitor what does and does not help.
- Talk about it with a friend.
- Swim, run, walk fast or try yoga for exercise.
- Try relaxation techniques.
- Eat frequent small meals.
- Try having an evening meal high in carbohydrates. This may work by altering the serotonin levels in the brain.
- Try cutting out sweets, coffee and alcohol. Women who drink excess alcohol tend to have more severe PMS than those who do not.
- Give up smoking. There is some evidence that there may be a link between PMS and smoking.
- Try taking vitamins and minerals. Calcium, vitamins B6 and E and magnesium have all been recommended and there have even been a few trials to see how effective they really are. However, the results have been rather disappointing. They are certainly not miracle cures though some women swear by them. There is no harm in trying them as long as you follow the recommended dosage. If you do decide to take vitamin B supplements, the dose should be 10 milligrams a day. Larger doses have been found to cause damage to the nerves in your hands and feet if you take them for a long time.
- Take oil of evening primrose (gamma-linoleic acid) which is available without prescription. It helps to alleviate breast pain.
- Try a well-fitting sports bra if breast tenderness is a particular problem.

Tracey Berry, Beauty Therapist: *Starflower oil. I always find for me that it helps with mood swings, any tenderness in the breasts and just helps you feel much better in yourself ... with the pains and PMS you feel quite tense, you feel quite moody. My boyfriend calls me his little monster ... and the oil really does help. It does seem to even out your temperament. You get the same effect with evening primrose oil but you get more of it with the starflower oil.*

What the Doctor Can Do for You

If the self-help options have not helped, you may wish to see your doctor for advice.

For General PMS Symptoms

Many women complain that their doctors seem unsympathetic when they make an appointment to talk about PMS. This could be related to the lack of effective treatments. If your doctor is not sympathetic, see another. Persevere, and take your coping chart with you once you have kept it for three months. If your PMS is bad, it is worth trying the various treatments to see if any of them works for you. Many of the treatments involve hormones. Although we are still not sure why and how PMS occurs, changing the balance of hormones does seem to help some women. Your doctor could prescribe the combined oral contraceptive pill, oestrogen patches, an intrauterine progestogen coil, danazol, progesterone, progestogens or fluoxetine (Prozac). But all these drugs have advantages and disadvantages. Which you decide to take and whether you take them at all, will depend on the severity of your PMS.

The combined oral contraceptive pill gets rid of PMS for some women, whilst for others it seems to make matters worse. If this happens, try another brand. If you need contraception anyway the pill might be a good option. Sometimes taking the pills for a few months without a break helps. Recent studies show that PMS can be helped by using the oestrogen patches that are usually used for HRT (hormone replacement therapy). But you will also need to take progestogen tablets for ten days a month to stop any dangerous build-up in the lining of the uterus which could lead to cancer (see page 64). Different types of progestogens are used for PMS. One of the most popular, and particularly advocated by the British doctor and author Katherina Dalton who put PMS on the medical map, is natural progesterone (cyclogest) taken as a suppository in your rectum or vagina for twelve days at the end of each menstrual cycle. Although some women find it helps, proper scientific trials have not shown it to be effective.

More recently the natural progesterone creams have gained popularity. Progest is the one most easily available. It is claimed that it is effective and free from side effects and many women say it is helpful. Natural progesterone is derived from Mexican wild yam root which contains a chemical, diosgenin, which apparently gets converted into human progesterone. So far there have not been any decent trials to properly evaluate natural progesterones. Studies are now underway, and better information should be available soon. At the present time it is not licensed in the UK. Very few doctors prescribe it, so most women who want to try natural progesterone cream get it themselves by mail order (see page 390).

The intrauterine progestogen coil called Mirena (see page 36) gets rid of periods altogether in over 60 per cent of women and therefore stops the PMS. It is likely to be used more widely in the future. It also acts as a contraceptive but the downside is you can get a light period for several months after it is first put in. This bleeding nearly always stops.

Danazol stops ovulation and gets rid of the periods and the PMS. But it is being used less frequently because of the often intolerable side effects. Many women put on weight, get acne, feel bloated, and get hot flushes so it is only worth trying if your PMS is severe. Other drugs called GnRH agonists work on the ovaries and reduce the level of oestrogen, stopping the menstrual cycle and hence the PMS. But it is suggested that it only be used short term. It is not a good idea to have low oestrogen levels for a long time as it can lead to osteoporosis in later life (see pages 323–7). Fluoxetine (Prozac) and the other SSRI drugs (see pages 107–8) used to treat depression increase serotonin levels in the brain. Recent studies have shown that these drugs do help to alleviate PMS if taken continually. Studies are now looking at whether they continue to work if you start taking them just before your period as most women may not want to be on them indefinitely.

For Breast Pain
Bromocriptine on prescription reduces cyclical breast pain if taken in the second half of the cycle but side effects include nausea, vomiting, headaches, constipation and dizziness.

Fluid Retention and Bloating
A prescription for the diuretic, spironolactone, taken in the second half of the cycle may help. Other diuretics, including herbal formulas, have not been demonstrated to be helpful in research though individual women may find them so.

Pelvic Pain
For a discussion of pelvic pain associated with periods or dysmenorrhoea, see page 38.

PMS and Psychology

Counselling, psychotherapy and hypnotherapy might help you to cope with PMS. But since they have not been properly studied we do not know how good they are. Recently cognitive therapy has been tried and it looks promising (see also Chapter 5). This therapy tries to get you to think differently – and more positively – about your symptoms. This is thought to help you alter your emotional and physical response to PMS. Remember, these therapies may help you cope with the symptoms of PMS rather than get rid of them.

PMS and the Law

Courts of law have considered PMS as a factor in a woman's behaviour, although it does not stand alone as a defence. It is possible to argue a defence of diminished responsibility because of PMS.

Toxic Shock Syndrome

Toxic shock syndrome or TSS is a *very rare* disease but in the late 1980s and 1990s there was a lot of publicity about it. It is not clear why women are more at risk of toxic shock during their periods but the use of a tampon does seem to be associated with it. Men can get TSS too through an open wound. Women who do not use tampons are at very low risk. Since 1980 there have been 150 serious cases and 12 deaths in the UK. In all of these cases a tampon triggered the syndrome by altering the vaginal environment. This allowed the normally harmless staphylococcal bacteria to produce a toxin in large quantities causing fever, dizziness, fainting, rash, diarrhoea, sore throat, muscle aches and headache. Treatment is with antibiotics. Young women seem to be most at risk. This may be because older woman are much more likely to have been exposed to the toxin in the past and will already have built-in protection against it. Since teenagers and women in their early twenties are unlikely to have been exposed before, they have no antibodies and therefore can be overwhelmed by the toxin. It is not a good idea to leave in a tampon for too long for personal hygiene reasons and some people think that leaving a tampon in too long is linked with toxic shock. However, there is no need to change tampons more frequently than every four to six hours during the day and you can leave one in overnight. Leaflets inside tampon packets in the UK now list TSS symptoms and advise using the lowest absorbency necessary. In the USA a clear warning is printed on the outside of the packet.

> **Simmey, 16:** *I was in boarding school and my housemistress knew that I was very lazy getting up in the mornings so when she came in to get me up she wouldn't believe me that there was something wrong. Then I noticed all these black blotches all over my skin and when my housemistress saw this she realized I wasn't pretending and she took me straight down to sickbay. I had constant diarrhoea, vomiting, headaches, dehydration – I remember that very well, I was just constantly thirsty all the time.*

chapter 3

the menopause

Halina, 50: The most important thing I find for all of us to get into our thick heads is that menopause is not a disease. Women have been having menopause since the beginning of time, we will continue, we're not going to die from menopause.

The menopause has an image problem. It is renowned for making women feel hot, then cold, tired and crabby, depressed and old. So if the menopause could hire a public relations consultant she would surely turn to these next voices for help, for they are women who found themselves not over the hill at the change, but over the moon.

Diana Quick, Actress: *I feel that my second half century is going to be a period in which I take charge of my life in a way that I probably haven't done in my first half century. And I feel liberated by having no more periods to deal with.*

Connie: *I can't see why this is seen as anything other than another stage in getting older. I'm going to a city gym ... to classes with young men and young women in them and I can keep up with them.*

Edith: *It's a signpost and I think we're really lucky to have it. Men don't have that signpost. It means that you've been given a little nudge to think about your own mortality and that old age is inevitable.*

There is, of course, another side.

Vicki: *I had my last period when I was thirty-nine and a half. All of a sudden I ... realized the finality of it and I was so sad ... I don't have children. I don't have a boyfriend and I don't have a husband.*

Etta: *It's like saying I'm past it ... past my sell-by date ... no longer sexually attractive ... no longer worth employing ... This is what we menopausal women have got to counteract. We are still a force. We are still acceptable people.*

Tani: *I remember coming to this country as a young woman and the kind of attention one gets as a young woman is very different to the indifference that descends when you are menopausal. But when I go to India I feel good because ... I'm being treated as a woman once again as older age is venerated.*

Some women zoom through the menopause and barely notice it, while for others the change of life represents sleepless nights and the end of youth. In this chapter we examine the menopause in all its glorious detail, from hot flush to hormone replacement therapy – HRT. We consider what you can do about the menopause – if you choose to do anything at all – and we also hear from women who have opted for a 'natural' menopause and find out what gets them through the night.

Talk About the Menopause

In the past decade menopause has come into vogue. It is featured in magazines and not just those for women only. It was fiercely debated on radio and television with the arrival of Germaine Greer's book *The Change* in 1991, as if the menopause were something new. What is new is that the menopause is now a suitable topic of conversation, even in mixed company. It is funny, sad and sometimes painful. But we no longer only hear about it just when something has gone wrong. All women get it. Menopause is not a disease. It is a rite of passage. In spite of the communication barriers, men are talking about the menopause, not only ours but theirs. When we asked men for their thoughts on the menopause some of them automatically took the question to be about their own change:

> **Marc, 42:** *The male menopause? A turning-point that's what comes to mind ... Moods change, attitudes change. Mine I'm a little nervous about ... I'm only forty-two but I've seen it in other men who are older ... From what I can gather from colleagues and friends it's a loss of confidence. It's a question about where they are in their lives. Perhaps they were happier if they misbehaved or behaved like they did when they were twenty. There's a yearning for something they can no longer have. I think with men it's all psychological, for women it's also a change in cycles.*

> **Michael, 54:** *A lot of women my age are going through the menopause and it seems to me to be more in their own perception of what they're going through rather than my reaction to them. One woman I know – if she feels that she's irrational about something – she blames it on going through menopause. But I don't think men sit around saying my God so and so's really going through menopause. From the outside it's more women volunteering that they're in that state and that they're experiencing emotional and physiological changes.*

What is the Menopause?

The word menopause simply means cessation of periods. But we use the word to refer to everything that happens in the years just before and after our periods stop. The menopause usually arrives in the life of a woman between the ages of forty-five and fifty-five, but one per cent of women have had their menopause by the age of forty and occasionally a woman will have a premature menopause in her thirties (0.1 percent) and, very rarely in her twenties. This probably means her childbearing years are over, but newer fertility treatment may be able to help in a few cases (see Chapter 12).

Menopause does not mark the beginning of old age. Ageing is already underway long before our periods stop! Most women at menopause still have one-third or more of their lives to live. Menopause can arrive abruptly or it can sneak up, taking you months – even years – to realize your experience of it has begun. It may come with a wide range of symptoms or it may arrive and depart with barely a flutter. For a few of us the passage will be traumatic. But for most women, its time will bring both mild relief and minor inconvenience. And, as with our periods, the enormous variation from woman to woman is normal.

Hormonal Changes at Menopause

The seeds of the menopause are laid down at the time of conception. We are born with two ovaries, each containing about one million eggs. Ovarian activity is governed by hormones produced in the brain. The ovaries turn on at puberty when our periods start and ovulation begins with our ovaries releasing their monthly egg or ovum. Our ovaries turn off at the menopause and stop releasing eggs. At the same time the ovaries produce smaller amounts of hormones and it is this shortage of hormones – especially oestrogen, progesterone and, to a lesser extent, testosterone – which accounts for so many symptoms of the menopause. The lower testosterone levels, for example, may be linked to a fall off in our sexual drive at this time. Some oestrogen is still produced elsewhere in the body after the menopause.

We do not know precisely what makes the menopause happen. But common sense tells us why we have it. Babies born to women after the age of thirty-five do have a greater risk of Down's syndrome. The risk to a mother's health in pregnancy also increases with age. Evolution has created a genetic mechanism to bring on the menopause when the time to stop having children is right, most of the time. The average age for onset of the menopause is fifty. Nature makes mistakes, of course, and menopause sometimes comes before a woman is ready for it.

The menopause also involves the brain's pituitary gland which orchestrates most of our hormones. One of them, the FSH (follicular stimulating hormone), goes up at the time of menopause in one last attempt to make our ovaries produce eggs. Testing for high levels of this hormone in the blood can help some women identify whether they are at the menopause or not, though a normal level does not exclude the possibility as around the menopause the levels may fluctuate.

How You Know the Menopause Has Arrived

It can be difficult to know. Your periods might just stop but more than likely you will notice other symptoms first. The list of symptoms is long. You might sense a few or you might be unlucky and get the whole lot: hot flushes and night sweats, dryness in the vagina, tiredness, depression, insomnia, palpitations, anxiety, clumsiness, feeling insecure, low self-esteem, loss of interest in sex, irregular periods, no periods, heavy periods, cystitis, weight gain, joint pains, forgetfulness and feeling unattractive.

Hot Flushes

Hot flushes and night sweats are the most common menopausal symptom women experience and complain about. A hot flush is a sudden rush of heat which you might feel flooding upward from your chest and arms to your face. You think your face must be beet red yet see nothing in the mirror. Other women actually look flushed. You may sweat or stay dry. But it is a dramatic heatwave lasting for a few seconds or several minutes. Flushes might come a few times a day or every hour (or more frequently) and they come without warning. Hot flushes may start before your periods stop. Night sweats are equally dramatic.

> **Valma, 49:** *God, hot sweats at night, you'd think someone had thrown a bucket of water over me ... I just get up and I take everything off ... At work I sit in my office there and I feel the old sweats coming on and I'm sweating hot and everyone else is saying 'oh it's not that hot in here', but I've got my flash fan behind my desk and I turn it on whenever I get a hot flush.*

Tiny blood capillaries regulate our body temperature, controlling how much heat is let in and let out. Oestrogen appears to help control heat loss through our skin to keep us from overheating. Under normal circumstances this is our body's physiological cooling mechanism. At the menopause there seems to be a change in the body's thermostat, that means hot flushes are triggered off by the body trying to get rid of heat when it is at a lower temperature than before the onset of menopause.

Harriet, 44: *Mine arrived two weeks ago. I was away on business. My body was just burning up but I didn't feel ill. I reached over to check the radiator under the hotel window and couldn't believe it when it felt ice cold. I had several episodes like that through the night and the next day before I realized this is my menopause!*

Vaginal Dryness and Urinary Problems

The cells that line your vagina need oestrogen to help make the vagina flexible, moist and receptive for sex. When you lose oestrogen around the time of the menopause these cells wither and the lining of the vagina thins. Because there are fewer secretions the vagina feels rather dry, and sex can sometimes be uncomfortable or painful. But even when sex is not the issue a moist vagina feels more comfortable.

After the menopause women sometimes need to use lubricating jelly or cream to help with this dryness, especially if they start a sexual relationship after a gap perhaps due to divorce or bereavement. Women who have regular sex seem to have less trouble with vaginal dryness. Taking more time over foreplay helps too.

The cells of the urethra (the tube which carries urine from our bladders) also depend on oestrogen and they too lose some of their elasticity during the menopause. Sometimes this leads to incontinence problems or a feeling of needing to pee a lot.

Vicki, 41: *The worst part of the menopause, aside from not having children, is this frequent urination problem and the feeling of loss of bladder control. It's not really loss of control but you feel like you've got to pee all the time ... It just feels like I'm going to wet my pants all the time...*

Depression, Tiredness and Mood Swings

Mary: *I suddenly sort of flare up and start crying and say I can't cope and yet I am coping because I'm doing more than I ought to do. And I feel sort of sorry for myself. I'm so angry! I've had headaches and a bit of giddiness. The flushes I can deal with. I sort of giggle about them. I feel absolutely awful, all in a turmoil inside.*

Mood swings are incredibly common and like all the other symptoms, they are normal. Other challenging life events often conspire to coincide with the menopause simply by virtue of our age. Elderly parents need looking after, our children need guidance and many marriages find themselves in crisis at mid-life. All of these worries may magnify the problems of the menopause.

Sex and Attractiveness

A decrease in sexual interest is very common around the menopause. We may feel too tired, unattractive, or too dry. The lowering of testosterone levels which occurs in most women may also affect libido. It may return after the menopause, or it may not. On the other hand, some women feel freer than ever to enjoy sex since contraception is no longer a worry. Others are relieved to find they have more energy for other things.

> **Helen:** *When I entered the menopause, my libido died overnight. I went to bed with it one night and I woke up without it the next morning. Great relief. I felt like I'd gained a lot of time. It was the same feeling as when I gave up smoking. Suddenly the day was longer and I had a lot more energy to devote to things I wanted to do because, God knows, a sexual appetite takes up a lot of time and energy.*

Yet the grey hair, the wrinkles, the bulge around the middle – all of which arrive around the menopause – can work together to make us feel insecure and unattractive.

> **Sandy:** *All of a sudden you find yourself at a party being chatted up by a perfectly nice man but you look at him and you think it's going to be an awful lot of work if it comes to it. On the one hand it's nice to be out with a man. On the other hand I'd just as soon eat another Mars bar.*

If you do feel down about your appearance, do something about it. Think about your best assets – make the most of them. Treat yourself to a new haircut, a new hair colour, buy a hat! Have a massage or a manicure. We are often too hard on ourselves and overly critical of the way we look, so be good to yourself and try to think positively.

Periods

One definition of the menopause is when you have not had a period for twelve months. The end of our periods is the most tangible symptom of menopause and the one that comes to us all. Our periods leave us in as varied a way as their arrival. They may stop suddenly and forever. The cycle can change with our periods coming closer together, or further apart, or becoming lighter or much heavier. Sometimes they gradually become less frequent and then stop. Many women miss a few, think they are gone for good and then find they restart.

> **Kate, 52:** *I have experienced heavier and heavier bleeding. It has left me exceedingly fatigued and very tired which is a tremendous disadvantage as I have a very stressful job so I have to put a very brave face on it and keep going. I think because I work with men one of my worst fears is that I'm going to sort of leave a trail of blood all over the floor or something. It is very distressing.*

If your periods are very heavy it may be related to the menopause or there may be some other reason. Get it checked. If it is just to do with the menopause it can usually be helped by taking tablets such as mefenamic acid or tranexamic acid during your period (see page 35) or by taking HRT (see pages 60–8). If at any time you bleed between periods you should always check this out with your doctor (see also pages 43–5).

Planning for the Menopause

Menopause is an event that is worth preparing for. There are choices to make about possible treatments and it helps to be well-informed. To start with, though, it will make the menopause easier if your health is in the best possible state.

- Diet: It is all a matter of balance. Being too overweight increases your risk of heart disease but women who are a bit heavier do make more of their own oestrogen in their bodies which helps prevent osteoporosis (see pages 323–6). Make sure you get enough calcium and vitamin D in your diet to help keep your bones strong and prevent fractures.
- Relaxation: Learn to relax with yoga, meditation, or other stress-reducing exercises to fight off the depression and anxieties that sometimes accompany the menopause.
- Exercise: This helps build bone mass which protects against osteoporosis. Weight bearing exercises are best for this: jogging, aerobics, walking, cycling and skipping. One study found that hot flushes were reduced by 50 per cent in a group of women who actively exercised compared with those who did not.
- Stop smoking: Smokers have an earlier menopause and are more likely to develop osteoporosis. If you stop smoking even as late as the menopause you can still reduce the risk of hip fractures.

the menopause

Treating the Menopause

If menopause is not an illness, why is there so much treatment for it? Medicine helps to alleviate the unpleasant symptoms of the menopause. But medicine nowadays has a prize greater than the ability to see off an irritating hot flush. The big new hope, Hormone Replacement Therapy or HRT, even promises longer life. But, as with all medical revolutions, there are hitches. There are as many different opinions on the benefits or potential dangers of HRT as there are doctors.

> **Ann, 50:** *As soon as I started missing my periods I jumped on this thing. I had a couple of hot flushes and that was it. My doctor is very pro and he had been talking to me about it for quite some time. So for ten years I had been thinking when it came time I would try it.*

But experts in alternative medicine like journalist Halina St James are not so sure.

> **Halina, 50:** *We're being controlled by people whose goals are not your health but their profit margins. I am not categorically opposed to HRT. I think every woman has to decide for herself. She's got to be informed and she's got to have a doctor that's also informed and open. Doctors are overwhelmed with information in this information age. Your doctor may not know everything, your doctor is not God, but use your doctor as a resource. Go to the Chinese herbalist, go to the naturopath, go to the Internet and go to the book store ...*

The battle over the menopause began in the eighteenth century when doctors began treating it. At first they tried to make our periods continue and by the most gruesome methods: blood-letting, cutting veins and actually applying leeches to women's genitals. Menstrual blood was considered a poison which must be released monthly. Early in the twentieth century doctors were looking into a way that would prolong our periods, and hopefully prolong life. The HRT revolution began in 1938 with the discovery of synthetic oestrogen. Today one in five menopausal women in Britain is on HRT and the number is climbing. Many women feel their lives are transformed with treatment.

> **Enid, 60:** *I started HRT in the late 1970s. I'm sixty now and I finished treatment three years ago. It was an absolute miracle for me. It was like a fairy waving a magic wand and so many of my troubles disappeared and I could live a practically normal life after that.*

What is HRT?

HRT replaces the oestrogen normally produced by our ovaries, but which is greatly reduced at menopause. The ovaries and adrenal glands continue to secrete some oestrogen, but there is a dramatic fall in the level. This accounts for many of the symptoms of the menopause. Women produce different types of oestrogen in their bodies including oestradiol, oestradiol valerate, oestrone and oestriol. These are described as natural oestrogens. The ones we take as HRT are the same chemicals but produced in a laboratory. Some HRT comes from the urine of pregnant mares. These oestrogens, oestrone sulphate and equine oestrogens, are also natural even though they do not come from human beings. Synthetic oestrogens (ethinyl oestradiol and mestranol) do not occur in our bodies naturally and are produced in the laboratory.

It can be difficult to know when and whether to start taking HRT. Some women start taking it at the first sign of menopause, others wait for their periods to stop. You can begin once any of the symptoms of menopause are underway. HRT helps combat hot flushes, night sweats, loss of libido, vaginal dryness, depression, and low energy levels. But now even women with a problem-free menopause are turning to HRT for the long-term benefits it promises: protection from osteoporosis and heart disease.

The Short-term Benefits of HRT

Hot Flushes and Night Sweats
HRT stops hot flushes. Ninety per cent of women report improvement, with their heat 'thermostats' being set back to normal. Hot flushes may disappear within two to three days of beginning HRT, although in some cases it can take up to three months before it works properly. Women also report a significant decrease in night sweats.

Depression and Tiredness
These may be the result of hot flushes and night sweats, which disrupt sleep. Mood swings also often lessen with HRT.

> **Ann, 50:** *I feel more energetic. I feel more positive about life. I'm sleeping better. I just feel an overall sense of healthiness. My memory is better, no question about that.*

Sex and HRT
HRT helps many women resume a healthy sex life if sex has become less pleasurable at menopause because of vaginal dryness.

HRT also helps alleviate the cystitis you may suffer during menopause (see page 192–3).

Beauty and HRT

Finally there is some evidence that HRT improves the skin's collagen, the protein which gives skin its elasticity and helps to slow the ageing process. Some women take HRT purely for cosmetic reasons.

The Long-term Benefits of HRT

Osteoporosis

We all lose bone density as we age but this accelerates at the time of menopause due to the drop in oestrogen. This can lead to osteoporosis. Women most at risk are: thin women, women whose mothers have had osteoporosis, heavy smokers, women who do not exercise, women who exercise excessively, women who have used steroids and those who had severe anorexia nervosa when young. However, just because you have a major risk factor does not mean you *will* develop the disease, it just makes it a bit more likely. At the menopause, women lose bone density at the rate of 1–3 per cent a year since old bone breaks down faster than new bone grows. HRT reduces the risk of osteoporosis whilst you are taking it as it appears to slow down bone loss. When you stop HRT your bones start to thin again until after several months they get back to how they would have been if you had not taken HRT at all. This means that to get the full osteoporosis protection from HRT you have to continue to take it for many years.

Heart Disease

Heart disease is the most common cause of death in women and the risk of dying from it increases with age. Fifty per cent of women over the age of fifty develop heart disease eventually. The average age a woman will get a heart attack is in her seventies. This is probably associated with changes in levels of lipids (fats) in the blood and clotting factors causing atherosclerosis, a build-up in the artery created by fatty deposits. It is thought that HRT helps women who have heart disease and may also reduce the risk of women developing heart disease while they are on HRT by up to 35 per cent. However, other experts claim that between 100 and 200 women will need to take HRT for ten years to prevent one heart attack occuring.

Alzheimer's Disease

A recent study suggests that HRT significantly delays or reduces the risk of Alzheimer's (see pages 329–30) in menopausal women. Oestrogen might affect the neurotransmitter chemicals which are impaired in Alzheimer's. The results look promising but more studies are needed to establish a definite connection.

A Cautionary Note

Some of the positive effects of HRT may actually be due to the behaviour of the woman, rather than the characteristics of the treatment. For instance, women who take HRT are less likely to smoke and are more likely to come from a higher economic group. They are women who are more likely to pursue good health actively. They are also more likely to eat properly and exercise regularly so even without HRT they would have a lower mortality rate from heart disease, for example. How much 'good' HRT is actually responsible for is unclear.

The Worries About HRT

Up to 70 per cent of women drop out of taking HRT within a year. This may be because they are discouraged by the negative things they hear about HRT or because these women have unpleasant side effects. The main reasons women give for stopping HRT are weight gain, being fed up with periods (and HRT can bring on heavy ones), breast tenderness, worries about cancer and not wanting to take pills indefinitely because they are not natural.

> **Sadie, 86:** *I didn't want to be on pills for the rest of my life and I was worried about the side effects. I wanted to do it naturally, after all the menopause is not a disease. From what I've read I think the answer to healthy bones is to eat well, sleep well and keep moving.*

Weight gain

Many doctors claim that research shows HRT does not cause weight gain. But since so many women say the opposite – and also note a weight loss when they go off HRT – their observations cannot be ignored. Sometimes one preparation can cause weight gain whereas another does not, so ask to try another prescription if this is a problem for you.

Cancer of the Uterus

If you have not had a hysterectomy and use oestrogen-only HRT, the lining of the uterus can build up and occasionally a cancer will develop (endometrial cancer). You need to take progestogen with the oestrogen to remove the risk of this cancer developing. You can take progestogen in different ways. The most common way is to take pills which contain oestrogen for sixteen days of the month and pills containing oestrogen and progestogen for the remaining twelve days of the month. This is called the 'period' type of HRT. When you stop the pills with the progestogen *and* oestrogen you have a 'period'. These HRT 'periods' are not real periods but rather bleeds caused by the change in hormones you are taking.

You can also have a no-bleed HRT which is also a mixture of oestrogen and progestogen. The dose of the hormones is adjusted to stop you having periods and at the same time prevent any build-up of the lining of the uterus. But it is advisable to wait a year after your real periods have stopped before taking this type of HRT, otherwise you are likely to get slight continuous bleeding for several months until the lining of the uterus gets less sensitive to the hormones you are taking. During the time before you start on the 'no bleed' type of HRT you can take the 'period' HRT.

If you have had a hysterectomy you need only take oestrogen and do not need to take progestogen as there is no worry about uterine cancer, and you will not have periods.

Breast Tenderness

Breast tenderness and swelling can be a problem. It often improves after three months on HRT, but, if it does not, try a different preparation.

Premenstrual Syndrome (PMS) Symptoms

Sometimes women find they have symptoms similar to those that come with PMS when they take the progestogen preparation in HRT. If this happens you could try another preparation with a different progestogen e.g. levonorgestrol instead of norethisterone. A further alternative is having a progestogen coil (IUS) fitted into your uterus, which gives off a very low dose of progestogen over a long period of time (see also page 36), and you can get your oestrogen by pill or patch.

> **Janice, 50:** *I tried all the different types of HRT pills. Whilst I was on the oestrogen-only pills it was fine. The minute I started on the progestogen as well as the oestrogen it was a nightmare. Palpitations, tender breasts, mood swings – I had the lot.*

Headaches

Some women complain of headaches on HRT. Usually trying a different preparation of HRT solves this problem but a few women cannot find one that suits them.

Breast Cancer

The evidence so far is that there is a small increase in breast cancer after five years of HRT use with up to a 50 per cent increase after ten years. However, it looks as though it might not have quite the mortality rate of breast cancer in women who did not take HRT.

> **Ann, 52:** *I always wondered if the HRT could have played a part. I'd only taken it for a year when I found the lump and it was a cancer. They said I had not been on it long enough but you do just wonder.*

Women who have a family history of breast cancer may be particularly concerned about the HRT connection. We do not know whether these women may be more likely to get breast cancer if they take HRT. Most doctors would not recommend HRT to women who have had breast cancer as many breast cancers appear to be linked to oestrogen. However, studies are underway to see just how dangerous it is (or not) since some women who have had breast cancer do get very bad menopausal symptoms, often associated with the treatment for the cancer, and do need some treatment for the menopause.

Thrombosis

As with the contraceptive pill, there is a risk (but an even smaller one) of getting a blood clot in a vein. If you are not taking HRT your risk of dying from a blood clot is very small: one in a million women per year. If you are taking HRT it is three in a million.

Other Concerns

Gallstones are more likely to develop in women on HRT. Endometriosis (see pages 38–40) may flare up and fibroids (see pages 36–7) may also get bigger.

> **Carole, 54:** *I went through different variations of HRT and they [periods] got progressively worse and having been assured that none of them would start my periods again it was a bit of a shock. The worst morning, it was busy in the office, I had arrived at 8 o'clock with eight Tampax and eight towels and by 11:30 I had nothing left ... I went straight back to the doctor and said this just isn't on, I'm going to stop taking anything. I've been off for eighteen months and I was fine until a few months ago when my periods started again completely out of the blue. So the doctor referred me then to a gynaecologist ... fibroids were causing the trouble.*

the menopause

Women Who Should Consider HRT

- Women whose mothers have or have had severe osteoporosis.
- Women with early menopause.
- Women who have had their ovaries removed before menopause.
- Women on corticosteroid treatment (e.g. prednisolone) which causes our bones to thin.
- Women at high risk of heart disease.

Women Who Should Not Take HRT

There are probably no absolutes, but most experts think that women who have or have had breast cancer or endometrial cancer and women with a history of thrombosis should not take HRT. However, if you have had any of these problems, discuss the relative risks and advantages with an expert.

Which Hormone Combination for You?

- If you still have your uterus you need to take a combined oestrogen and progestogen preparation. Progestogen eliminates the otherwise increased risk of cancer of the lining of the womb caused by oestrogen alone (see page 64).
- If you have had a hysterectomy you need only take oestrogen.
- If your periods have not yet stopped, you need a combination which gives you periods each month – e.g. Prempack C, Nuvelle, or a combination which will give you a period every three months, e.g. Tridestra.
- If your periods have stopped for a year you can take a combination which gives you no periods, e.g. Kliofem. If you try this before your periods have stopped you may get continuous bleeding.

How to Take HRT

HRT comes in many different forms, most commonly tablets, but also conveniently as patches, gels, pessaries, creams and implants. You might need to try a few to see which one suits you best. Do not be afraid to discuss this thoroughly with your doctor. No one knows which is the best way to take the oestrogen in HRT but most of the studies looking at what happens over many years have been done using HRT taken as a pill.

If you take HRT as a pill by mouth, the oestrogen is absorbed and taken by the bloodstream to the liver. Some of the dose you take becomes inactivated during this process. Taking oestrogen by mouth reduces the bad cholesterol, the LDL, involved in heart disease (see page 386–7), more than if you take oestrogen via a patch on your skin. But the oral route increases the level of fats also involved in heart disease, the triglycerides. The skin route reduces or has no effect on the triglycerides. All the oestrogens you take eventually get taken to the liver via the bloodstream.

- Tablets – come either as oestrogen alone, or as a combination of oestrogen and progestogen taken daily, or oestrogen continuously with a progestogen tablet added for ten to twelve days each month.
- Patches – usually contain only oestrogen as oestradiol but some now come in combination as oestrogen and progestogen patches, or as a pack of oestrogen patches and progestogen pills. The patches are round or square and about an inch across. You stick them on your buttocks or abdomen for three, four or seven days depending on the type. You can bath with them on. Sometimes they cause skin irritation.
- Gel – contains the oestrogen oestradiol. It is rubbed into and absorbed through the skin daily, usually on your arms or thighs. It is easy to use, though some women find it a bit messy.
- Implants – are pellets of oestradiol inserted under the skin around your navel using a little local anaesthetic. They are usually put in by a doctor at the hospital, although a few GPs are trained to insert them. The oestrogen is gradually released into the body. They need to be replaced every three to six months. They are usually inserted at the time of a hysterectomy especially if your ovaries have been removed.
- Oestrogen vaginal creams and pessaries – are usually used by much older women in their seventies to treat vaginal dryness and urinary problems. They do not counteract hot flushes as very little of the oestrogen is absorbed. You need to use them two to three times a week.

Most women start with tablets and then switch to patches, gels, creams or another form of preparation if they have problems.

How Long to Stay on HRT

The answer depends on whether you are taking the HRT to stop menopausal symptoms or to prevent heart disease or osteoporosis.

For the Menopause
The majority of women take treatment anywhere from a few months to two years to stop the immediate symptoms of menopause – especially hot flushes, insomnia, depression, joint pains, fatigue and dryness in the vagina. If you have an early menopause (before forty-five) you should consider taking it for longer.

It is difficult to know when to stop HRT if you are taking it for menopausal symptoms rather than to help prevent osteoporosis or heart disease. Menopausal symptoms will revisit most women when they stop it although they are not usually as severe as before and do settle down in time. HRT simply helps bridge the years of change but you will not really know whether you have crossed the bridge until you stop taking HRT.

For Prevention of Heart Disease and Osteoporosis

If you want the additional protection HRT is thought to provide against osteoporosis and heart disease, you will need to take it for many years, perhaps forever. You may decide the protection is worth the increased risk of breast cancer. Heart disease, and fractures relating to osteoporosis, are more common than breast cancer. It is an individual choice you need to make – weighing all the benefits and risks, including the hoped for improvement in quality of life from taking HRT.

Alternative Treatments

There are other approaches to dealing with the menopause without recourse to HRT including diet, acupuncture, homoeopathy and, more recently, natural progesterones. Many women use a combination of these treatments with or without HRT. Those with few or no symptoms at all may take nothing at all. Very few alternative treatments have been properly evaluated.

Natural Progesterone

This is a substance which acts like the progesterone our bodies produce. It is found in Mexican yams and carefully processed mistletoe. Its proponents claim the substance, rubbed into our skin, gets rid of hot flushes, can increase bone density and alleviate other menopausal symptoms. They say it has fewer side effects than synthetic progestogens. However, definitive research to prove these claims has yet to be done (see page 49–50). Trials have started in the UK. One problem is to find a drug company willing to invest in natural progesterone when there is not much money to be made from it as it cannot be patented. You can buy it in some health shops in the UK, although there is not yet a medical licence for its use as a drug here.

> **Halina, 50:** *I've been using [natural] progesterone cream and it has made a real difference to me ... I put a very small amount on the soft parts of my body, less than a quarter of a teaspoon. I put it on my arms, inner thighs, my breasts and my belly. I rotate where I put it and I do this twice a day. For seven days a month I don't use the cream at all. It comes with instructions for use and here's what I've found. No more mood swings, lots of energy, feeling very positive, severity of headaches gone, still get some headaches but not as badly.*

Joan, 48: *I did have a great deal of pain in my right hip. I was unable to walk. I was unable to put my foot on the ground ... So I started to use this cream. I applied it on my breasts, tummy, around the thighs and the hips, the ankles and inside the arm and around the wrists. Within a fortnight I noticed the pain started to subside but it did take a lot longer than that ... I had a bone scan... and having only used this cream for between a year and eighteen months I'm almost back to normal.*

Diet, Vitamins and Trace Elements

Dr Jean Coope, Editor, *Journal of the British Menopause Society*: *In Japan women don't seem to get hot flushes. They eat more soya foods there which contain oestrogen but I think they have a very different outlook on life. I think the women live for the family and they are extremely important. Their role doesn't change in midlife because they are absolutely key members of the family who are needed to look after the old and the young.*

A good diet will help your health, menopause or no menopause, but the most important ingredient in the menopause diet – for the prevention of osteoporosis – is calcium. Calcium is important in your diet throughout life. Studies show that 1500 milligrams of calcium a day is all it takes to reduce hip fractures by 25 per cent (see pages 324–5 for more information on calcium-rich foods).

Trials have shown that vitamin E and ginseng help to reduce hot flushes. How often women get hot flushes and other menopausal symptoms varies between countries. This is also true for osteoporosis and hip fractures. There must be some explanation for these variations which can give us a clue on how best to treat these problems in a 'natural way'. Diet, exercise, and sunlight may all play a significant role. Women in Asian countries get fewer hot flushes and their diet is high in soya products. This may be cause and effect, but it may also be due to other factors to do with genetics and lifestyle. There is particular interest in the effects of soya and linseed oil. A small study gave a group of women, who had reached the menopause, dietary supplements of soya flour and linseed for six weeks. At the end of this time the linings of their vaginas were tested and found to be thicker, looking as though they had taken oestrogen as in HRT. This has led to more interest in how hormones in soya, and other naturally occurring hormones such as progesterone in wild yams, affect the balance of oestrogen and progesterone in our bodies.

Halina, 50: *I am supplementing my diet with a lot of oestrogen-rich foods ... eating tofu, soya milk, flax seed, and soya flour products. When you look at Japanese and Chinese women there is no word in their vocabulary for hot flushes because they don't have any because they're already eating a diet high in soya products.*

We do not understand why there is such variation in the way women of different nationalities experience the menopause. Studies show that whilst 70–80 per cent of women in Europe complain of hot flushes, the figure is 18 per cent in China, 14 per cent in Singapore and 57 per cent in Malaysia. Race, build, lifestyle, patterns of fertility and diet all play a part.

Magnesium, B vitamins and the right balance of fatty acids also seem to help our hormone balances. So try to make foods high in these nutrients part of your diet. You can also try cutting down on tea, coffee and alcohol and avoid hot spicy foods. This may reduce the number of flushes you have. Some women find that herbal teas, such as sage, help with the sweats and anxiety. They have never been properly evaluated but may be worth a try.

Melba Wilson, Writer on black women's health: *Amongst the black women I know who are menopausal or who have undergone it there is a sense that they don't want to have HRT. And I must admit I never really thought I would have HRT until I started talking with some of my white women friends who raised it as a possibility. My friend Beryl who comes from Guyana uses sarsaparilla root to cope with her hot flushes. My mother uses herbal teas. I think I'll probably go that route too.*

Stories Our Mothers Told Us

The way we approach our own menopause is bound to be influenced by how our mothers and grandmothers saw theirs, and by what they told us.

Anna: *My mother had this endlessly pessimistic view of the next stage of life ... you wait till you reach my age ... you're going to be miserable about the menopause. She was totally despairing and that's part of the reason I felt dread about it ... but every inch of the way I realized she was offering me a chance not to be like that.*

Jane: *Menopause to me is my mother's menopause. I was in the middle of puberty when I remember her becoming strange to men, suspicious and having a lot of problems with temper.*

Ilona: *My mother had an awful time during her menopause mostly due to the fact that her older male GP thought the menopause was something women made up to get attention. So when she went to see him he told her to pull herself together and stop being silly, not very helpful at all. She had the lot – hot flushes, dizzy spells, funny heads, very heavy bleeding. It was awful and mum says that at the time she was also very emotional.*

Edith: *My mother is a very liberal and noble woman and she found the menopause a walkover and I've no doubt at all that's what helped me.*

The menopause is just one of the stages along the way in our continuous ageing process.

Halina, 50: *The most important thing I find for all of us to get into our thick heads is that menopause is not a disease. Women have been having menopause since the beginning of time, we will continue, we're not going to die from menopause. It's only when people start fooling around with Mother Nature that we are going to get into trouble. The baby boomer women are heading into menopause and that means one thing for the big multi-national pharmaceuticals – money. And to that end they will push and promote HRT. They will try and promote as many synthetic hormone products as they can.*

Menopause means something different to each of us. Our bodies and our minds will influence our course. We may choose to ride out the change with Mother Nature as our guide or opt for the latest brand of HRT. Treatments come with risks. But so does suffering with what can be unbearable symptoms. Each of us can consider the risks, and come up with a strategy. There are no rules and no guarantees but women have more choices now than at any other time. By making informed decisions we may find ourselves over the moon, at least some of the time.

chapter 4

on the surface

Sue, 42: I'm a cream person ... I buy sun creams, factor 2, 3, 4, 6, 8, 10, and after-sun, special anti-wrinkle cream to go around my eyes and I buy this stick block to go around my eyes and lips. I'm a body-cream freak.

Mrs Cavendish's *Manual of Home Beauty*, 1882, advice to a new young bride:
Never be tempted to go without the discipline of corset and stays. Like an untended plant the unrestricted figure rapidly reverts to an unpleasing state. Always retain the fat skimmed from mutton broth; mixed with cornflour and applied nightly to the skin around the eyes, it wards off blemishing wrinkles. Goose fat may also be used but store neither longer than three days as the smell becomes offensive.

Imagine a 1990s version of Mrs Cavendish's regime. The modern woman would probably skip the corset and she would certainly reject the fat of mutton or goose. But like Mrs Cavendish she tries to hold back the wrinkles. Our daily routine, more than a century on, might well include the use of a cleanser, toner, exfoliator, moisturizer, hydrator, rejuvenator, repair serum, eye cream, day cream, night cream, neck cream – even bust cream – as well as all over body cream. So much choice, so much promise, so much money.

Sue, 42: *Every morning I go through at least five rituals in my bathroom. Soap and water never touch my face and ... it's the usual cleansing and toning but then there's a special one for the eyes and a special one I use three days a week and there's one I use every day. But I don't think I'm out of the ordinary.*

Honor Blackman, 70, Actress: *One was made up at seven o'clock in the morning and sometimes, on television films, one worked until ten o'clock at night ... one sat under the dryer for an hour ... and then the lights all day. So when you got home at night it was so embedded and I must say I've always been fanatical about cleaning my face off.*

The fact is, for many women, when we look our best we feel our best, and vice versa. In this chapter we examine how to get the best from our skin, hair, and nails. And we offer suggestions for the treatment of a range of problems from sun damage to the inevitable wrinkle.

Skin – a Brilliant Design

Skin is our body's largest organ. It is not just a covering. Skin comprises several layers which form our entire body's outer shell. It is made of cells, both living and dead, an intricate network of tiny blood vessels, hair, oil and sweat glands, fatty tissues, and muscle fibres as well as pain and pleasure receptors. Our skin is tough and protective, but at the same time it is delicate and sensitive. The outermost layer, the epidermis, is made up of keratin (a softer version of the same substance which makes our hair and nails), and dead cells which continuously slough off. Keratin varies in strength depending on which part of our body it is covering. The soles of our feet and the palms of our hands have the thickest keratin, our armpits and groin the softest. Keratin also keeps the surface pliable and crack free. Our living skin cells are underneath the epidermis.

Our skin is also sensitive to pressure and temperature. Tiny blood capillaries near the surface of our skin help to control our body temperature. Skin protects our body from invading irritants and infections. It also controls what is released. The critical substance in this process is sebum, a mixture of wax and oils produced by the sebaceous glands which are just under our outer skin layer. Sebum lets in moisture and also controls how much water is allowed to evaporate when we perspire. Without it we would dry out. We produce sebum most efficiently when we do not wash too vigorously with detergents, soaps and shower gels.

Although we need to drink about two to three litres of fluids – water, fruit juices, tea, coffee (but not including alcohol) – every day to sustain and nourish our bodies, there is no evidence that drinking more water does anything to purify our bodies or enhance our complexions in spite of such claims. Skin, as we noted above, is made to conserve the water we give it very efficiently. In fact, even if you do become dehydrated it does not show on the surface unless the condition is extreme.

Skin: the Body Barometer?

Our looks are about skin because skin is what people see. The condition of our skin sometimes – but not always – reflects the state of health we are in. Many women believe they can see the results of healthy living on their faces. A good night's rest and a healthy diet shows. But if we have a skin problem like acne or eczema, no matter how we live our skin may let us down, even though we might be very healthy inside. And there are always those mystery women who live on junk food and look terrific all the time.

Some women with skin problems can be slaves to diets and creams and still be disappointed with the results. There are things all of us can do to give our looks their best chance but some things we cannot easily change. A rested face usually looks better than a tired face but some people just have 'bags' under their eyes no matter what they do. Smokers and drinkers do tend to have more lines on their faces.

> **Jennifer, 44:** *OK, this morning. I woke up after having a solid night's sleep for the first time in weeks and looked in the mirror and thought 'Hey, I don't look bad today'.*

Skin is designed to look after itself, up to a point. Even moisturizer is not usually necessary until we reach the age of thirty or so – and even then, whether or not you really need it depends on your skin. Apart from maintaining good hygiene, the one area where nature alone cannot do the work for us is when we are under the sun. It is important, especially for pale-skinned people, to make full use of sun creams and hats to protect our skin from day one. Debra Hutton, health editor of *Vogue* magazine, gave her top skin tip to *Woman's Hour*:

> **Debra:** *Know what the skin does and how valuable it is and to protect it with a really good sun screen is the number one and not to unnecessarily distress it with all the exfoliants. A little bit of healthy respect.*

Our skin starts to need more help – beyond protection against the sun – when our oestrogen levels begin to fall. Oestrogen helps to keep skin elastic and looking young. Around the time of the menopause our skin may become flaky and dry. Moisturizers should help. If you choose hormone replacement therapy (see Chapter 3) to deal with other symptoms of the menopause, this should help your skin become more pliable and smooth.

> **Marge, 24:** *When you're my age looking good is fun, it's not a race against time. It's about buying purple lipstick, not wrinkle cream. You know it's the last few years of your life when you can easily do these things.*

Moisturizers

Moisturizers vary, like our skin, from creamy to greasy. Test different moisturizers on your skin – there are endless free samples at make-up counters – your skin will soon tell you what it likes. Start with one for normal skin unless you are aware your skin is either too dry or too oily. Lanolin, made from sheep wool, is closest to our own natural oils and may be useful if you are very dry. It is important to keep our skin moist and sealed because cracked skin itches and allows environmental irritants and allergens to get in more easily. The more we shower and bathe the more moisturizer we will need to counteract the drying effects.

A cheap moisturizer is probably just as effective as an expensive one. Professor Terence Ryan, an Oxford dermatologist, has tested some of the market's most expensive skin creams, yet he relies on one of the cheapest for himself. But if you want to spend money on your face, try not to be fooled by sales gimmicks. Cosmetic representatives sometimes encourage women to buy more than one moisturizer, claiming that it is good for our skin to have a rest from a particular cream. But there is no evidence that rotating beauty creams is good for your skin. Your skin will tell you when it is time to change.

Freckles

A freckle is a pigmented area of skin. Some women hate their freckles. Others wish they had them.

> **Catherine:** *Freckles always look quite cute I suppose. They're generally associated with youth and younger women and I suppose it gives the impression that you live this kind of outdoor semi-healthy fresh air existence.*
>
> **Michelle:** *The first time I knew freckles were a problem? In* Jackie *magazine there was an article about how to bleach your freckles with lemon juice and I thought, 'oh no, they must be really ugly'.*

The Wrinkle and the Wonder Creams

The cosmetic companies and their followers believe there has been progress on the wrinkle front. And arguably there has been. If you have the inclination to fight the inevitable you do need dedication and money. The cosmetic industry promotes youth, playing on women's anxieties about ageing. Having a wrinkled skin is supposed to be unattractive but many women are quite comfortable about changes in their face and body.

> **Francesca, 42:** *Even though I see the lines coming, somehow I don't feel so badly about them because I feel that's an inevitable part of life. It's the parts that I feel I can control that I worry about.*

The 'wonder products' are expensive. They also need to be approached with caution. Many claims have been made about antioxidants – these are supposed to fight the free radicals which eventually lead to the destruction of our body's tissues inside and out. When you hear people talking about vitamin E as a sort of fountain of youth, it is the antioxidant bandwagon you are listening to. Research on vitamin E and other supplements looks promising, but more needs to be done.

AHAs – alpha hydroxy acids, also known as fruity acids – are now available in lots of creams. When they first appeared in moisturizers they were considered a major anti-ageing breakthrough because of the way they attack dead skin, penetrating through to expose a more youthful fresh skin below. They do create a temporary glowing effect in many women, but AHAs can also damage sensitive skin and cause redness.

The cosmetics industry has an ever-changing vocabulary of its own and you need to understand it to make the best choices for yourself and to be able to figure out which of the many claims to believe. For instance, would you know whether to spend money on a liposome? Liposomes are minuscule moisture sacs which apparently transport special moisturizing ingredients through our outer epidermis, to take them literally under our skin. The deeper a moisturizer goes the better its chance of working to our benefit.

> **Rona Mackie, Professor of Dermatology, Glasgow University:** *The outer part of our skin is composed of between twelve and twenty layers of cells and I would calculate that liposome-delivered moisturizer might get down to about layer fifteen, whereas if it wasn't delivered in a liposome it might only get down to layer ten ... our skin is losing moisture all the time and skin cells are 90 per cent made up of water so the actual moisturizing base in which some of these supposedly miracle ingredients are contained can be very helpful. What they should only be allowed to claim is that the treatments only go as deep as the outer layer of skin, what we call the epidermis.*

There might be something in the liposome then, and cosmetics companies are working overtime to show us. Digitized image analysis lets scientists take an extremely close look at our skin, to examine the effects of the new super creams. There seems to be something in it. The trouble is you have to keep at it to keep up appearances.

> **Rona Mackie:** *Many of these new cosmetics do have a plumping up effect on the skin as long as one goes on using them and I'm sure digitized image analysis will show that minor wrinkles are smoothed out. Usually the absolute factor though is that one must go on using the relevant cosmetic forever.*

A problem with trying these products is the price: you can pay £75 for a tiny pot of cream to dot around your eyes for what may only be minuscule – and temporary – improvement. Many cosmetics companies offer samples, so ask for some before you invest. Very expensive cosmetic lines are often quite happy to give away samples, especially if you buy something small like a lipstick and let the beauty consultant know you are interested in her line. If you do want to try a regime, take time to browse from counter to counter to make yourself an expert. Ingredients are constantly changing. By shopping around you can check out the terminology, who has what and compare price and sales pitch.

If you ever wondered why department stores devote their ground floors to cosmetics in cities around the world, it is because this is where most of our money is spent: on the way to other more mundane corners of the store. According to a 1997 report by Euromonitor which tracks consumer spending, women in the UK spend £17.50 per year on make-up and colour cosmetics, much less than many of us might expect. We are just behind French women in this category. The analysts also found that British women spend on average £18 per year on skin care products.

> **Sue, 42:** *I wouldn't dream of having a bath without covering myself with cream, from top to toe. If I was forced to do that it would be torture for the whole day. I would turn into an old potato if I didn't ... I do believe my skin is better for having spent more money on it over the years.*

Top Skin Tips
- Moisturize. Especially after the age of thirty.
- Exercise helps to keep skin elastic and prevent water from collecting and causing cellulite.
- Minimize sun damage by covering up and using protective creams and wearing a hat.
- Stop smoking or smoke less to lessen wrinkling.
- Alcohol makes blushers blush more. Drinking cold drinks instead of hot ones may help keep your face from flushing.
- Keep your skin clean, but do not dry it out by over-washing.
- Check the water supply in your area for soft or hard water. If you live in Manchester, where the water is soft, you need less soap and shampoo. In London where water is hard you need more. Don't use more than you need.
- If your skin is dry, shampoo your hair in the sink instead of the shower since shampoo dries the skin.
- Vitamin E is an antioxidant. Oxidation is a natural process which damages cells and there is increasing evidence to suggest that vitamin E plays an important part in keeping the skin healthy and preventing damage. Taking a vitamin E supplement may be helpful.

Skin Problems

The sun, the source of so much pleasure, causes many of our serious skin problems. The more exposure you have to it without protection, the faster the ageing process will be. If you let yourself burn in the sun you increase your risk of skin cancer. Two bands of ultra-violet rays are singled out as being the culprits. UVA rays penetrate the deepest and are thought to be the ones that make our skin prematurely wrinkled and leathery. The other band, UVB, attacks the outer layers of our skin and is blamed for skin cancer.

Sun Damage and Skin Cancers

Elizabeth, 37: *I have what my dermatologist says is solar keratosis and that's the fancy name for sun-damaged skin. Damage was done to my skin between ten and thirty years ago. I never in my life had a blistering sunburn. But as a child and as a young adult I spent an enormous amount of time outdoors ... I kind of grew up in that era where the best thing you could put on your body was baby oil maybe mixed with a little iodine. It was the early equivalent of fake tan!*

Sun damage and skin cancers are on the increase largely because we spend so much of our lives in the sun without sufficient protection. In 1996, the Health Education Authority found that 40 per cent of women aged 16–24 had suffered sunburn. The thinning of the ozone layer also means that we are subject to more intense UV rays. The best protection is to cover up, especially between the hours of eleven and three when the sun's rays are most damaging. Wear a hat with a brim to keep the sun off your face and use sun creams.

Most sun blocks help cut out UVB light and stop sunburn. The higher the number the better the protection. The creams are given an SPF (sun protection factor) number which gives some indication of the degree of protection being offered. A number 30 block on your skin means that it should take thirty times longer for it to turn red and burn than it would normally take without any cream. Although these creams help, they do not offer total protection. There is no such thing as a total sun block. The grading is done in laboratories where tests are often conducted with more cream applied than many people actually use. Sun blocks can give you a false sense of security because we do not know how much they really do protect our skin from sun damage and slow the ageing process. The fairer your skin the higher the SPF number you need and the more frequently you need to put on the cream to try to prevent burning. Titanium dioxide is a chemical included in some of the creams available over the counter and on prescription, and it helps to block UVA.

Elizabeth's skin condition – solar keratosis, a form of sun damage – was detected early:

Elizabeth: *I had this one spot on my face, itchy and irritating, and I had this other spot on my upper lip... It would come and go. I thought it was a weird kind of pimple. And then about six months ago my mother was visiting me and... one morning at breakfast she peered at my face and said... you need to see the dermatologist... he said you have to deal with this. It's a very slow progression. If left untreated it will result in cancer at some point in the future.*

Elizabeth consulted three dermatologists and eventually decided on a prescription cream called Efudix which gets rid of the solar keratosis. Efudix takes several days and sometimes weeks to do its work. It identifies abnormal cells and brings them out, turning them bright red. It may even cause blistering and bleeding, not just in a few spots but in dozens of areas depending on the degree of skin damage. People who have had this early stage of skin damage must avoid the sun or use extreme caution when they are in it.

Most, but not all, skin cancers can be completely cured if they are caught early. Almost all of them are linked to exposure to the sun. Women most at risk have quite white or pink skin which burns easily. Often they are redheads or blondes. There are three types of skin cancer – basal cell, squamous cell and melanomas. If you think you have any type of skin cancer, see your doctor right away.

Basal Cell Cancers

Often known as rodent ulcers, these are the most common and least worrying. Like all skin cancers, they are most common on skin which gets regular exposure to the sun. A basal cell cancer often looks pearly white around the edge. It spreads slowly and gradually into the surrounding skin. These cancers can be treated easily by scraping them off under local anaesthetic or by freezing them. Sometimes they return and require further treatment. If you leave them untreated they spread locally, but it may take many years for them to become very large.

Squamous Cell Cancers

These start in the epidermis of the skin and mostly affect women over the age of sixty. Once again they are most likely to affect skin which is exposed to the sun. Squamous cells appear like red roughened areas of skin. Cutting out the cancer under local anaesthetic is the treatment. These cancers can spread if they are not treated early.

Malignant Melanomas

These are cancers of the skin pigment cells – melanocytes – which normally produce the pigment melanin. Dark-skinned races are less likely to get skin cancer because of the melanin already in their skin, whilst in light-skinned people melanin is produced in response to the sun and normally helps protect against the ultraviolet sun rays. However, the melanocytes sometimes over-react and become cancerous. If caught early and cut out under an anaesthetic, when the cancer is very small and thin (less than 7 millimetres deep), it can usually be cured. The thicker the melanoma the more likely it is to spread. Even if it has spread, there is still much that can be done to improve the prognosis with new types of chemotherapy and virus cell targeting treatments. However, in some instances it will be fatal. Malignant melanomas are twice as common in women than in men.

Moles

Although most of us are born without any moles, they gradually develop through childhood. How many we have is in part genetically determined. Usually moles are not a problem but they can be dangerous. People with more than 100 moles need to be more aware of melanoma. If a mole changes get it checked, especially if it darkens, bleeds, alters in shape or develops an irregular outline, as it could be developing into a cancerous malignant melanoma. Larger moles – more than 7 millimetres in diameter – are more likely to become cancerous so always get them checked if they change. Such changes do not necessarily mean they have become cancerous but this can be easily checked by removing them and looking at them under a microscope. Doctors can sometimes have difficulty diagnosing them just by looking at them. If a mole is found to be a melanoma, a larger excision may be necessary.

Acne

Just about everyone has some experience with acne, and the variation of experience is very wide. Acne ranges from a few annoying pimples to debilitating cases where the entire face, neck, back and upper arms may be covered. Acne usually develops when we are in puberty. It is set off by hormonal changes and imbalances in our skin's surface oils and grease. Our oiliness and dryness is inherited and very oily skin is more prone to acne. Some women find acne gets worse just before periods, others when they are stressed. It usually disappears after a few years but in 10 per cent of women it may persist into adulthood.

A range of creams and cleansers is available to treat acne with or without prescription. The only non-prescription treatments definitely shown to help contain benzyl peroxide. These can cause irritation and redness of the skin. Antibiotics are sometimes prescribed but some people are resistant to them. Those usually prescribed are: erythromycin, tetracycline, minocycline (which can cause pigmentation of the skin) and vibramycin. They need to be taken for at least six weeks before any significant improvement will be seen. Antibiotics can cause side effects such as diarrhoea or thrush (see pages 180–2). There are also antibiotics which can be used on the skin in the form of a lotion. Some contraceptive pills can exacerbate acne but others help, one of which, Dianette, is regularly used in the treatment of acne. If none of these measures works then you may need something stronger. Retin A which comes as a cream, lotion or gel is more frequently used in North America as a kind of fountain of youth cream. It can be used for acne but it may cause side effects such as redness, scaling and irritation.

Rona Mackie: *One of the things that retin A does, is it makes the skin very much more sensitive to sunlight, and American women ... have had to agree that if they're going to use retin A they must completely give up not just sunbathing but sitting out in the sun even. Retin A can induce a little bit of dermatitis, a rather fine red scaling of the skin which isn't always terribly attractive.*

Another alternative is the prescription drug isoretinoin (roaccutane) which should only be used if the acne is very bad. It is not an antibiotic and you take it for a few months. It may cause your skin to become too dry. And there is a greater danger. You must *not* take it if you are pregnant, or trying to get pregnant, since it can lead to malformations in the foetus. Many other side effects can occur including damage to the liver, eyes, kidneys and white blood cells.

Serious cases of acne should be treated early to try to avoid permanent scarring and to reduce the anxiety sufferers experience. People with extreme acne can suffer discrimination at school, in work and in relationships. It may be difficult to talk about your feelings but it is important to discuss them. Tell your doctor and those close to you. Many people complain that doctors do not take the problem seriously. If you feel this is the case, see another doctor. The anxiety created by a bad case of acne may make the problem worse.

Eczema

There are several types of eczema. The symptoms are dry, cracked, scaly skin or patches of rashes, very often on arms and legs. Eczema can be related to hay fever or asthma, which is known as atopic eczema and is usually inherited. One in eight children has this. It may be an allergic reaction to something such as elastic, or laundry detergent. Eczema can also be caused by things in your environment such as soap, house mites, pets, perfume, or bath oil when it is known as contact eczema. See your doctor about getting tested to help find the cause. Sometimes it is difficult to distinguish between allergic and contact eczema. If you think you may be allergic, keep a diary of what you eat and wear – clothing and jewellery. If your eczema is caused by nickel in jewellery, for example, stop wearing it. Allergies may come and go and are not fully understood. For some people the condition worsens with stress.

> **Anne:** *I developed eczema when I was twenty-one. I was mugged and about four weeks after that I realized I was starting to get a bit itchy especially on my arms ... I later went on to develop boils which was very nasty. I started to get hot – suddenly very hot. Hot flare-ups and the skin would get very itchy.*

Anne attributes her eczema to the stress created by the mugging, although it is not known how much a role stress plays in the onset of eczema. As for the symptoms, most of hers are typical as Tina Funnel of the National Eczema Society told *Woman's Hour*:

> **Tina:** *Spots and infected sores are very common ... the classical hallmark is very hot itchy skin. It can range from just a patch of dry skin, through to people's bodies being affected on every part, with sore, itchy skin that's often bleeding or weeping and infected.*

Anne: *It makes it very difficult especially with housework. I have to wear gloves to do any polishing or any cleaning but again even wearing gloves your hands are going to get hot, and you're going to get itchy and ... it starts it all off again ... the bedroom is a disaster area because as soon as I get into bed I warm up and get too hot and then I itch and get scratchy.*

A study carried out by the National Eczema Society (see Useful Addresses on page 390) found that 19 per cent of those surveyed believed eczema affected their sex lives.

In minor cases, keeping the skin moisturized may be enough to prevent cracking. This is vital since cracked skin is more susceptible to irritation. A good all-over body cream is E45 or aqueous cream, available without prescription. It is much cheaper than any of the heavily perfumed body lotions. For small, irritable patches you can use a light hydrocortisone cream such as Hc45, available without prescription, but only use small amounts, and not for more than seven days at a time, especially if using it on your face. Higher powered cortisone creams are available with prescription but must only be used very sparingly as with long-term use these creams can thin the skin, particularly the delicate skin of your face.

There is no real cure for eczema, unless you have the contact variety. In this case, you remove whatever it is that is causing the irritation, assuming you can find it. It can be extremely difficult to discover the source of the problem. Sometimes you can use something for years – a particular soap or laundry powder – without any problem at all and then suddenly develop eczema from contact with it. But for most people, eczema, whatever the cause, can be well controlled.

Rosacea

This facial condition makes your cheeks inflamed, red and blotchy and it usually affects older women. People who suffer from it are often mistakenly labelled drinkers, although it is true that alcohol can aggravate it.

Sonja: *I was on holiday in the sunshine and I couldn't understand why the spots on my cheeks, either side of my nose, wouldn't go away with normal treatment. But it wasn't until a couple of years after that I showed them to my doctor and he was able to diagnose rosacea straightaway. I've always had a slightly red face and I tend to blush easily when I get nervous or tense, when I drink alcohol, and eating certain foods causes a flush. But the spots ... looked like teenage acne spots but different and didn't go away.*

Women who get it are often blushers to begin with, but with rosacea the 'blush' becomes permanent. The spots can be deep and painful or they might dot the surface of the skin. In extreme cases the nose becomes red and distorted, the mislabelled 'alcoholic's nose'.

> **Olivia:** *It's very upsetting to feel that your face looks as though you hit the bottle all the time ... But when you have any condition on your face which makes you feel self-conscious, you feel bad about yourself and your confidence levels drop and so I find when I have a flare-up I slap on more and more make-up which probably makes it look worse.*

Treatments for rosacea include antibiotics either as pills or cream. Try to identify particular foods and drinks which affect you. Chocolate, red wine, sherry and spicy foods set off an attack in Olivia, so she has cut them out.

Cellulite

Cellulite is mainly a fat problem. The fatter you are, the less mobile you are and the more cellulite you will have. It collects in certain areas of our bodies. The rippling orange peel look is created by protrusions of fat, forming pockets under our skin. The amount of cellulite relates to water accumulation just under the skin. Cellulite commonly occurs in breasts, stomachs, thighs and around the tops of our knees. It can become very painful in extreme cases.

> **Professor Terence Ryan, Oxford Dermatologist:** *Mobility is absolutely essential if the skin's going to do a number of things. Not collect water. If it's going to maintain its elasticity and collagen content, it needs movement. People who are overweight get more and more immobile and their metabolism gets less and less. They burn up less fat but they also don't redistribute their fluid in the way they should. And fluid collects in these big legs, big tummies and big breasts.*

Treatments

The best treatment for cellulite is to eat less fatty food (see page 138), lose weight, and exercise. Keep your skin moving so water does not get the chance to accumulate. Even gentle massage helps. A lot of exercise might help to reduce cellulite but you will probably never get rid of it altogether. Activity and a proper diet should help prevent more from developing. You can buy a range of motorized devices to strap on and shake the cellulite-prone corners of your body, but if you are that desperate will you actually have the energy to get up and attach yourself to the torture chamber?

Liposuction is a procedure which sucks out fat but it is not safe and can result in scarring. Dieting and exercise are much safer. Still many women go for liposuction, seduced by advertisements which promise 'a new walk-in, walk-out day procedure that instantly and permanently removes unwanted fat within a few hours and requires no overnight stay'.

Liposuction involves sucking fat from the target area – usually the abdomen or thighs – through a plastic tube with the use of a liposucter. This is tantamount to vacuuming out unwanted bits of your insides. It is supposed to alter the contour of your body, restoring the more desirable shapely curves. The success of this procedure depends on the skill of the operator and the state your body is in before the suction takes place. The older you are the less your skin can adapt to its new shape. Since only small amounts of fat can be removed in one operation, the results can be disappointing. But if too much fat, blood, and other body fluids are carelessly removed, serious complications can arise and, rarely, it can be fatal. Liposuction is major surgery. Think carefully before going ahead with it, check the operator's record and if you do go ahead make sure you are in good condition – a difficult order since presumably if you are really tempted by it, you are not in the best of shape.

Warts and Verrucae

Warts and verrucae are really the same. We call the ones which usually appear on fingers warts, and those on the soles of our feet, verrucae or plantar warts. There are also genital warts (see pages 185–6). They are caused by wart viruses and are very common. Verrucae can be picked up from swimming pools or shared shower facilities. Eventually, they will go away on their own although this may take months or years. If they do not cause you any problem you can leave them. If they are a bother, try one of the many wart-removing gels or creams available without prescription. If they persist, your GP may be able to freeze them with liquid nitrogen quickly and usually without too much pain. Very occasionally you may be referred to a dermatologist. Sometimes the procedure can be painful and may in the case of a stubborn plantar wart, take many months to heal. If you have warts on your face or any sensitive skin area, see your doctor before attempting to deal with them.

Fungal Infection

Athlete's foot is caused by fungal infections which like to live in warm moist places. Drying thoroughly between your toes can help prevent it. Fingernails and toenails can also get infected, becoming wrinkled, deformed and yellowish in colour. Athlete's foot is easy to treat with various antifungal creams or powders available without prescription. Nails present more of a problem. You can get tablets on prescription but you need to take them for several months. The newer ones are expensive and some doctors are therefore not keen to prescribe them on the NHS.

on the surface

New Treatment, New Hope

Recent progress in laser treatment offers hope to women with certain skin problems. A laser allows surgery to be much more precise. A surgeon can aim the laser directly at the unwanted bit, whether it is a cancerous lesion, a tattoo, or a birthmark, reducing the impact on neighbouring good cells. Even tiny veins can be targeted. The procedure gives a tingling sensation but is not painful. It leaves a small purple stain which disappears after a few days. Laser treatment is not routinely available on the NHS but it may be where you live. If you have an obvious birthmark and it distresses you, your doctor may be able to make a case for the NHS to pay for its removal. The most troublesome birthmarks seem to be the deep purple so-called port wine stains. These can also be camouflaged by special make-up (ask your doctor and ask at make-up counters) or removed by other means such as radiotherapy or surgery.

Cosmetic Surgery

Negative images and cosmetic surgery often go together. This is partly because plenty of cosmetic surgery is unnecessary. It is also due to the horror stories that one hears about cosmetic surgery. Society also makes fun of people who have evidently had cosmetic surgery. You can spot elderly women – or men – who have had their faces lifted so tightly (or so many times) that they wear a kind of permanent surprised look.

Very few of us wake up every morning thinking that we are physically perfect. We have seen the models, the magazines, and the film stars all portraying society's idols, and we are not like them. Most of us accept this and do nothing radical about it. But occasionally we may become obsessed with one of our physical features and want to change it, to improve our appearance and perhaps our confidence. We may feel that our ears stick out, our nose is too crooked, our eyes too baggy, breasts too big or small. Sometimes we decide to have our appearance altered in the hope that it will change our lives for the better. Most of us learn to accept ourselves as we are, realizing that having a new nose or larger bust will not solve the other problems we may have in our lives.

But when we have a genuine physical abnormality we may be discriminated against, made fun of, ignored or stared at. We can have trouble forming relationships and getting a job. In such cases, or for example if you have huge breasts which cause you severe pain, the NHS may pay for cosmetic surgery.

Cosmetic surgery, whether you need it or not, carries all the risks that go with any major surgery. Many cosmetic operations are successful, a few fail and occasionally you are worse off than you were before. Very occasionally someone dies. Less dramatically you may go through with an operation and find you do not look that much different than you did before. With cosmetic surgery you can have any part of your anatomy changed. Here are some of the popular alterations you can have:

- Face lifted.
- Nose altered.
- Bottom tucked.
- Breasts enlarged or made smaller (see Chapter 10).
- Tummy tucked.
- Ears reduced.
- Lips enlarged.
- Bags removed from under your eyes.
- Blemish removed.

If you feel you cannot live with yourself as you are, see your doctor and ask for a referral to a plastic surgeon. Try to talk to people who have had the same operation. Do as much research as possible to become informed about the procedure before going ahead.

Hair

Linda, 50: *When I've had my hair cut ... and my hair is alright I feel better about myself than I do at any other time. I look at my hair and I think well that's not too bad and I think perhaps you're not such a bad old bag after all.*

Hair is keratin produced by the fastest-growing epidermis (see pages 73–4). In most people it grows about half an inch per month. The kind of hair we have – its colour, curl, thickness, even when we will turn grey – is genetically programmed from conception. We turn grey when our bodies stop producing melanin, the pigment which gives our hair its colour.

What is 'fashionably correct' for our hair these days is very flexible. Any colour goes – from shocking neon shades to highlights and lowlights to gentle overall colour to cover grey or just for fun. We spend a fortune on shampoos and conditioners, mousse and spritzers, gel, fudge, and wax. Some of these hair products probably replace our own natural oils removed through too vigorous washing. We buy sprays for thicker, bouncier, supposedly sexier hair, slickers to make hair shine, spray to make it hold. Women consistently put having their hair done high on their list of enjoyable things to do.

To keep on top of a carefully styled cut, you need to see a hairdresser about once every two months. The information analysts, Euromonitor, track what we do with our hair. British women colour their hair less frequently and spend less on their hair generally than women in France and Germany, for example. A colour treatment in a mid-range salon costs about £50. If you have all-over colour, it needs re-doing every four to eight weeks. There are of course plenty of hair dyes available that you can apply yourself at home, which are much cheaper.

> **Stephen, 40, Hair colourist:** *Women have their hair coloured because it makes them feel better and that makes them look better. It makes them more alluring, gives them more confidence. But I don't feel women or men have a very realistic view of how they look. Sometimes someone puts on a colour that's too blonde for them, but they like the idea of having that colour so they go for it. I think nice shiny hair is quite sexy in itself. Always use conditioner, always have it well cut, and have a colour that suits your complexion.*

Of course, there are always those who are either not concerned, or for whom style comes effortlessly.

> **Joanna Lumley, on her character, Patsy, in *Absolutely Fabulous*:** *Patsy doesn't care ... She doesn't give a hang what she looks like or what people think about her. She's got no interest in beauty at all. She has her hair piled up high on top of her head because at the moment she admires Ivana Trump ... she's effortlessly good looking ... but ... she decays rapidly every day.*

Dry Hair

Too much shampoo may reduce the important natural greases which both protect our scalp and make our hair shiny. Our hair may then become brittle and our scalp dry which can produce unwanted white specks (bits of flaking skin from our scalp). Conditioners do moisturize the scalp and hair, so use one if you have dry hair. There is no evidence that wax and oil treatments give lasting results but they may make you feel better and give brief relief from a problem condition.

Oily Hair

It is possible that too much washing has the opposite effect to the drying problem above: that in scrubbing vigorously you remove the grease, thus making your scalp work all the harder to produce more grease, leaving you with overly greasy lanky hair. Dermatologist Terence Ryan says that people who complain of greasy scalps are often the most vigorous washers. He points out that in France some dermatologists tell their patients to stop washing altogether until their scalps recover their ability to produce the right amount of grease.

If you want to wash your hair every day, there is a huge range of frequent-use shampoos for sale. But, as with skin cream, experiment, and stick with the one your head seems most happy with.

Dandruff

What causes this heavy flaking of skin from our scalps is not fully understood, but it is related to oil production in the sebaceous glands. Sometimes there can also be a fungal infection in the scalp. Non-prescription shampoos should help, including one containing the anti-fungal ketoconazole. But if it is still a problem, see your doctor as other skin conditions such as psoriasis can cause 'dandruff' which will not go away without treatment.

Unwanted Hair

> *Midsummer Night's Dream*, **Shakespeare**:
> *Nay, faith, let me not play a woman; I have a beard coming.*

But when you are a woman and you have a beard coming it is something else.

> **Elizabeth, 74:** *The unwanted hair on my chin drives me insane. The hair on my upper lip and my chin is one of the biggest sources of annoyance for me and it doesn't matter how often you go to have them removed by the best of technicians they keep returning and it's the most annoying experience for me. It's very expensive just to go for electrolysis and have a few hairs removed.*

There are many reasons for unwanted hair. Hairiness can be inherited. It can be related to a hormonal change in your body which is why menopausal women often notice new hairs appearing on their faces. The birth control pill and hormone replacement drugs used to treat menopausal symptoms (see Chapter 3) may also increase hair growth. The novelist Sara Maitland manages to put a positive spin on it: *'I've got a moustache! It's one of my gains.'* You can put up with body hair, leave it – as many continental European women do – or you can get rid of it. There are several approaches.

Shaving

Many women shave their underarms and legs. You have to do it regularly to maintain smoothness but the frequency varies from woman to woman. Shaving to rid your face of unwanted hair is not a good idea since hair does grow back rougher than before.

Waxing

Hot wax can be used to shape your eyebrows, remove unwanted hair from your face, lower legs or bikini line – that is the hair along the top of your legs by the panty line. The wax is applied to the area of treatment, a cloth strip is placed over it, and it is then removed quickly, pulling the hairs out with it. After a wax treatment, the hair usually does not grow back for a couple of months. The advantages are that it is quick and therefore the pain on removal short, and the hairlessness lasts longer than shaving. If you think the wax feels too hot, speak up because it can cause a minor burn especially in sensitive areas.

Ingrown hairs after a bikini wax can be a problem. Using an exfoliator or a loofah can help prevent these. Exfoliators – usually a grainy cream mixed with water – are massaged into the skin and rinsed off. They are supposed to loosen the outer layer of dead cells, slough them off and expose the new layer of living cells below.

Plucking

This method of hair removal is not at all permanent and it is time-consuming. Some women also say the hair regrowth is tougher after plucking compared to waxing.

Bleaching

This may help camouflage a moustache, but get professional advice from a beautician or at the cosmetic counter because some dyes may leave your hair too bleached out or yellowy and therefore noticeable anyway.

Electrolysis

This procedure involves a licensed operator (they work in most large beauty salons) using a needle through which a very mild electric current passes. The charge is supposed to burn the base of the hair follicle so the hairs do not grow back. However, hairs often return and need removing again. Some women find the procedure painful, others do not. It is more painful in more sensitive areas, the upper lip being more sensitive than the chin. Depending on how much hair you want to lose, if the hairs grow back and how quickly, and how much treatment you can tolerate and afford, you may see an operator once a week or once every few months. Operators recommend visiting as soon as you notice the hair coming through. This is the time when permanent removal is supposedly most successful. All reputable operators use a new needle for each appointment. Make sure your operator follows this practice to avoid any kind of infection.

Not Enough Hair

The formal name for this is alopecia. Women with thin hair are usually simply unlucky. They are at the thin end of the normal range of hair thicknesses. If you have a problem with overly thin hair, ask your doctor to check your thyroid or check for a possible iron deficiency which could be causing the problem. Thyroid conditions can be detected with a blood test. If you do not produce enough thyroid hormone, your skin may be dry and your hair thin. But this is easily treatable with thyroid tablets. Women can start to lose their hair in their middle years, in a similar way to men, because of genetic factors. Oestrogen protects us from balding during our fertile years and it is normal to have some thinning around the time of menopause when oestrogen levels fall (see Chapter 3). Some women find their hair falls out after a serious illness, a stressful event or pregnancy, but it nearly always grows back. A good hair style can help conceal a problem, as can scarves, hats and wigs. Sometimes women get patches of baldness called alopecia areata. We do not know why this happens but the hair nearly always grows back.

Chemotherapy and Hair Loss

Chemotherapy used to treat both benign and cancerous tumours may make you lose your hair (although it does grow back and sometimes curlier). How we handle this depends on each individual. The British politician Mo Mowlam was able to laugh off her hair loss – at least in public – within weeks of her appointment as Minister for Northern Ireland in 1997. She lost her hair after chemotherapy treatment for a benign tumour and created a sensation by removing her wig in public.

Nails

Like our hair, our nails are made of keratin, the same protective substance which covers our whole body. Nails are tough and resilient and a calcium-rich diet will help keep them strong.

Manicures and Pedicures

These treatments involve trimming, shaping, and polishing nails, as well as a massage for the hands and feet. You can do it yourself or better still have someone else do it for you. It can be very relaxing. Having a manicure for your hands or a pedicure for your feet is a treat but it can also do damage. Make sure the seal between your cuticle and nail is not broken. This seal keeps out irritants which can cause dermatitis (inflammation of the skin). This condition is painful and can lead to irregular patterns in later nail growth.

The cuticle is the slim flap of skin which makes the seal between the base of the nail and the skin of the fingers and toes. If you do want to push it back to tidy up the appearance of your nails, wait until after you have had a bath or shower. Do it gently with a towel when the skin around your nails is softened. If you want to give yourself a manicure and are using a little stick to push back the cuticle, cover the stick with cotton wool and push very gently.

Nails also need moisture so use hand lotion if you notice dryness. Nails should be trimmed by cutting straight across, rather than in a pronounced oval shape around the top. Cutting too short and close to your skin can also lead to an infection. Nail varnish does not usually offer protection but, again, research on this is yet to be done.

Feet

Vera, 66: *And I tell you, what I like is having my feet done. Oh it's heaven. To have them massaged and seen to and any callouses, give 'em a real good going over. I've got good feet if I have it done twice a year.*

Gwen, 81: *I enjoy going, I went a fortnight ago. Have your nails cut and a little bit of hard skin on the bottom removed and it puts you nice and tidy.*

Our feet are good at retaining moisture, again thanks to the keratin. The most serious damage to our feet is caused by footwear. Nothing is more uncomfortable than the wrong shoe and the wrong size shoe. Err on the large size – but not too large or you will trip. Throw out old ideas about the shoe stretching to fit the foot. It will only stretch as much as it has to. If your toe touches the inside front of the shoe it is probably too small.

Bunions and corns usually appear as we age – corns on the outside of your little toe and bunions on the side of the joint below your big toe. Corns are thickened skin, often the result of a badly fitting shoe. Bunions occur when the big toe turns outwards. The toe is no longer straight and the skin over the bone at the base of the big toe sticks out, making it difficult to find suitable shoes. The skin rubs against your shoe and forms a bunion. Bunions seem to run in families but they are made worse by too tight shoes. Podiatrists can help deal with these problems, but for bunions that get really bad you may need a small operation.

Professor Ryan, Dermatologist: *Fashion footwear is a tremendous strain on the foot ... most women get one toe beginning to come up above the rest and this is entirely due to footwear and then it gets in the way and then it gets a corn on top of it.*

The modern materials shoes are made of now sometimes also cause problems. Children, and sometimes adults, get friction dermatitis when they wear nylon socks and synthetic running shoes which fail to absorb their sweat. It is a good idea to wear cotton socks and leather shoes to prevent this.

The Last Word on Make-up

In the beauty business there is probably nothing more individual or controversial than make-up. Wearing make-up – or not – is no longer reliably a statement about feminism or anything else. But if you want to wear it and are unsure, shop around, try it out and wear what feels right. Ask for samples. Sometimes spending a little more gets you a less gloopy mascara and spending less gets you just as nice a glitter.

Make-up is in constant revolution. Purple lips and purple painted fingertips are no longer far out. Eyeshadows and lash lines are more soft than bold these days, but fashions in make-up come round in cycles too. We give the last word on looks to Dusty Springfield:

> **Dusty Springfield:** *About every five years or so there's this sort of sixties retro and I sort of leap out and go, 'look! see!' It doesn't look that dated after all. Actually I think it was a great look. It took so much effort though.*

She admits she really did use to sleep in her eye make-up and kept it on for a week:

> **Dusty Springfield:** *I still have a tendency to do it. You will get that marvellous build-up if you do that. There was so much on, it would take an awful lot to get it off – a few hammers and spanners and things – so between that and the beehive … I used to sleep bolt upright.*

on the surface

the state you're in

Susan, 41: If there is one thing I could have done differently it would be not to have worried about men so much. When you're young you spend so much time fretting ... about whether you will meet someone and when you do ... whether he will call again and whether he likes you.

Our emotions, feelings, moods, egos, hearts and minds have been scrutinized throughout the twentieth century, from Freud onwards. The seventies were the boom years for psychologists, psychiatrists and therapists, group therapy and gestalt therapy, 'I'm OK you're OK', transactional analysis, transcendental meditation, psychoanalysis, psychotherapy, hypnotherapy – to name just a few of the methods on offer. People have always had problems but we clearly live in a time when we want to do something about them.

> **Dorothy Rowe, Psychologist:** *People are very unhappy. The amount of misery in the world is immense and particularly with people who know that they have got the basic things in life which ought to make them happy – job, home, family – and increasingly they want to know why.*

Our mind and body health are interdependent. The state our body is in affects the state our mind is in and vice versa, no matter how great or minor the change in either. There is no such thing as a state of absolute well-being, but rather an endless gradient between feeling really good and really bad.

No matter how well-adjusted we are, the likelihood is we will come face-to-face with crisis at some point in our lives, and quite possibly more than once. We may experience insecurity, self-doubt, low self-esteem, the break up of a marriage, an identity crisis, serious illness, and certainly – unless we die early ourselves – the death of a loved one. Crises can arise over ageing parents and ageing children, infidelity (yours or your partner's), fear of flying and other phobias, alcohol, drug, or sexual abuse. If you have not yet been acquainted with any of these, you may have the fear of one. In this chapter we travel the roller coaster of life's anxieties. We try to reassure and suggest ways to go forward, leaving troubles behind.

Anxiety and Depression

Many more women than men ask for help with anxiety and depression. Men also have problems with anxiety and depression but they are less likely to admit it. They may deal with their problems by denying they have a problem at all, as do some women. The way we handle our psychological ups and downs depends on our self-confidence and self-esteem, and how adaptable we are to trying situations. At one level bad moods are appropriate and even helpful, but they can also be crippling, and that is when they are at their most destructive.

Anxiety

Everyone has some anxiety. Anxieties can be attached to tangible events. The way we perceive a situation can also make us anxious even though our interpretation may not be accurate. When women talked to us about their own private anxieties, financial worries and personal security popped up again and again, as did worries about how others see us.

Amy, 30: *Financial difficulties, job insecurity. I think those are the two main ones. Especially now that I have a daughter to support.*

Gertie, 42: *That I won't be around to see my children grow. That's my biggest fear. To think that my children would be orphaned while they're growing up, while they need me, actually makes me feel sick.*

Mary, 72: *I think there are some things we can never absolutely get rid of or cure, a childhood hurt ... it's just an anxiety that will never leave me ... I was the one that could be left at home, left out of things. I think it has just left me with this anxiety that I've spent my whole life trying to get rid of. It's close to what I would call fear. A fear of being left alone. I can be surrounded with people and still have this anxiety.*

Panic Attacks

Panic attacks are an extreme form of anxiety. When you are having one – and depending on the intensity of it – you may feel a range of symptoms: heart palpitations, insecurity, breathlessness, fear, uncertainty, confusion, a sense that there is no way out. You may feel there is no solution to the problem, while you may not even be sure what the problem is. You may feel disoriented, uncertain of taking the smallest step, like which way to turn in the street. One way of dealing with these feelings – again depending on the severity – is to try to wait it out. Stand still, close your eyes and concentrate on breathing. The feeling will pass, eventually. If you are actually hyperventilating, you should try breathing into a brown paper bag (*not* a plastic bag which could cause suffocation). If you feel so out of control that you cannot tolerate the situation tell someone you trust and feel safe with, or ask your doctor for help. Panic attacks are not uncommon and vary enormously in their intensity and duration.

Margaret, 58: *It was a feeling that I couldn't do anything. All I wanted to do was to get into bed and pull the covers over my head and the thought of getting up and even going to have a shower and wash my hair made me panic and I couldn't do anything.*

Linda, 50: *I found it hard to come into work. I'd go to bed, go to sleep, wake up about three o'clock in the morning in a panic and I'd lay there thinking, 'I've got to go to work. I've got to go on the bus. I might be sick on the bus'. And the more I laid there thinking about it the worse it became.*

Helen: *There comes a sort of final straw ... mine was a matter of moving from an area that I'd lived in for thirty years and it was bitterly cold. It was winter ... I started to have one panic attack after another ... and it was like heat going from my feet up my body and into my head and not only that. I had this feeling of ants or insects crawling all over me ... it's just horrible. You know you just want to die.*

When Anxiety is Good: In small quantities anxiety can actually be a positive force.
- It forces you to get things done.
- It concentrates your mind on something, and gives you drive.

When Anxiety is Bad: In large quantities it makes you:
- Less confident.
- Feel out of control.
- Think the worst.
- Feel tired and unwell.
- Indecisive.
- Unable to concentrate.
- Unable to cope.
- Have frequent headaches.
- Experience other physical symptoms of stress (i.e. eczema, irritable bowel syndrome).

Common Stresses Causing Anxiety:
- Friction in relationships at home or work.
- Changing jobs.
- Moving house.
- Divorce.
- Children.
- Bereavement.
- Pregnancy and childbirth.
- Retirement.
- Unemployment.
- Money problems.
- Illness.
- Pressures of work.

Stress-inducing events sometimes come in clusters, guaranteeing trouble:

> **Linda, 50:** *I had the hysterectomy one year, then I got divorced the following year, then I started my job as a receptionist and I'd never done it before and it was completely different to what I'd been doing which was working in a shop. I just found everything suddenly caught up on me and I was very anxious.*

Manifestations of Anxiety

Common signs of anxiety are sleeplessness, bad temper, humourlessness, overeating or undereating.

> **Lydia, 45:** *I always know when I'm really anxious. Instead of laughing when my family tease me I get really cross and we all end up shouting at each other which makes me feel even more anxious and stressed.*

The more extreme forms of anxiety may have more serious consequences and may cause you to harm yourself, or even attempt suicide (see pages 111–13). However, there are some very practical things you can try to help cope with anxiety.

Managing Anxiety

- Make a list of your anxieties.
- Share your anxieties with other people.
- Think about what is making you anxious and break it into manageable parts, so you can face it bit by bit and not feel so overwhelmed.
- Do something you really enjoy to give yourself a break from it.
- Take some exercise – walk, swim, run, anything.

> **Barbara, Yoga Teacher:** *By stretching the body to get rid of tension, by energizing the body by very, very deep breathing and by making the body feel great you get this marvellous feeling of radiant health.*

- Make a plan to improve things, and try to be realistic about it, then act on what you can to begin to decrease the total burden.
- Avoid situations or thoughts which you know trigger anxiety.
- Face your anxiety when you are feeling strong and try to consider the worst scenario – it is frequently not as frightening as you expect. Uncertainty is a major cause of anxiety so recognizing the uncertainty for what it is helps.

- Avoid caffeine (in coffee, soft drinks, chocolate etc.) because it can make you feel jumpy.
- Alcohol can make you sleep poorly and feel depressed which will feed negatively into your anxiety.
- Ask friends for help with practical things like babysitting or food shopping. You may be able to set up an exchange with a neighbour or friend where you help one another.
- You can try to relax by making time for yourself, even if it is just for a few minutes. Time of your own to lie down or sit still, to enjoy the quiet, to read a book, to listen to music which relaxes you. For tips on sleep see pages 117–19.

> **Kath, 20:** *I ... concentrate on the good things about myself ... take time out to go for a walk, go to a museum, go to a concert, do something I enjoy and remind myself of what it is about me that makes me enjoy it.*
>
> **Annie, 44:** *I have developed a whole repertoire of things that make me feel good and I'm constantly looking for new things. Massage is one of them ... I would sometimes plan my massages around things I knew that were going to be stressful. Like my mother has Alzheimer's and so if I was going to visit my mother then I would book a massage for after ... so that I could sort of try and get rid of it. And there was actually one time I was on the massage table and I just lay there and I just was flooded with tears ... but that was also good. It was relaxing because I have a problem with crying. I can't cry if I'm deeply upset. So that released something.*
>
> **Mary, 72:** *I've just started to wake up to the fact that it's such a waste of energy to be spending life being anxious instead of letting myself enjoy some peace and quiet. I am just discovering that I can sit quietly and not be anxious.*

Some people are more anxious than others and cope with stress better. Anxiety is something we help to create inside us, often by placing great expectations on ourselves. The stresses are different at different stages of our lives. Exams, dieting, health concerns can all cause stress and anxiety. Many of us now juggle full-time work with full-time child-rearing. This often means full-time hassle. Arranging childcare can be a nightmare. It is often so expensive we worry whether being out of the house is worth it. For many women it certainly is, although independence comes with a financial and emotional price. When we eventually do find the childcare we need it can still be a challenge to manage. The child gets sick and cannot go to the nursery. Sometimes the children do not like the carer, the carer does not like the children, or the beloved carer decides it is time to move on just when everything is running smoothly. In the middle of this an ageing parent becomes ill, an errant husband leaves, someone else gets the promotion at work. The other option – of staying at home with the children, by choice or enforced – is not without its pressures. Twenty-four-hour childcare is stressful and there are none of those positive inputs from colleagues at work. Gillian Butler and Tony Hope, co-authors of *The Mental Fitness Guide: Manage Your Mind,* suggest trying to look at things differently:

Instead of Thinking:	Try Thinking:
• I have to do this perfectly.	• I can only do my best.
• I'm a failure if I need help.	• Asking for help isn't a failing.
• This must be finished today.	• I'll get it done as soon as I can.
• My friends cope better than me.	• I do cope well with some things.
• It's all too much.	• I can deal with it if I take it in steps.

Really out of Control?

When stress and anxiety become too much to handle by ourselves there is help out there. As always friends and family may be the first to give support. Just sharing the problem can often ease a stressful situation. It is important to keep your friendships healthy – let your friends know when you are stressed so they can understand your irritability. But there is only so much listening and supporting a friend can do and if your anxiety begins to feel unmanageable, you may want to seek outside help – talking to someone completely detached from your situation can help put things in perspective. You may choose to talk first with your doctor who may treat you or refer you to a counsellor. A range of counselling (see pages 104–6) is available sometimes at the doctor's practice, in a separate NHS clinic or hospital, or privately. Sometimes when anxiety or depression overwhelm us to this extent, it is known as a nervous breakdown.

There are also drugs which may help with anxiety in the short term but most of them, such as diazepam (Valium) are addictive if used for more than a few weeks, so doctors are more cautious now about prescribing these drugs after their liberal use in the sixties and seventies. Then, prescriptions were handed out freely, and the drug companies claimed the pills were non-addictive. The withdrawal symptoms associated with Valium are similar to the feelings of anxiety for which you may have taken the drug in the first place. You may experience heart palpitations, dryness in your mouth, have difficulty swallowing, and feel sweaty then cold. The intensity of the symptoms depends on the quantity of drugs you have taken and for how long. If you have been addicted for years, the withdrawal may take years. Ask about the side effects of withdrawal and check out the recommended guidelines. Do some research yourself. If you think you are hooked and headed for trouble, see your doctor or find out if there is a self-help group in your area. Do not delay.

Beta-blockers, such as propranolol, available on prescription, are sometimes used to help attacks of anxiety especially when they are linked to exams, a musical performance or a driving test. These drugs are usually used in the treatment of high blood pressure but they do help block the nervous fast heart rate and trembling hands which could ruin a driving test or violin solo. They are not addictive but can make you feel rather flat and lacking in emotion if taken continually. They are not suitable if you suffer from asthma as they can precipitate an attack and can also make your fingers and toes feel rather numb and cold. If panic attacks and anxiety continue to affect your life, other approaches such as cognitive therapies (see page 105) may be more useful in the long term.

Depression

There is all the difference between a few days of feeling sad, which everyone goes through, and being depressed. Everyone experiences sadness. Depression is markedly persistent and all-pervasive. There is nothing that can cheer you up. Your energy is sapped, your sense of humour non-existent. You probably wake early and cannot get back to sleep, yet you are unable to get up and be productive. You lose interest in food and find it hard to concentrate. You dwell on yourself, full of self-blame, convinced of your worthlessness. If this is the state you are in, you need help and you are not alone. Depression affects one in twenty people at some time in their lives badly enough for them to need help. Yet it is estimated that 70 per cent of depression goes untreated.

> **Rosemary:** *It's a sadness that continues and never lifts and with it comes a feeling of hopelessness and helplessness. You don't want to face anything, don't want to get up in the morning. I just want to shut myself away and I feel with that comes low self-esteem and lack of confidence, not wanting to face people, feeling alone even though I'm with people. It's an internal aloneness that nothing and no one can relieve. When I'm not depressed I'm confident, outgoing, want to achieve, don't doubt myself at all.*

Depression can occur any time in your life. It can strike over the death of someone close, the break-up of a relationship, the pressures of exams or exam failure. It is obvious that at times like this we will feel down, but for some, however, the response is more severe. Depression can also occur after what should be a happy event like having a baby. Most new mums experience postnatal depression to varying degrees (see Chapter 11).

Sometimes depression seems to come from nowhere. Experts are divided over what causes depression. Some see social factors as being at the root of it, others believe it is chemical – something in our make-up which predisposes us to depression. In women, our hormone levels are often blamed for our ups and downs. Psychologist Gerrylin Smith leans towards social explanations:

> *I think the reproductive cycle is important in terms of how women understand their depression, but on balance I think there are other explanations which are related to the social position of women that are, for me as a woman, much more compelling as to why more women are depressed than men. I think it's important to look at women's place in society ... the ways that they derive their self-esteem are often connected to relationships and giving care to other people and in doing that they often don't take care of themselves and often aren't valued for the things that they do – mothering for instance being something that's extremely important but not carrying with it very much status.*

It is likely that depression involves an interaction between social and biological factors. In severe depressions associated with a manic depressive illness, it has long been known that there is a strong genetic link. There is increasing evidence that more mild depressions – and the ease with which people become depressed – also run in the family.

Dealing with Depression
Eighty per cent of depressions appear to get better in three to six months – even without treatment – but this will seem like an eternity to the sufferer and to close family and friends. One of the problems about being depressed is that it leads to a downward spiral – those you love most may find it difficult to be around you since you are not your usual self, and because you may be very focused on your own problems. They may feel there is nothing they can do to help and have difficulty themselves coping with the sadness they see in you. You may be made to feel weak and pathetic, amplifying the negative image of yourself you already have. If you have cancer, people rush round to help, whereas when you are depressed you may be less likely to get support from friends and relatives.

If you learn to recognize the very early signs of depression, it is much easier to turn things around. One of the first signs of depression is in the way you think about yourself. When you are depressed you think negatively about your life. Try to swap these thoughts for positive ones, putting the brakes on your fall. Try to look outward rather than dwelling on yourself. Keep a diary of what you do each day, noting what makes you feel good or bad, and what times of the day and night are better or worse for you. It can also help to think about or write down positive statements, or 'affirmations', about yourself.

> **Jennifer, 44:** *I write almost every day in a notebook in the morning when I get up or I will sometimes take a break at lunch hour and just go off and sit in the park and write. Sometimes it's how I'm feeling and sometimes it's affirmations which a friend recommended to me a couple of years ago.*

Exercise Physical activity often helps to lift depression, even though the depression itself probably makes you feel you cannot even start to do any exercise. But try. Exercise releases endorphins, hormone-like chemicals, which are related to our sensations of pain and pleasure. Exactly how this happy, feel-good substance is released and how it works is not fully understood. When people talk about the great feeling they get from exercise, this may be related to the kick they get from the endorphins. You do not have to run the marathon to get the kick either. A brisk walk or any vigorous household task is enough to release this substance.

> **Jennifer, 44:** *I started exercising because I got hit badly with depression ... and it really did help. An hour after I had exercised it was like the depression would physically lift. So for the last twelve years I have used it as a way of getting rid of stress. I actually don't know how people don't do it because if I didn't do it I think I'd go bonkers. Then the side benefit is that I think I am physically fit.*

Going for Help Never be afraid to ask for help. Everyone feels low and needs support at times. As with anxiety, try talking to friends and family. If you have tried the self-help strategies (see pages 98–9 and 127) and they have not worked, look for other help. When you are depressed, it is sometimes difficult to know when and whether to seek professional help. There are no absolutes but it is time to seek help if your depression:

- Interferes with your work.
- Severely affects your home and family relationships.
- Severely affects your relationships away from home.
- Interferes with your sleep and appetite.
- Causes you to drink heavily.
- Causes you to consider suicide or harming yourself.

Asking for help and following through can be an extremely difficult step to take. If you have never felt the need to ask for help before, you may feel it is a sign of weakness or a sign that you are out of control. You may feel resentful and angry and convinced you can take care of yourself by yourself so you soldier on, alone. This is often the most painful stage in the process, because you are on your own.

the state you're in

Asking for help is a positive step which takes courage, and when you finally do get your nerve there is still the problem of who to go to. Your GP is a good first call, provided you feel comfortable with your doctor. For many women, a few visits to the GP will start to get you back on track. If you prefer not to talk to your doctor, you can ask your GP for a referral to see a counsellor, or you can make enquiries yourself by getting in touch with one of the psychological associations or help lines listed on page 390. Finding the right therapist can be a very difficult process, but it is important to keep looking if you are not happy with your first choice.

Mild depression is often more easily treated with counselling and other psychological approaches rather than drugs. Self-help groups also work for some people. A combination of approaches often proves the most successful. More severe depression may require anti-depressant drugs, long-term psychiatric help and, in extreme cases, admission to hospital.

Talking about It There are many types of approaches to talking about depression. How to choose which treatment is the best one for you depends on the problem, and what is available. The availability of counselling, psychotherapy and psychoanalysis on the NHS varies. Many women who want one of these therapies will have to pay for it, although some medical practices do have counsellors attached to them. Practice resources may only allow for a few sessions. It is difficult to sort out the differences between therapists and what they have to offer, and the usefulness of talking therapy and counselling continues to be debated.

Counselling is a loose term referring to a range of psychological therapies. It can be anything from a single chat with your GP to a series of sessions with a GP, therapist, psychologist or psychiatrist spanning months or years. GPs vary in their ability to provide psychological counselling and you will have to make a decision about your own GP based on your experience with him or her. Professionals involved in psychological treatments, whether they be called counsellors, psychotherapists, psychologists, analysts or psychiatrists, also vary enormously in their training, talent and experience. Counsellor training ranges from a minimum of several weeks – as in the case of mediators trained to work with divorcing couples – to many years in the case of psychiatrists and psychologists.

A variety of counselling is available on the NHS. If you decide to see someone privately you might pay anywhere between £20 and £50 for a session and possibly much more. Finding the right person for you can be an exasperating and frustrating experience. Going for therapy is an individual, subjective, and private matter. The counsellor who suits one person may turn off the next. There are hundreds of different approaches to counselling. The British Association for Counselling (BAC) tries to monitor them. When choosing a counsellor, check to see if he or she is a member of the BAC as membership ensures some training standards, although this may not be true of older counsellors who have been working for many years. It is very important when you are looking for a counsellor that you 'try them out'. If you see one and are not happy, try another. There is nothing wrong with this. It is a healthy, but sometimes difficult part of the procedure, particularly if you are feeling desperate and needy. But if none of them seems right, it may be that this approach to your problems is not going to help. Still, try not to be turned off altogether if you do not like a particular counsellor's approach. You can also ask trusted friends if they know of anyone. If your depression is related to a particular problem in your life, there might be an organization near you which can suggest ways of coping, in confidence.

Psychiatrists are medical doctors who have done further training in the diagnosis and treatment of mental illness. They deal mainly with drug and hospital treatment, although there are also community psychiatrists who work with specially trained nurses and GPs in the community. A psychiatrist may or may not have taken a further qualification in psychotherapy. Only professionals who are qualified as doctors may prescribe prescription drugs as part of your treatment.

A clinical psychologist is someone who has done a degree in psychology, followed by a three-year training course and supervised work in many different NHS settings – for example with the elderly, children, or individuals with learning difficulties. The training teaches cognitive and behavioural therapy in which clients are taught strategies for altering their attitudes and behaviours. This approach attempts to retrain your mind and is especially useful for treating anxiety and phobias (see pages 118–20). Various experiments and trials have shown that this type of treatment can work.

A psychotherapist does not need to be medically qualified and is trained in one of many schools of psychotherapy. It takes a minimum of three years to qualify, including the analysis of the trainee who takes on patients under supervision. There is no legal register of training, but several qualifications are well recognized such as those from the London Centre for Psychotherapy, and the British Association for Psychotherapy.

Psychotherapy involves sessions lasting about fifty minutes. They may be once or several times a week and carry on for a year or more. During the sessions you sit up and talk, although in some therapies you are encouraged to recline while you talk. You can talk about anything you want. You may be there to discuss ways of coping with your depression, or there may be particular areas of your life, or patterns of behaviour that you are unhappy about and which you would like to explore further and ultimately resolve. You are likely to talk about your childhood, your feelings about your parents, friends, partner, former partner, the partner

the state you're in

you wish you had, colleagues at work, the neighbours – anyone! You will probably talk about your loves and hates, fantasies and fears. Focal psychotherapy may last for a shorter time and focuses on a special area intensively whilst the rest of your personality is not explored.

A psychoanalyst is a graduate of one of the internationally recognized institutes such as the Institute of Psychoanalysis or the Tavistock Institute. Psychoanalysis may take years to complete and is not available on the NHS. Psychoanalysis takes so long because of the territory it covers. You are going back over your life, not once but again and again, interweaving the past with the present. It is like the layers of an onion – there is always another layer of skin to peel off. It can be painful but exciting and full of revelation. In a way it disassembles you and puts you back together again. Ending long-term therapy is part of the therapeutic process. The patient and therapist work together towards the ending, over many months, preparing for the separation so that it does not bring new trauma to the patient's life. Some people, however, never leave.

There are many different schools of psychoanalysis based on various theories. The main ones are Freudian (based on Freud's study and treatment of neuroses), Jungian (based on Jung who put greater emphasis on enlightenment and spirituality and less emphasis on symptoms and illness), Kleinian (with a special interest in early infancy and the baby's fantasy life), and Existential (based on Laing who had a philosophical and political bias).

Almost all analysts have appointments lasting fifty minutes during which you sit or lie on a couch and talk about whatever is on your mind. The analyst may direct the discussion to make the links between what is happening in your life now and events in your childhood which may influence your present behaviour. Analysis has never been evaluated to see how effective it is and some people are sceptical about its worth.

> **Judy, 39:** *When I first went to see a psychiatrist I was I think ashamed, and felt weak. Then I discovered how many of my friends had been. Friends I respected. One told me, 'It's strong people who do this' and I now believe this to be true as there is a lot of very hard stuff you have to deal with in the process.*

Judy usually sees her therapist once a week and she has been seeing him over several years, but with long breaks (up to a year) in treatment. She returns to therapy when she feels the need. Judy is slowly sorting out a variety of concerns she has about herself and her family and her place in the family.

Judy: *I believe in the process, as I believe I am ultimately a more peaceful, self-aware person. If I hadn't gone through this I am sure I would have continued to make the same mistakes, and have repeated the same problems, because I wasn't aware of the patterns and cycles I was in.*

Alternative treatments such as acupuncture, aromatherapy and hypnotherapy may also prove helpful in the treatment of depression. It may be that the time spent talking to a therapist is as important as the technique itself.

Drug Treatments Almost twice as many women as men are prescribed antidepressant drugs. This may be because they are more likely to get depressed, but it could also be that they are more likely to seek help, or that doctors are more likely to prescribe antidepressants to women. For some women with depression, drug therapies will enable them to get back to their previous level of functioning. With depression we may have no appetite, be unable to sleep, and generally lose interest in caring for ourselves. In these cases drug therapies can provide a kind of emergency treatment to get us up and operating more or less normally. We may then have a better chance of solving our problems or at least come to terms with some of them. Other drug therapies provide a window of opportunity to start making changes which is when psychological therapies can be helpful in addition to the drugs. Unfortunately there is no drug treatment that does not potentially have side effects, though not everyone who takes antidepressants has problems.

There are two main groups of antidepressant drugs: the tricyclic group such as amitryptiline and dotheipin, and the newer SSRIs (selective serotonin re-uptake inhibitors) which include fluoxetine (Prozac). These drugs act on the chemicals in your brain. The problem in the past with older tricyclic treatments was that some people developed side effects and stopped the drugs before they reaped the benefits. Possible side effects of the older antidepressants are dry mouth, constipation, blurry vision or urinary problems but they are not addictive and may be especially helpful if insomnia is a big problem. Another disadvantage is that they can also kill you if taken in overdose.

Prozac and other SSRIs also cause side effects, such as nausea, insomnia, restlessness and impotence, but they are usually better tolerated. SSRIs are also less likely to kill you if taken in overdose than the tricyclic treatments They are expensive which may be one reason a doctor does not prescribe them. It is claimed by the manufacturers that they are not addictive but as they have only been used for a relatively short time, it is not yet known. Patients are beginning to report difficulties in withdrawing from these drugs. The drug Valium was said to be non-addictive when it first came out in the sixties, but since then it has been shown to be very addictive with severe withdrawal symptoms on stopping (see page 100).

the state you're in

Two million prescriptions were issued for Prozac in the UK in 1995 and the majority were for women. Prozac is also being prescribed for lesser problems, especially in the United States. Women are taking it to cope with loneliness, low self-esteem, and even to ease the struggle of getting back to work on Monday morning. It is also being prescribed for quite minor depression and eating disorders. Peter Kramer, the author of *Listening to Prozac*, has coined a new phrase for this nineties drug: 'plastic surgery for the personality'.

> **Rosa:** *Suddenly you start to feel strong. Prozac's not a happy pill ... it's a strong pill. It makes you cope. It just saved my life.*

Prozac, or any other SSRI, should start to work within two weeks, slightly more quickly than the tricyclic antidepressants, but can take a couple of months to take full effect, a drawback for someone desperate for relief from depression. Once you feel better, it is tempting to stop the pills but it is a good idea to keep taking them for about six months to reduce the chance of the depression striking again. Prozac does seem to lift depression completely in some people. For others it is a complete failure. You usually take it in pill form once a day in the morning. If you take it before you go to bed, it is more likely to interfere with your sleep and cause insomnia which will make you feel even worse.

> **Judith:** *I took it for about three weeks or so ... After two weeks I felt absolutely wretched. I started to tremble. I couldn't even lift a cup up I was shaking so much and my concentration went completely and I just felt I was in a complete daze all day long ... I could certainly tell that these side effects were not my depression. They were much more physical than that.*

Alcoholism

> **Jane, 50:** *I drank for more than one reason. I found I was a different person. I could be more outgoing and bolder. Music and dancing seemed more fun. I was shy and non-assertive and I could do more speaking ... Drinking ... helped me to feel better, so I thought.*

Drinking alcohol is one way of *not* dealing with your problems. It gave Jane a confidence in public she had never known before. But it nearly cost her her life:

Jane: *I remember lying and I remember now that I can't remember things. I had blackouts and things are gone forever. The spiral was never ending ... I was in and out of hospitals. My own doctor said that he would be finished with me if I didn't take the help but this didn't work. I kept on and on. My husband left me at points throughout ... my family would have group meetings to try to help. I just wanted to drink and die. I could see no other way.*

Women who drink heavily have a high divorce rate. Nine out of ten marriages where alcohol is abused break down. Women drinkers are more likely to be victims of violence and to be violent themselves. We argue more when we drink because we misjudge situations. We try to use alcohol to solve problems but it often makes situations worse.

Alcohol ravages our bodies. Heavy drinking can be associated with cirrhosis of the liver, cancers of the liver, mouth and oesophagus, mental illness, depression, high blood pressure and brain damage. Heavy drinking in pregnancy can be devastating for the baby and can cause foetal alcohol syndrome, retarding the baby's physical and mental growth. What causes alcoholism is not fully understood. Some scientists think the tendency may be inherited. Children of alcoholics often become alcoholics, so while there may be a genetic component there is certainly a social component. If your parents deal with problems through alcohol there is a chance you will try to, too. Or you may go the other way, rebelling against the unhappiness created by alcohol you witnessed as a child. Alcohol is heavily promoted in our society, in advertising and throughout our social life. Dinner parties, cocktail parties, receptions, welcomes, goodbyes, all almost always revolve around drink. A great deal of mystery still surrounds who will be the woman who can find the inner strength to recover from alcoholism. How recovery is made is also a puzzle. Groups like Alcoholics Anonymous can help. Jane recovered without them, although she did have counselling.

Jane, 50: *I remember someone saying you should go to AA and I was horrified ... I remember I was beginning to become assertive. I was now able to make my own decisions. I didn't need someone to tell me what to do. It was like a turning point for me ... My counsellor told me I was punishing myself. She told me to stop saying I was an alcoholic, that I had already admitted it, and I was on the road to recovery and she could see that in my personality it was no longer necessary. And the more I called myself an alcoholic the more it was keeping my self-esteem low, and rubbing it in.*

Jane found there are no rules. Each recovering alcoholic must find the way that is right for her or him.

Jane: *I find it really hard to say exactly how I stopped ... I would promise myself that when I got out of hospital I would only have one or two drinks but of course it never worked ... I fell into the trap again and again until finally reaching a hospital that in a sense was under 'lock and key' ... I had so much hell that something happened to me that last time ... It truly was some kind of miracle. I think I could suddenly feel all the sadness that I could see in everyone's eyes who loved me and who had supported me. It was time to try. I remember calling my mum ... and telling her, 'Mum it will be OK'.*

You probably have a problem with drink if you:

• Are obsessed with when and where you will get your next drink.
• Feel the need to drink every day.
• Start drinking early in the day, say in the morning.
• Feel you need to hide your drinking from those close to you.
• Regularly notice you drink more than everyone else.
• Do a lot of drinking alone.
• Notice that drinking interferes with your physical and mental well-being.
• Feel the need to drink to face difficult or frightening situations.

If alcohol is interfering with your life, try to get up the courage to ask for help. You can also try following these guidelines to help stop heavy drinking:

• Have two or three drink-free days every week.
• Try other ways of relaxing, such as through exercise.
• Sip the drink rather than gulping it.
• Put the glass down between sips.
• Alternate the alcohol with non-alcoholic drinks.
• Keep a drinks diary so you know how much you are really drinking.

Living with an alcoholic is also traumatic. Problem drinkers often lie, sneak, and manipulate situations and relationships to try to avoid being caught. If you live with an alcoholic and want to help him or her – as well as yourself – here are some things you can do:

• Do not collaborate in their cover-up.
• Do not start a discussion about the problem when the drinker is drunk. It will not do any good, you will both probably get upset and it will likely end in an argument.
• Consider your own safety and the safety of others. Sometimes people become violent when they drink. Do not put yourself in jeopardy.

- Do not let the drinker blame you for their alcohol problem.
- Try to negotiate a contract about the drinking. It may be that the non-drinker will put up with some drinking, at certain times or occasions.
- See a doctor yourself to get support for yourself and advice on how to deal with the partner, child, parent or friend who has the drinking problem. Many communities have self-help groups for the relatives and friends of alcoholics. You can call Al-Anon, the support group for families and friends of alcoholics, or Drinkline (numbers on page 390).

Suicide

Feeling suicidal is an extension of feeling depressed. Teenage girls attempt suicide more than any other group, but happily they seldom succeed. Relationship problems are the most common reason for the suicide attempt. Most girls take an overdose of a non-prescription drug like the painkiller paracetamol (which is very damaging to the liver), sometimes mixing it with alcohol. They may call for help or be discovered by friends or family. Often they do not really want to kill themselves – the act is more a cry for help – but they may end up damaging their bodies. The figures for attempted suicide rates are unreliable because only a tiny fraction of cases get to hospital, making it hard to judge the extent of the problem. When someone really wants to kill themselves they often hide. Boys and men attempt suicide less frequently, but when they do they are more likely to succeed and they take their lives by more violent methods. The suicide rate among young men is increasing all over Europe.

If you have suicidal feelings, the first and most important step to take is to tell someone. If you do not want to tell someone you know – and many do not – ring the Samaritans (see Useful Addresses on page 390). Many people find talking to another human voice helps and it is often easier to do this by telephone with someone you have never met. As low as you feel, try to remember that suicidal feelings, like depression, do lift. There seems no way out when you have suicidal feelings, but they do pass and you can later feel completely different. Even a day, or a week or two can make a huge difference. The tragedy is that sometimes people attempt suicide perhaps not really meaning to kill themselves, but do. With the help of counselling and perhaps antidepressant drugs your self-esteem will improve and you will feel more able to address your problems. It is very important to see your doctor or another health professional. They do not see suicidal thoughts or suicide attempts as a weakness and they will help you.

Look for alternatives to make yourself feel good when you are low. Write down your negative feelings – it often helps to discard them. Try to exercise, walk, read light material. But if you feel bad about the way you look, stay away from the magazines that make you feel even worse. Try to be good to yourself. Most of us have suicidal thoughts at some time. It is quite normal.

It often falls to doctors to try to assess the level of a person's suicide intent. Managing attempted suicide is difficult. One in four people who attempt suicide will try again.

> **Kath, 20, is taking a peer support counselling course at her university:** *At the course they tell us if someone seems to be indicating that they might be contemplating some form of suicide or taking an overdose you should actually spell it out, you should actually say 'Are you feeling suicidal?' because the chances are they are quite likely to respond to that. If you stay on the periphery and say something like 'You're not thinking of doing anything stupid?' you might make them clam up and be defensive.*

Self-mutilation

Women tend to turn their anger inward more often than men do and even inflict harm on themselves in acts of self-mutilation. About 10,000 people are hospitalized every year in Britain because of this and there are undoubtedly many others who do not seek treatment at all. Victims may stab, cut or burn their bodies to punish themselves, but it is also a way to seek attention, which ultimately is a cry for help.

> **Pat:** *I had no way of expressing it other than by cutting myself ... it was a way of survival. If I hadn't cut myself I think I would've done something much worse.*

Some women find that when they tire of harming themselves they inadvertently find someone else to do it for them:

> **Christine:** *I entered into several violent and abusive relationships which I think – for me – was linked to self-injury. It actually meant I didn't have to injure myself because other people would do it for me and it then reinforced my own feelings of worthlessness and that I needed punishment and that was all I was good for was to be hurt and used and abused but I still did self-injure in several ways. I began taking overdoses – very carefully controlled overdoses, again not to kill myself. I used drink to blot out feeling too.*

Having thoughts about self-harm or suicide can be frightening and you may feel ashamed to tell anyone. Try to do things to turn yourself outward. Once again do not be afraid to seek help from friends, a doctor or counsellor. You may be surprised to find you have company.

Fatigue

Many women complain about feeling tired all the time and this is often a reflection of low mood. If you feel down, tiredness goes along with it. Perpetual tiredness may be related to physical illness, like viral infections or less commonly cancer and heart problems. It can also be related to depression, anxiety and stress, ME or chronic fatigue syndrome, and SAD (seasonal affective disorder) syndrome which is triggered by low levels of light in winter.

Chronic Fatigue Syndrome (ME)

There has been much debate as to whether there is such a thing as chronic fatigue or ME (myalgic encephalitis) syndrome. Most doctors now accept it is real. It is defined as a severe disabling fatigue lasting for at least six months, and made worse by minimal physical and mental exertion. An adequate medical explanation is lacking for this condition. It can be associated with the virus which causes glandular fever, but to date other viruses have not been linked with it. Though it is thought to be caused by a complex interplay of factors and not a psychiatric disease, antidepressants – especially the newer SSRIs – do seem to help sufferers, as do some of the cognitive behavioural therapies used to manage anxiety and depression. Total rest for this condition is harmful and a programme of gradually increasing exercise helps.

SAD (Seasonal Affective Disorder) Syndrome

Some people feel depressed, anxious and lethargic when the days are shortest. January and February are considered to be the worst months for SAD syndrome because sunlight is limited and low light levels are believed to trigger the depression. SAD syndrome is thought to be linked to the hormone melatonin which the body normally produces at night to make us sleep. Melatonin is secreted from the pineal gland in the brain in large amounts in response to the lack of light. Women are more likely to suffer from SAD syndrome. Sitting opposite a special light box for several hours a day is supposed to help alleviate the symptoms (see Useful Addresses on page 390, or ask at your local health store).

the state you're in

113

Love

We get some of our best and our worst feelings from love. When it is at its best we feel good about ourselves, attractive, and healthy. We feel needed and important. We enjoy giving our love and receiving it from another. Love takes a lot of our energy but it also energizes. Our first tingling intense relationships thrill, but with an intensity it is impossible to sustain. One in three marriages ends in divorce. For some women it feels like a bereavement, for others it brings relief.

Frances Campbell, Oxford Psychotherapist and Marital Counsellor: *At the turn of the century I'm told the average length of marriage was fifteen years because one or the other died. I think we have to grow up about divorce – if you marry somebody at twenty now you're quite likely to be married to them at eighty. Sixty years later. Falling in love is developmental, part of growing up. Divorce is giving people another chance. I've found people often fall in love more deeply, more profoundly, in later life. I really do think sex is for grown ups. You need a certain amount of ego strength to abandon yourself to love, and when you're young you don't have it. I tell kids you think sex is for teenagers, but the older you are on the whole the better your sex is likely to be.*

Anna Massey, Actress, on her late marriage: *I love it. I love it. I think that a life with the wrong person is very, very bleak and a single life is better than that, but a life with the right person ... everything seems to fall into place and it's very, very enjoyable.*

But whenever love goes wrong it can be horrible. The break-up of a relationship is one of the most stressful events that can happen in one's life. Some men 'trade in' their wives and marry younger women. Novelist Olivia Goldsmith calls them 'trophy wives'.

> **Olivia:** *There are some photographs of men and their new wives and the previous wife is very often just an ageing replica ... men have often or always had younger women or been attracted to them but they maintained their marriages. I'm not talking about divorce being morally wrong. What I am talking about are the kind of disgusting betrayals that have gone on publicly now and without any kind of retribution for the man.*

Mary recalls her feelings on her fortieth birthday when her husband of twenty years announced he was leaving for a younger woman.

> **Mary:** *Confused and bewildered and shattered and pulverized and bereaved because it's a bit like being a widow without the respectability ... I tried very hard because you're committed to that person and you want them, come what may ... you're determined just to accept what's happening and ... you hope it will pass and that ... it will just be a bad phase and everything will blow over.*

Olivia herself had experienced the same loss.

> **Olivia:** *I was desolate ... it wouldn't be fair to say I just turned over and I wrote this book and then everything was lovely ... no, I had two or three years of true depression, but the women in the book decide that anger that's expressed is much better than anger that is withheld ... There are a lot of depressed women out there who if they examined it are essentially angry.*

> **Mary:** *After the bruises have gone it's a lot better and then in fact you are the envy of some of your friends who frequently are married to boring bigots.*

Relationship breakdown is traumatic and the healing process can be long and painful but, as Mary discovered, you can come out much stronger in the end and this is exhilarating. You feel in control of your life, often more so than ever before. You may find a new confidence and the energy to pursue new goals. If you can pull it off, you have a self-sufficiency and self-reliance your friends truly will envy. But it can be a battle getting there.

Relationship Breakdown Survival Guide

- After a relationship breakdown we often suffer a loss of identity, especially when our identity is closely linked with our partner's. So look for ways to build your own new identity. New friends, new job, new volunteer work, new hobbies. Are there things you always put off doing because your partner was not interested? Now can be the time to take action.

- You may have done everything with your partner. Now you have to find company. Loneliness is a common feeling after breakdown, although remember loneliness inside a bad relationship is also very painful. You could get involved in a sport. Join a club. Would you like to try a group holiday? The Ramblers Association has great cheap walking holidays for all sorts of people at all stages of fitness levels. Or you could try a singles package holiday to a sunny destination.

- Are there some single friends you have ignored because you were caught up in a couples' world? Try to build a bridge back to old friends and acquaintances you may have dropped for no good reason. You might find you have a lot to learn from them.

- You may be dropped from the couples' circuit too, so be prepared to do some entertaining yourself. And when you assemble your new social list, try to mix it up a bit with young and old, couples and singles, male and female. Such an eclectic group will probably be more interesting anyway.

- How are you with money? Who paid the bills? You may benefit from a course in finance.

- If you have not been working but want to get a job now, find out about local retraining programmes.

- At first you might miss having sex. But you might not. When we are broken-hearted our sex drives often take a dive. When you feel ready for sex again, take it easy and make sure you feel comfortable with your new partner.

- Try not to think negative thoughts like 'I'll never have another love' or 'I'm too old to find another' or 'Who would ever want me?'. You are bound to have such thoughts but push them away. Take one day at a time. Take an hour at a time.

- Sort yourself out. It usually takes two to end a relationship. You may benefit from exploring through counselling what went wrong and what your own role in it was, rather than blaming your partner (even if your partner was a nightmare – you were there for some reason!). What were your expectations of the relationship? How did you participate in it? What emotional baggage did you bring into the marriage or relationship? Where is the baggage now? This is the time to take a look at what you carry around inside you so you take a different suitcase next time – and find a more suitable partner.

- The breakdown of a relationship can be like a bereavement. Getting over it does take time and you will go through different feelings and emotional ups and downs. You may feel stunned and not believe it. You may feel sad and depressed. You then may feel angry, hateful and full of revenge. Gradually you come to terms with it and feel better.

Insomnia

Karen, 44: *It's awful. I'm more used to it now and I don't panic. But when I first started to have insomnia I think that the worst was the fear that somehow not sleeping I was going to crack up or die. And now I'm so used to having it I know I can get through so it's not as bad. There's nothing quite so luscious to an insomniac as having a solid night's sleep. You just feel like a different person.*

May, 71: *Nights are so long ... You don't sleep ... During the day you try to do something and then when you go to bed you get overtired and just can't seem to rest.*

People vary in how much sleep they need. The average is about seven and a half hours each night, but some of us feel great on four hours where others feel they need ten. In general you need less sleep as you get older, but this does not apply to everyone. Insomnia and sleep problems are often, but not always, linked to stress and anxiety.

Amy, 30: *Sometimes when I am really stressed about something happening the next day I'll have a hard time sleeping but that's it. I try reading because that usually knocks me out, or hot milk but usually it doesn't work.*

Margaret, 58: *I go to sleep very easily but I do wake up about half-past four in the morning and I find if it's my early morning to come to work when I have to get up at about 6.15 I often don't go back to sleep again. If I don't have to get up early I will go back to sleep again, so it's a sort of tension thing I think.*

Tips for Treating Your Insomnia:

- Avoid stimulants like alcohol and caffeine in the evening.
- Exercise during the day.
- Have a hot drink – a herbal tea or warm milk.
- Try a herbal remedy, such as valerian, available without prescription.
- Try relaxation techniques and counting games to try to block worrying thoughts.
- Stop working at least an hour before going to bed, and try to relax.
- Try reading something light before going to sleep.
- Listen to relaxing music or try a relaxation tape.
- Use your bedroom as a place for sleeping and not working.
- Develop a routine for bed and try to keep to it.

If you have insomnia try not to fight against it. This can make it worse. If you cannot sleep, give in to it and do something with the time. There is contradictory evidence about how lack of sleep affects our performance the next day. Some scientists say a person who has not slept properly functions just as well at intellectual tasks as someone who has had a good night's sleep. Recently, however, American researchers reported evidence that our moods and thinking abilities are badly affected after loss of sleep.

> **Karen, 44**: *I'll get up and have a glass of milk and take something to eat back to bed, just a little snack and I'll read a book and try and relax about it and say, 'OK I'm going to be awake for a while'. I used to get up and watch TV but I don't do that anymore because I find that TV's stimulating for me as opposed to putting me to sleep. And try not to read too interesting a book. Like a murder mystery or something like that – I want to know who did it – so I'll read until the end!*

All sleeping pills are potentially addictive so they should not be used night after night. Most doctors suggest taking them for a few nights to break a pattern of insomnia or to help get through a crisis.

Phobias

> **Sue, 42**: *Up until I was about thirty-two I used to fly around the world ... and after I had my first child I suddenly developed a slight fear ... and over a period of about ten years my fear of flying became more and more apparent with each trip that I did ... and I've got to the point where I can barely get on a plane at the moment.*

Sue is now at the point where her fear of flying interferes with her life, which is what happens with phobias. We do not know why some people have irrational fears. In some instances a fear occurs because of a bad experience in the past. If you have been bitten by a Rottweiler it is not surprising if you feel fearful of them in the future. But if you feel fearful of all dogs and panic when you see one, then a fear has become a phobia. The feelings are out of proportion to the risk. Phobias can be very irritating to friends and family as they rarely understand why you feel as you do. But the feelings are real. They prevent you from doing things you need or want to do. Sue's trouble with flying starts as soon as she has booked her flight.

> **Sue:** *Then when I go my stomach starts to churn, I get diarrhoea and ... if there's a delay and they say there's something wrong with the incoming plane that's it. That plane is going to crash with me on it ... I cannot control my thoughts.*

Sue took a fear of flying course to try to overcome her phobia.

> *It was comforting because there were 200 other people on that course, a lot of them a lot worse than me. The majority of them were women ... the men who were on the course were the worst ... one man stood up to try and run off the plane ... I'm a little bit better because I understand that when a plane lands all the tyres could burst and the plane can still taxi on the runway. If an engine breaks down you can still fly ... in fact even if all the engines break down you can glide for thirty minutes, I discovered, which gives me a little bit of comfort. Now you've got to find an airport in thirty minutes to land the damn thing on. If you're over the Atlantic forget it. But what happens if the pilot dies? Well the co-pilot, what happens if he dies? Paranoid! It's the control. I'm a control freak anyway and where I lose control – certainly over what I think is my life – I cannot cope.*

The worst thing to do with a phobia is to consistently avoid it. So the first step is to confront the fear. Make an appointment to see your doctor to talk about it. Avoidance makes a phobia even more difficult to overcome.

Agoraphobia

A very common phobia for women is fear of going outside or agoraphobia (literally 'fear of the marketplace'). A shopping trip, even to the corner store, is a terrifying journey if you have this condition.

The common stages of this phobia are:

- A feeling of panic comes over you when you contemplate visiting your regular supermarket, for example, but you drag yourself there anyway. The panic grows, however, until you can no longer face going at all.
- Instead you visit the smaller local shops. This begins to limit your horizons.
- Soon the local shops fill you with panic too so you must go with a friend or get someone else to go for you. Your isolation is beginning.

- You are alone at home now. You do not go out at all. You are isolated. You know it is a problem but you are paralysed by the phobia.
- It is destructive to you and your relationships. And you start to think about getting help. Others around you prod you to do something.

Overcoming the Phobia
- You get up the nerve to call your doctor. You may even cancel the appointment for fear of going out, but eventually you do get there with help from a friend or partner.
- Your doctor will help you formulate a step-by-step plan of liberation from your agoraphobia. It will consist of a set of tasks of increasing difficulty. Sometimes it will help to start the process with a friend. The first might be to step outside your front door, then walk to the street, then to the corner, then round the block.
- Gradually you will change your thinking from, 'I can't do this' to, 'How can I do this?'

Progress may be slow and there may be set-backs. If this happens, do not give up but retrace your steps and build up slowly again. You need to break the vicious circle where you avoid the thing that gives you fear.

Compulsive Helping

Some people, women in particular, have a great urge to help others and in the more extreme cases it is destructive. Doctors called it compulsive helping. People who have it have a desperate need to be needed and it interferes with their lives.

> **Sally:** *I've always been aware that I tend to go out of my way. I pick up waifs and strays and I want to help and I'm staying up late at night when I'm supposed to be studying and I'm on the phone. The phone bills, I'm talking 200 pounds ... I'm a student. I can't afford to pay phone bills like this but yet I'm doing it because I want people to like me in a way. I want to help them feel good about themselves because in some way it feeds me. It gives me my self-esteem.*

Sally became a pest to her friends, ringing up daily to see how they were, sending advice through the post, telling them how to live their lives. She eventually went for help and learned that far from wanting to help her friends she was trying to dominate them. What she was doing went far beyond caring even though what she thought she was doing was helping to make her friends feel good about themselves. She went into group therapy where she met Frances who was diagnosed as having a submissive form of compulsive helping.

Frances: *I do find in my relationships with my boyfriends it's impossible for me to break up with them and I am always at their beck and call. They can phone my house any time and I put everything down to deal with their needs. And really I don't look after myself. I always make sure they're OK ... Perhaps it was something to do with my upbringing. Very strict convent school where it was instilled in all of us to put other people's needs before our own. It was always think of others first and then of course that a woman's role was really to look after the men.*

Women, and occasionally men, who are compulsive helpers do get pleasure from helping. But often the compulsive activity is just a cover for what is really troubling them underneath. The Promis Recovery Centres (see Useful Addresses on page 390) in London and in Kent treat women for all kinds of addictions. It uses the twelve-step Alcoholics Anonymous programme to fight compulsive helping. Step number one is to admit you are powerless, that you cannot in fact make other people happy.

Margaret: *I've been married for thirty-five years and certainly I think I was care-taking for other people way back into my early teens. My father was alcoholic and I was always very attuned to his moods and I married somebody who was a gambler and who had an eating disorder although I didn't realize it or recognize it for many years and again I was totally attuned to his needs and wants to the self-denial of my own. I felt better when he felt good. If he came home in a good mood then I was in a good mood. If he came home miserable and unhappy then I was miserable and unhappy and crept around and looked after things and just hoped for him to feel better. I would be always trying to fix it and try and put on an appearance for the outside world that we were a so-called normal family ... I was painting a false picture both to the outside world and in fact to myself and it was when I actually faced up to that that I started to recognize that there was more to life than looking after everybody else, that I had to actually start looking after me.*

Bereavement

Mary: *I didn't leave the house for eight weeks. I just sat in one seat in the lounge looking out of the window. I didn't know what time of day it was. I couldn't cook. I couldn't do the general cleaning of the house.*

Gwen, 81: *I found Billy dead beside me in bed in the night you know. It was a shock. Then you got to think well you're there by yourself. Think of your home and all the rest of it. Be thankful for small mercies and be thankful you've got your health to carry on like that. That next fortnight I had a big blast come out on my face. What from? 'Shock', the doctor said and gradually it went but then you've got to look after yourself.*

Mandy was just twelve weeks pregnant when her thirty-seven-year-old husband Charlie died of a heart attack.

Mandy: *The one person I wanted to talk to was the one person who wasn't there ... Charlie ... the one thought that kept going through my mind was that Charlie would never meet my little boy – because I soon found out that I was going to have a boy ... I was just so devastated at the thought that he would never meet his dad ... The one thing I would have loved is a photograph of the three of us together.*

Life's greatest sadness is unpreventable and inevitable: the loss of a loved one. This can be so profound it takes time even to accept it has happened. It is accepted that there are four stages of bereavement: shock and disbelief, sadness, anger, and finally acceptance. How long each stage lasts varies from person to person and depends on individual circumstances.

Jane, 54, when her husband died after 22 years of marriage: *I just couldn't take it in when they told me that he had died. For weeks I kept expecting him to be there when I came in from work. The children were devastated. All the neighbours were fantastic – bringing food and calling – almost too much. Then I started to feel really angry with him. To die and leave me on my own, it seemed really selfish. He'd always driven too fast and though the police said it was one of those freak things I've always wondered. But it's difficult to tell even my friends how cross I feel.*

Even when you are prepared for a death, or have watched someone die in great pain, losing someone close to you can be extremely difficult to cope with.

> **Rosy:** *My father had been ill for four years having had several strokes. In many ways for me he died with that first stroke as he was never that same person again. Some of my grieving started then but it was still a shock when he died and I saw him dead lying on the settee in the lounge. My mother wanted him to stay overnight and wait before the undertakers came. She kept going in and talking to him as though he was still with her.*

Occasionally grief can be so debilitating that it becomes a depression for which you need treatment (see pages 101–8). Sometimes it takes years before we are ready to deal with a bereavement.

> **Carla, 28:** *My father died when I was eight. He was thirty-seven and died of a heart attack – very sudden, unexpected. And then I was in a road accident with my mother when I was fourteen and she was killed outright.*

Fourteen years later Carla turned to a counsellor for help with her depression:

> **Carla:** *She really helped me to get to the root of my feelings. She felt that I'd bottled up my grief and I'd tried to go out there and be a together person that could get on with her life. You know, I've been through this so I can go through anything and then unfortunately your body rebels after a while because you can't.*

Stillbirth

Hospitals are much better prepared to support bereaved parents of stillborn babies than they used to be. Parents are encouraged to name their child, to hold the baby, take a photo, and a funeral can be arranged. The time after leaving hospital can be the most difficult. Mums will be returning to a home where a room is ready for a new baby, where the family and friends who were prepared to welcome a new life will instead be greeting bereaved parents.

> **Janet:** *Just as soon as he was born we held him. Beforehand I was very worried ... but at the time it was just lovely. He was all warm and cuddly and it was just as if there was nothing wrong. We didn't want to let go.*

> **Sharon:** *Every little bit about him is so clear in my mind and I can remember him lying at the end of the bed just lifeless but absolutely perfect in every way.*

Some hospitals have local support groups for those who have lost a baby or had a miscarriage. It often helps to talk – if only by telephone – to someone who has been through the same experience. SANDS (Stillbirth and Neonatal Death Society) provides information and a national network of support groups for bereaved parents (see page 390).

Children's Grief

Diane Briggs counsels bereaved children with Marie Curie Cancer Care in Penarth, South Wales:

Diane: *With younger children they will sort of re-enact the cause of the death. They might re-enact the funeral which parents can find quite distressing, and keep asking questions ... 'Is Daddy coming home?' And it takes them a long time to work through that so that then they stop asking the questions and can actually become quite withdrawn. Middle children – seven, eight, nine, ten year olds – often their behaviour changes quite dramatically. They can become quite angry and often have temper tantrums.*

Kiley, 8, joined a counselling group two months after her mother died of cancer: *We sat around in a circle and we talked about ourselves and about the person who died. I got a bit upset sometimes. I cried a little bit.*

Pat, Kiley's grandmother: *She told me she was crying the night before, 'I was thinking of Mum', and of course it does us good to cry because you get that heavy feeling out of your system and I think it was good for Kiley to meet other children and to have their feelings ... to help Kiley cope with the situation.*

Diane: *With teenagers what they want is to be one of the group, to be in with their peers and a death actually isolates them tremendously ... they have difficulty in expressing how they're feeling and their behaviour can alter dramatically ... It can be that they resort to stealing, to missing school, to becoming very aggressive with their teachers ... to actually just looking and feeling very angry and very sullen teenagers.*

Diane on memory objects: *We have memory objects at one session. They bring an object in from the person who's died and they tell us all about it and what it means to them. We've had bars of chocolate in because it was Dad's favourite chocolate and that taste was really important to the child. The memories are still there and they're good memories. And as we pass them round the group ... they begin to talk more about their feelings and they begin to talk about their bad memories as well as their good memories.*

the state you're in

124

A Mother's Death

> **Hope Edelman, Author of *Motherless Daughters*:** *Older women lose a friend. They say they lose not only their mother but an adult who they consulted for woman to woman issues and problems and advice and that's a huge loss for them as well. Even if her mother was a source of stress to her she had patterned her life around coping with the stress, if they had a feisty relationship.*

Losing our parents is a turning point in life. But losing our mother marks the end of possibly the most significant relationship of our life.

> **Rohan:** *I was thirty-four when my mother died. I think my mother's death was absolutely a milestone in my life. I think that although I knew she was going to die the realization that she had died and that I no longer had the chance to have the relationship with her that I'd always wanted, that was devastating.*
>
> **Liz:** *Even now I can remember the sensation in that bedroom was extraordinary. It was as if symbolically the windows were all open because she had gone. There was nothing there.*
>
> **Rebecca:** *I felt liberated and then I thought, 'Oh goodness what a thing to feel when somebody has died, somebody as important to you as your mother'.*
>
> **Debbie:** *When she died I wanted to phone her up and talk to her about it and of course she wasn't there.*
>
> **Victoria:** *You're suddenly faced with your own death when you suffer the death of somebody else close to you. You realize death is ever-present.*

Coming to Terms with Death

It is virtually impossible to get through life without brushing with someone else's death – someone close to you or close to someone you know. And facing up to that is a healthy thing. It is the first step towards coming to terms with death and dying. When someone experiences a loss there is nothing more hurtful than having others fail to acknowledge it. Just a few words can mean a lot.

Marion, 44: *I've been through a number of bereavements ... I try not to judge people who don't say anything but it's difficult. And I try not to judge them because I know if you haven't been through it it's just hard to know what it's about. But there are some people who just ignore it and it ... gives me a sense of the kind of person they are, that they're not comfortable with their emotions or they're scared of it themselves, maybe their own parents' or their own death.*

For all women, but especially older women, getting through bereavement can take a long time. Anniversaries of the death, marriage, and birthdays may be painful. Women who have led isolated lives with their partners are particularly vulnerable. They may struggle with their identity and discover they have not developed interests of their own. Often just filling time is the challenge. There are parallels with the readjustment after divorce. And many of the same survival tips after marriage breakdown apply (see page 116).

Sadie, 86, a few months after the death of her husband: *I nursed him for the last five years. Now things are difficult, how to deal with the time on your hands? Life is a bit empty. I've got friends, not girlfriends exactly. Most of my friends have still got their husbands. I was so involved with my husband. We were fifty-one years married.*

Sadie, one year on, at 87: *I'm better in the sense that I've tried to do things ... I'm interested in music so I go to a music appreciation class. I'm learning French so that helps a bit and I try to visit my friends and since last year I've been going to a university course. I do try to get out as often as possible. It's difficult to make new friends at my age – most of them have (still) got their partners and it depends on what they're interested in and some of them are not so able ... I've got a nice family and lovely grandchildren I see from time to time. I still get lonely because it's hard being on your own and ... you can't meet somebody every day. Fortunately there's the radio and television.*

The Empty Nest

Sometimes we grieve even when no one has died. The empty nest syndrome, when our children leave home, is often a time of great sadness mixed with joy. It is also linked with other major life changes – menopause, retirement and caring for elderly parents.

Ginny: *I had things from when the children were very small that went on the Christmas tree each year which was a routine so I took them all and I went down the garden and I put them all on the bonfire and burned them and sort of sent them off with my love and thanked them for being a pleasure all the time. It might sound silly but that's what I did. And that worked for me. I felt sort of a freedom afterward and a sense of exhilaration really.*

Valerie: *I had a real physical sense of loss when she left. I felt like somebody had cut my arm off and it wasn't there any more. I was very surprised at what a great loss it was and how much grief I felt.*

Managing the State You're in

We close this chapter with a few basic steps you can follow – no matter what state you are in. You can call on them any time. Add a few of your own, and drop the ones you do not like, to help sort yourself out when you are feeling down or simply overwhelmed.

- Identify the problem and develop a strategy to deal with it – right at the very beginning of feeling down.
- Be good to yourself and look after yourself.
- Organize your life so as to avoid situations which make you feel depressed.
- Try to build up your self-esteem by spending time with the friends you like to be around.
- Do work that you want to do.
- Develop interests outside work that you enjoy and make you feel good.
- Learn specific ways to help yourself to relax using exercise, going for walks, reading, yoga, etc.
- Take time to concentrate on these things because they are really important if you want to change or keep your moods healthy.
- When you need outside help don't be afraid to ask for it.

chapter 6

the shape you're in

Madelaine, 41: Maybe it's our attitude towards being in shape. We put it up on some sort of pedestal and it's this unattainable goal and so that becomes self-fulfilling.

There are those who love exercise.

> **Margo, 40:** *I'm one of these keeno exercisers ... I need to do it for how it makes me feel about myself. After I've exercised I feel healthy, I feel younger, I feel that I look younger. I feel clear-headed and stronger and I feel more in control of myself. My idea of a good weekend is Saturday definitely doing some exercise, but on Sunday it's to spend the day outside doing something physical and if I don't do that I just feel cheated.*

And those who would love to love exercise.

> **Madelaine, 41:** *I get into these periodic bursts of I'm going to be fit, like I went out two weeks ago and bought some jogging shoes and made it sort of almost all the way around the park and I haven't done it since! I don't find it a lot of fun. Partly too I think it's a habit. Exercise is a habit and if you can get into the habit then you can probably sustain it. In those few times in my life where I've actually been relatively in shape I think, 'Hey I'm in shape! I don't have to do anything now!' Several months later you're in terrible shape again and you're down in a rut and it's difficult to get out.*

And in between the Margos and the Madelaines there are all kinds of variations. On average, however, the British woman is under-exercised and overfed. We are out of shape. This means that most of us would fall short of perfection should we decide to take a fitness test. This does not, however, spell disaster. What it does mean, though, is that at every turn there is someone waiting to sell us a fitness video, a diet book, membership to a gym, dumb-bells, skipping ropes, stationary bicycle, trampoline, weight-reduction machine ...

> **Clare Longrigg, Editor, *Guardian* woman's page 1994–96:** *The gym is institutionalized torture. You cycle for miles without going anywhere, run upstairs without ever getting to the top and stare at the unpleasant sight of oneself in a lycra leotard. It seems to me the most demoralizing activity one can do.*

There are tremendous benefits to getting in shape and staying that way, but what you may need is something you cannot buy: a change in attitude. In this chapter we look at what it takes to get in shape. We discuss exercise, diet and problems we have with food.

the shape you're in

Fitness and Exercise

The 1990 Allied Dunbar National Fitness Survey is the most comprehensive look at 'the shape we're in' ever carried out in Great Britain. The study asked 6000 adults, selected randomly, what exercise they do and it found that even though we under-exercise, most of us falsely believe we are in good shape. More than one-third of women take little or no exercise. Fifty per cent of women over the age of sixty-five cannot get out of a chair without using their hands to lever them up. Only 5 per cent of women routinely participate in vigorous exercise. One in six people do nothing.

We eat less than we did ten years ago, but we weigh more. The queen of British health and fitness, Rosemary Conley, thinks people are out of shape because 'they're less active now than they were ten years ago and that's because of videos and because of cars and because of dangers in the street'.

The benefits of even just a little exercise are enormous. Barring serious illness and accident, people who exercise will almost certainly live longer. Exercise plays a role in fighting off disease, including heart attack and osteoporosis (see pages 323–7). It can also play a part in the way we look – just a little exercise shifts the water pockets just under our skin which create cellulite (see pages 84–5).

> **Andrea, Fitness Instructor, size 20:** *Fitness is not about thinness, it's about looking after your heart and lungs and looking after your body. Since starting the fitness programme, I feel a lot better – I sleep better at night, my heart and lungs are fitter, I can run miles without getting out of breath, I'm stronger and more supple.*

For most women exercise is about appearances: the Dunbar study found that women work out to look good and to control weight. Men exercise mainly for fun and relaxation.

> **Valma, 49:** *I play golf on Saturday and Sunday and I go to the gym at least two or three times a week. It makes me feel better. It tones my body up. It makes your mind work better. For an hour I'm not thinking about the office, I'm thinking about getting myself into shape and it's an hour that I spend for me, doing something totally for me and for no one else except for the fact that I look good to other people.*

The exercise philosophy of the nineties seems to be rather laid back. The emphasis now is on being active, naturally: walking instead of driving, using the stairs instead of the lift. Sweating your heart out has given way to warming up and getting just slightly out of breath – raising your pulse rate each time you exercise helps to improve stamina. Jogging, although still popular and beneficial, has given way to brisk walking and other more moderate kinds of exercise. The Health Education Authority recommends five exercise sessions per week, each lasting thirty minutes. Some experts say three times per week is enough.

Your pulse rate tells you how fit you are when you exercise. To tell whether or not you are fit, try walking a mile:

- If you are aged under forty you should be able to do this in fifteen minutes and your pulse should be below 130 beats per minute if you are fit.
- If you are aged forty to sixty you should be able to do this in seventeen minutes and your pulse should be below 119 beats per minute if you are fit.
- If you are over sixty you should be able to do this in twenty minutes and your pulse rate should be below 108 beats per minute if you are fit.

Why Exercise?

- Women who do not exercise at all have up to double the risk of heart disease compared to those who do.
- Exercise helps keeps us trim. Being overweight contributes to heart disease, strokes, cancer and mobility problems.
- Regular walking helps prevent osteoporosis. One in four women who lives to ninety can expect a hip fracture. Exercise reduces the odds.
- Regular exercise is a ticket to independence throughout our lives. If we maintain good muscle tone, flexible joints and mobility, we may not need to rely on assistance later on.
- Regular exercise sometimes helps to control blood pressure.

- Exercise improves stamina.
- Exercise reduces stress and helps us to relax.
- Exercise is more critical than ever before, because we are living longer than ever before. It is one way of enjoying better health in our old age.

The Quick Fix

Remarkably, six weeks is all the time it takes to transform from couch potato to active person, barring a serious medical problem. It is always advisable to check with your doctor before you embark on a major overhaul of your body, particularly if you have a medical condition.

The recipe is simple: six weeks of exercise five times a week. Each half-hour session should include five or ten minutes of warm-up and cool-down exercises on either side of your main fifteen-minute routine. Women just beginning an exercise regime should start slowly, exercising for five or ten minutes at a time each day. When you can comfortably manage more, move on to the next stage, and the benefits will become obvious more quickly. The more fit you are the less you will notice any improvement in your condition, because you are simply maintaining it, but you do need to exercise to maintain it.

Rosemary, 51, started running when she was 45: *When I started I couldn't run 200 yards. I've got a small block where I live and I couldn't get round it. I did gradually. I gradually did it walking and running, walking and running and I built up with lots of encouragement from friends and family. It's very slow. It is literally very slow and you've got to keep at it. It doesn't matter if it's fine, sunny ... or tipping down with rain but you have to get out and do it.*

First, the Warm-ups

Before you begin vigorous exercise it is important to do ten to fifteen minutes of gentle exercise to prepare your body. There are good reasons for this. Warm-ups stretch your muscles and literally warm them by getting the blood flowing to your muscles and improving circulation. If you exercise without doing warm-ups, your muscles will be tight and inflexible, to varying degrees. When muscles are loose and supple and warm they stretch as opposed to snapping. So you stand a greater chance of injury if you go straight into vigorous exercise without warm-ups. In addition to preventing injury, warming up also makes exercise more enjoyable because of the improved flexibility. A typical warm-up regime is stretching combined with something else, perhaps cycling on a stationary bicycle, or walking – before going on to the more strenuous exercise. Swimming, too, even though it is a low-impact sport (not weight-bearing) needs warm-ups. Swimmers stretch and bend before entering the water, and make windmill circles with their arms to limber up. Then, once in the water, it is advisable to swim several lengths slowly before beginning the push into the 'real' exercise part of your programme.

The Actual Exercise Session
Initially, if you cannot do twenty or thirty minutes in one go, split the routine into ten-minute sessions: brisk walking, dancing, concentrated hoovering – whatever. One benefit of doing a sustained thirty-minute workout is that fat burns more quickly after twenty minutes of moderate exercise.

Now, the Cool-down
After vigorous exercise your body needs help to return to a normal level of activity. Even though you warmed up and prepared your muscles in the first place, exercise can stress them. If you work with weights, for instance, doing leg lifts can make your thighs and calves very tight. Running, too, puts your leg muscles through a real test. Stretching at the end, for five to fifteen minutes (depending on the intensity of the workout) should bring back the flexibility you created with the warm-ups. Stretching, particularly in the cool-down phase, is excellent to help prevent stiffness and soreness. The older you are the longer you should give yourself for these limbering exercises, but everyone should do them to prevent injury.

Which Exercise?

Walking is terrific for looking after almost everything. It is a useful exercise since it gets us to our destination and can therefore be more easily fitted into our lives. It is excellent for the prevention of osteoporosis because it helps to increase bone mineral density, making bones stronger. What it does not do, unless you speed walk or you walk briskly and for long enough, is get your heartbeat going fast enough to give you that out of breath feeling needed to improve stamina and fitness.

Any weight-bearing exercise – activity which puts the weight on your feet – such as running, jogging, dancing, and walking helps to prevent osteoporosis. Swimming is good for circulation. The water pressure on your skin helps to disperse water inside your skin which, left to sit, helps to create cellulite. Aerobic exercise is almost anything you like doing as long as it gets you moving. It includes all out-of-breath activities, assuming you do them vigorously enough and long enough to get that benefit and build stamina: it can be dancing, running, skipping, or scrubbing floors!

the shape you're in

Age and Exercise

At menopause when oestrogen levels drop (see Chapter 3) our joints become stiff and we lose some of our flexibility. Keeping as active as possible helps to prevent some of this stiffness. Even making sure you never sit too long in one position will help. No matter how much exercise we do, our muscle strength and breathing capacity decrease with age. Regular exercise will, however, help to reduce this loss and to delay its onset. Heavy weightlifting, especially in older women, might be risky if you have never done it before because it raises blood pressure and increases the heartbeat. This type of arm exercise generally in older women should not be undertaken without guidance.

> **Rosemary, 51:** *I only run three times a week. It doesn't sort of rule me. Some people think you have got to do it every day of the week ... when I started I was only doing yards and then you sort of build up to a mile and it gets more and then I joined a club ... so I was running with people because you can chat to people. It's boring if you're running on your own.*

Rosemary went on to run the London marathon:

> *It was just brilliant from beginning to end, even getting up at four in the morning, I could never ever repeat it. It would be an anti-climax. And I ran every step of the way. I didn't walk at all ... four hours, thirteen minutes, twenty-six and a bit miles. The best bit of the marathon is when you're given your medal at the end. I looked at the medal, I turned it over, it says 'I came, I ran, I conquered' and I nearly burst into tears.*

Over-exercising

Although exercise is good, over-exercising is not, especially when it is associated with severe dieting. This can not only make our periods stop but also increases the risk of premature osteoporosis in young women (see pages 323–7). But it takes years for the damage to be done once the periods stop, so there is time to stop the damage before it becomes irreversible. This can be done by decreasing exercise and improving diet. Periods should then return within a few months.

Food and Dieting

The trend in dieting now is not to diet at all, but to eat differently. Vegetables, fruit and fish are in. Red meat and fatty foods are out. The philosophy is eat what you want and as much as you want, but choose from the right food list. This may sound like dieting, but its advocates say it is more of an approach, a shift away from counting calories.

Patricia: *I've done the F-plan diet. I've done the hip and thigh diet. I've tried fasting by eating only apples until you were sick of the sight of an apple. I've tried all those things and you lose a bit of weight and you feel like a saint.*

At least one in five of us is on a diet right now. Six out of ten women diet at some time in their lives. You can join Weight Watchers or buy diet books. You can do the baked potato high fibre diet, the bananas-all-day diet, high protein, low protein, food combining (Hay), eat-fat-to-get-thin diets. In desperation some women wire their jaws shut and resort to sucking yogurt through a straw. Others try detoxification for purification. You can eat eight tiny meals in a day, or three big ones. But diets only work in the short term.

The Genetic Factor

Have you noticed even people with the worst eating habits sometimes have the greatest shapes? Scientists are moving towards the idea that 'the shape we're in' has much to do with inheritance. In other words some people can live on hamburgers and chocolate and still look great. Others can eat properly, work out like crazy, and still feel they never look that good. The actress Honor Blackman believes she was given a good set of genes, but she also exercises and watches her diet, and at seventy it shows.

Honor Blackman, 70, Actress: *I have a sister who is skinnier than I am and I have a sister who is four times my size and I had an aunt who had to go through the door sideways ... I've always been very active and it is true to say that in this profession I play the sort of parts where it wouldn't be a good idea if I turned into a sort of great hefty creature. And I think a part of it is due to the way I was reared; I suppose I'm fairly good on self-discipline.*

Burning Calories

The exercise we get and the food we eat combine to make our shape. The weight-loss/weight-gain formula is no mystery. Exercise burns calories, so if we burn more calories than we take in we lose weight. It takes 3500 calories of energy output to burn off one pound of fat. Put the other way around, 3500 calories of energy (food) intake without any activity attached to it adds one pound in weight to your body. The table shows how much you have to do to use up calories. But the benefit does not just last whilst you are actually exercising. If you do exercise for twenty minutes, your metabolic rate will be raised for several hours afterwards, helping to burn up calories in your food more quickly.

However you choose to control your weight, there is no getting away from the fact that 'calories in' need to be used up, otherwise they are 'calories on'. Dieting without exercise is bad because we lose not just fat but muscle too. Many women try to crash diet, and they mainly fail. Weight that falls off slowly – two pounds per week for example – is weight that has a better chance of staying off.

What Exercise Do You Have to Do to Use up the Calories in 1 Digestive Biscuit of 80 kcals?

- Squash 5.5 minutes
- Moderate swimming 7 minutes
- Running 6.5 minutes
- Table tennis 17 minutes
- Scrubbing floor 14 minutes
- Digging 14 minutes
- Tennis 8.5 minutes
- Cycling 17 minutes
- Aerobics (low impact) 13 minutes
- Playing piano 26 minutes
- Office job 30 minutes
- Badminton 19 minutes
- Sitting around at home 1 hour 15 minutes

What to Eat

The 'experts' are always telling us to eat 'healthily', but it is difficult for us to know exactly what this means. The experts change their minds. What is a good diet one week is out the next. Most difficult is relating a 'good' diet to what we actually find on our kitchen shelves when it comes to cooking a meal.

It is not really a case of 'good' and 'bad' diet or foods, but rather 'how much' of any particular food that we actually eat. What we need is a balanced mixture of all different types of foods, the proteins, the carbohydrates, the fats, which will give us the right amount of calories. Generally, we need a diet that is relatively low in fat and high in roughage and contains the essential vitamins and minerals. For pleasure, any diet ought to be varied and taste good.

This seems simple, yet most of us in the UK do eat a diet that contains too much fat and sugar and therefore too many calories. This is not least because there are hidden fats and sugars in many of the foods we buy. For instance, most tins of baked beans contain sugar and many 'ready prepared' sauces are high in fat.

There is a debate over whether it is necessary routinely to take vitamin supplements. If you eat a healthy balanced diet you should get sufficient amounts. But some of us do not eat a healthy diet. We have insufficient fresh fruits and vegetables – excellent sources of many vitamins. Vitamin tablets are often expensive and it is probably better to spend your money on fresh fruit and vegetables. There is also concern that it is dangerous to take too much of some vitamins even though they are widely promoted. Too much vitamin A taken in pregnancy can cause abnormalities in the baby, too much vitamin D can cause kidney damage and too much vitamin B6 damages the nerves in the fingers and toes.

How Diet Affects Our Health

The red-meat industry has taken a battering with the BSE scares of the 1990s. And now scientists are beginning to link cancers with high intake of large amounts of red meat. But there is also evidence that vegetables and fruit protect you against getting cancer even if you are a heavy meat-eater. How much and how often you should eat red meat therefore remains controversial. Increasingly it is accepted that what we eat affects our health. High-fat diets are linked to an increased risk of heart disease. High-fat and high-sugar diets are linked to obesity which is linked to heart disease, high blood pressure and some cancers.

But the diet and cancer story is complicated. Apart from whether an individual food is good or bad, there are many additives used in food preparation. In research it is difficult to know precisely what people eat, so it is a challenge to understand the relationship between a food and an illness. There have been estimates that diet could be involved in anything from 10 per cent to 70 per cent of all deaths from cancer. The consistent message coming through all the many studies and reports about diet and health seems to be the importance of eating lots of fresh fruit and vegetables, not eating too much fat and not letting yourself become very overweight.

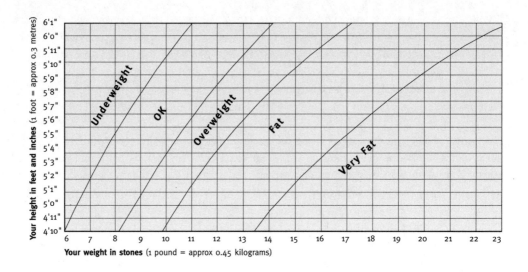

Your height in feet and inches (1 foot = approx 0.3 metres)

Underweight
OK
Overweight
Fat
Very Fat

Your weight in stones (1 pound = approx 0.45 kilograms)

A Guide to Fats in Your Diet

We need some fat in our diet but not as much as most of us eat. There are different types of fat in different foods. All fats are loaded with calories, so eating a low-fat diet will help you lose weight, or not put on weight. Forty per cent of the fat we eat comes from butter, margarine, oils, cakes and pastries. Twenty-five per cent comes from meat. The rest comes from milk, cream, eggs and cheese. Some fats are better for us than others.

- Saturated fat – is found in fats from red meat and in milk and cheese. These can raise blood cholesterol, and are the most important to reduce or avoid in your diet.
- Monounsaturated fat – is found in olive oil. It has no effect on cholesterol.
- Polyunsaturated fat – is found in most, but not all, vegetable oils. Corn, sunflower oil, polyunsaturated margarine and oily fish are all high in this type of fat. They do not raise blood cholesterol and may help lower it. Some of the cheaper vegetable oils and coconut oil are exceptions and are full of saturated fats, so check the labels when buying oils.
- Cholesterol – is found in egg yolks and offal and can also raise the cholesterol in your blood, but saturated fats may be more important in raising blood cholesterol.

How Many Calories a Day?

The energy in food is measured in kilocalories (kcal), often called calories.
- The estimated calorie need of a woman of average build is 1900 kcal per day and that of a man is 2500. If you are very tall, very energetic or your job is physically very demanding, you will need more calories, as you will if you are pregnant or breast-feeding.
- If you want to lose 1lb of weight a week, you need to eat 500 fewer kcal than your

average daily requirement. If you exercise you can eat more and still lose weight.
- Don't forget the calories in alcohol: 1 small glass wine 50 kcal, 1 standard measure of spirits 50 kcal, 1 small glass sherry 60 kcal, $\frac{1}{2}$ pint bitter, lager or cider 85 kcal, $\frac{1}{2}$ pint strong ale 205 kcal.

A Good Food Guide

Below we offer a guide to healthy foods along with a few good tips.

When Buying
- Buy a wide variety of fruit and vegetables, particularly the ones that you like.
- Buy low-fat foods including chicken (without skin) and fish.
- Read the labels for 'low fat', to check how low fat the products really are.
- Buy low-sugar drinks.
- Try to limit buying crisps, cakes, chocolate and biscuits so that they are not a temptation.
- Buy pasta, rice, and cereals.

When Cooking
- Grill or bake rather than fry.
- Use lemon juice on vegetables rather than fat or butter.
- Use lemon juice or vinegar instead of oils on salads.
- Use mustard or low-fat mayonnaise in sandwiches in place of butter or margarine.
- Use small amounts of olive oil or sunflower oil to cook in, rather than butter.
- Use semi-skimmed or skimmed milk.
- Use minimal salt.

When Eating
- Have five portions of fruit or vegetables each day.
- Eat pasta, rice, wholegrain breads and cereals.
- Don't add salt.
- Keep butter and spreads off the table.
- Drink only semi-skimmed or skimmed milk.
- Cut down on hard cheeses such as Cheddar and Edam.
- Limit cakes, biscuits, crisps, chocolates and pudding.
- Snack on fruit and vegetables.

Vegetarianism

Vegetarianism is especially popular among young women – about 17 per cent of women under twenty-one do not eat meat. Partial vegetarians may eat fish, chicken, dairy products or eggs but no red meat. Surveys show that this diet is usually chosen for health rather than moral reasons. Vegetarian diets are healthy because they are so high in roughage from vegetables and low in fat, unless the diet includes large amounts of hard (e.g. Cheddar) cheese. Care may be needed to achieve a balanced diet, especially in vegans who consume no animal products at all. Important vitamins may get missed, and some vegetarians are more prone to anaemia unless they take vitamin B and iron supplements.

> **Linda McCartney:** *I have never ever talked about my food being healthy. I have never pushed the health angle in vegetarianism even though a lot of doctors and nutritionists have ... I'm talking about a kinder way of eating and I think eating a pig sausage or a cow burger is very cruel and that is why I became a vegetarian.*

Slimming Pills

Private slimming clinics peddle pills to help you lose weight. Although they may initially make you lose a lot of weight fast, as soon as you stop taking them your weight goes straight up again. Slimming pills suppress our appetite by the action they have on the hypothalamus, the part of the brain which determines how hungry we feel. Some of the pills are similar to amphetamines. Two of the most popular pills, fenfluramine and dexfenfluramine, have been withdrawn from use, both here and in the USA, where they had been widely promoted in slimming clinics. These pills are potentially addictive, but much more worryingly they can damage the valves of the heart, in some cases causing death.

> **Ann, co-author of this book, visited an Oxford slimming clinic:** *When I arrived the doctor said, 'Hello, I've got just the thing for you'. He showed me a card with pills stuck on them and said they are recommended by doctors. When he said there were no problems with side effects he didn't ask me anything about my health but he did weigh me. It cost £30, and he gave me seven pills and said, 'See you next week'.*

Weight, Shape and the Media

It is no wonder that some women are attracted to slimming pills and heavily promoted slimming foods. Magazines and television continue to bombard us with images of how the looks industry thinks we should be. The image of woman changes from season to season, and decade to decade. Thin is in and curvy out, then curves are in and thin is out.

The mannequins of the 1920s were a size 14 compared to the sizes 8–10 used now. As we write, power shoulders and the micro-mini are making a comeback after a ten-year break. What do you do? Start work on those cellulite thighs this minute, or give yourself a break?

Fashion can be fun, inspirational, liberating. But frequently the look is unreal, and the demands it makes on most of us completely over the top. Our bodies come in myriad shapes and sizes and it is neither possible nor natural for every woman to be a size 8.

The look varies from season to season and from culture to culture.

Bola Olufunwa, Journalist: *It's funny that in the West they're now seeing women with a voluptuous figure as attractive because in Africa this has been the case for centuries ... In fact if you have a small figure you are actually seen as unattractive and the media proclaim the bigger woman as the more beautiful.*

Eating Disorders

Therese, 42: *I have always had trouble with my body image and how I feel about my body. I suspect I'll struggle with it all my life. I struggled with weight as a teenager. I lost weight. I gained weight. I was anorexic. I was very overweight. Body image and feelings about oneself – self-esteem – are so intimately bound up for me. When I feel thin I feel good about life and when I feel toned I feel confident about life. When I feel fat I feel frumpy. I feel there are no options in life. It's scary how much my weight dictates my psychological view of life.*

Eating problems are on the increase particularly among girls and young women, although the percentage is still small. Teenage anorexia is often initiated by dieting and over 70 per cent of teenage girls have dieted. Bingeing problems tend to develop later, and often in women who have recovered from anorexia. They do this when they lose control of their strict dieting patterns. But experts regard anyone unhappily preoccupied with dieting and weight-watching as having an eating disorder. In other words, you do not have to be an extreme anorexic or bulimic to have an eating disorder.

Eating disorders are usually only seen in our western culture where the ideal body image, the thin supermodel figure, is the measure of attractiveness. Dieting appears to trigger eating disorders in vulnerable personalities. Girls particularly at risk tend to have low self-esteem, lack self-confidence, be perfectionist, competitive and obsessional. Some studies have linked childhood sexual abuse with later eating problems. A family history of depression is also common. Mothers with eating problems are more likely to have daughters with eating problems and whether there is a genetic component is still under investigation.

Anorexia and bulimia are different but they do overlap. In both conditions women are extremely preoccupied with their size and shape and this completely dominates their lives. Both groups diet. Recent studies show that 2 per cent of women have anorexia and this figure has remained reasonably stable. Four per cent have bulimia and binge-eating problems. But the real figures are thought to be much higher, as women hide their eating problems, suffer alone, and rarely seek help.

Anorexia Nervosa

Anorexics understand how food interacts with their bodies in astonishing detail. They study their systems, what happens to the food they put in their mouths, and learn how to lose weight quickly. This is their goal and they 'achieve' it. Anorexics drop to less than 85 per cent of their recommended body weight, sometimes losing so much weight that their life is threatened. They often wear baggy clothing to try to hide this, but family and friends usually notice something is wrong. They become withdrawn, depressed and secretive. They are very reluctant to admit they have a problem. Even when a dangerously low weight is reached the anorexic girl or woman sees a fat person in the mirror.

Anorexics live on very little, avoiding all fattening foods, often eating only a piece of fruit or a carrot for a meal. This starvation dieting makes them lose their appetite. They avoid eating meals with other people. They get so thin their periods stop. They often exercise excessively – at least two to three hours per day. They are terrified of putting on weight.

Therese, 42: *I was quite overweight and I'm nervous to talk about this. At my height [5'4"], at my fattest, I was 180 pounds. Huge. I feel more shame about that than anything ... I've been 90 pounds ... I went on a diet when I was eighteen years old and I couldn't stop dieting. I stayed at 90 pounds for two and a half years and actually dipped down to 76 pounds. And I can really remember when I went up to 80 pounds I panicked ... I was insane at that time. Food obsessed me. I was terribly depressed. I had to order my life in the most minute ways. I was a miserable little creature who had no sexual feelings. By then I was in my twenties. I looked like a fifteen-year-old boy. I felt like a depressed fifteen-year-old boy and it wasn't until I gained some weight that I got my periods back and my feelings back, my feelings of being a woman but it took a long time.*

Bulimia Nervosa

Marge, 24: *Our society still hasn't accepted women being larger than men. It's not about fashion magazines and anorexic models. I didn't want to take up too much space in a room because women aren't supposed to do that. I don't know how to say it any better than that. You feel like a bumbling oaf. It's everything. People forgive small people for making mistakes because it's cute. Big people are serious. I am a big-boned muscular healthy person which was not acceptable to me. It's all about having this ideal and the ideal was all about being thin and waify and little. Little people. Big isn't a bad word now. Big now is strong. I don't know how I was made to feel that big was bad but I did. Throwing up was humiliating but it was a release.*

Women with bulimia, like those with anorexia, are preoccupied with size and shape. They also diet, but the difference is they are not so good at it. They tend to give in, lose control and eat a lot, sometimes massive amounts. This is called a binge and involves eating substantially more than any normal person would eat.

Diana, Princess of Wales made bulimia a topic for public discussion when she revealed her own struggle with it in her BBC TV interview with Martin Bashir:

I had bulimia for a number of years and that's like a secret disease. You inflict it upon yourself because your self-esteem is at a low ebb and you don't think you're worthy or valuable. You fill your stomach up four or five times a day. Some do it more and it gives you a feeling of comfort. It's like having a pair of arms around you but it's temporary ... you're very ashamed of yourself and you hate yourself. People think you're wasting food so you don't discuss it with people and the thing about bulimia is your weight always stays the same whereas with anorexia you visibly shrink so you can pretend the whole way through. There's no proof.

Margaret Duncan of the Eating Disorders Association assessed the impact of the Princess of Wales's revelation: 'It was a big help to a lot of people who thought, "Yes that's me. I'm going to do something about it." The other side are these people who don't want to believe eating disorders are a valid way of dealing with problems. Many people were scathing about what she was saying.'

Anxiety and depression are very common in women with bulimia. They do not feel good about themselves and are often full of self-loathing. They feel guilty, helpless and a failure. Some relieve the tension after bingeing by self-harm and cutting themselves. Five per cent of women asking for help for their bulimia have attempted suicide.

There are other things which happen to your body if you have bulimia. The vomiting and abuse of laxatives can affect the balance of salts in your body making you dizzy, thirsty, tired and lethargic. Constipation and tummy pains are very common. Eighty per cent of women with bulimia stop having periods for a few months and in half of them this will last up to a year or longer. Periods usually come back to normal when the bulimic phase stops.

A bulimic binge might include two litres of ice-cream, a loaf of bread, half a pound of cheese, two bars of chocolate, a litre of lemonade and a jar of peanut butter. Therese followed the typical course of many anorexics. Her anorexia merged into bulimia.

> **Therese, 42:** *I panicked. I would go on little binges. Then I would starve myself so that I would make sure I would lose the weight again but it got to the point where my physiological instincts to get the weight back on got the better of me and I literally ate all that weight back on. One day the floodgates opened and I just couldn't stop eating. I couldn't put the brakes on. I ate and ate and ate ...*

Bulimics feel desperate and guilty after a binge. Their method of compensation is to make themselves sick, an attempt to rid their bodies of the calories. Some resort to taking large amounts of laxatives, diuretics, or exercising excessively. But the binges work against their goal of being slim. Even with the vomiting they are mostly within the normal weight range for their height. Vomiting is not a good way to lose weight because you absorb half the calories you eat straightaway. You can also end up with very badly damaged teeth caused by the acid in vomit. Bulimics are very efficient at hiding their problem and it is more difficult to be sure that someone is behaving in this way.

What to Do about Eating Disorders

There are many reasons why women with eating disorders are reluctant to seek help. They feel ashamed and guilty about what they are doing and find it difficult to tell a doctor. They may have had a previous bad experience with a doctor who has been unsympathetic or just given them a diet to try, trivializing the problem. They hope and believe the problem will just go away on its own. They feel they have brought it on themselves and therefore they do not deserve help. They are frightened that the treatment will make them gain weight. It can be difficult to get treatment even if you want it. Not all GPs are equipped to cope with it. But see your GP first. Your doctor may be able to refer you to an expert or to a local clinic. You can also get in touch with the Eating Disorders Association who can help direct you to what is available (see Useful Addresses on page 390).

Coping with Anorexia

If you think you have anorexia or suspect someone close to you has a struggle with it, it is vital to get professional help as early as possible. Talk to your doctor first. Anorexia can become life-threatening and the earlier the treatment the better the success rate. Sufferers usually need intensive psychological help to bring about a change in their thinking and perception about their bodies and themselves. To recover they must gain weight, a hurdle made all the greater because it is the very thing they do not want. This is why treatment is so difficult. Some are treated in hospital for many months, although others manage to be successfully treated as outpatients. Force feeding is rarely used nowadays. Specialist units are the best way to deal with anorexia, although there are not many of these and waiting times tend to be long. Family therapy has been successful, especially when it is linked with cognitive therapy (see page 105). About 40 per cent of anorexics recover with this approach, 20 per cent carry on with anorexia throughout their lives. One in five women with severe anorexia dies from the condition. Women who manage a lifetime of anorexia sometimes survive simply because they manage to stay just above a critical line.

Living day-to-day with an anorexic is full of stress. Some of the following tips may help:

- Talk to a friend, doctor, or counsellor.
- Try not to blame yourself.
- Keep eating normally yourself.
- Have meals at regular times and sit down together.
- Do not force high-calorie food on to the anorexic.
- Be firm but supportive.
- Do not pretend it is not happening.
- Do not blame them and make them feel guilty.
- Continue to show affection.

Coping with Bulimia

The main problem with bulimia is the dieting and this needs to be stopped. It is difficult because it goes against the bulimic's philosophy. The best treatment is cognitive behavioural therapy though some psychotherapy works too. Cognitive therapy aims to change the abnormal thinking and behaviour. In mild cases education alone can work once the woman realizes the pattern she is following. There are also self-help books which can lead you through a step-by-step programme to recovery. Seek help from your GP or the Eating Disorders Association (see Useful Addresses on page 390).

the shape you're in

Before you can start to treat yourself and get better you need to understand that bulimia is a series of vicious circles. To stop the bulimia you need to break the circles. When you diet you impose strict rules on yourself. As long as you keep to these rules you feel good and in control. But as soon as you break a rule, even in a small way by eating a biscuit or a piece of chocolate, you over-react, give up all rules for the day and binge. Dieting and starving yourself means that you always feel hungry. Depending on your build and size you will need a diet of approximately 1900 calories a day to maintain a steady weight, so if you eat fewer than that the hunger drive will make you want to binge. This sets up another vicious circle.

Another circle is bingeing and vomiting. Women who binge feel that if they vomit they will get rid of all the calories in the binge so it does not matter what they eat. But vomiting, even immediately after a binge, only gets rid of 50 per cent of the calories. As an average binge is 2000 calories, 1000 calories will still be absorbed. This is why women who are bulimic do not tend to lose weight. It also means that if you stop bingeing and vomiting and start eating normal meals you will not put on weight. Women who have recovered from their bulimia tend to stay at their normal weight.

The last circle is linked to self-esteem. Women with eating problems and bulimia are preoccupied with their shape and weight and judge their self-worth and whole being in relation to these things. If they lose control and binge, they feel guilty and ashamed at their loss of willpower. This feeds back into their feelings of low esteem, perpetuating the disorder.

It is very difficult to make a decision to stop dieting and to realize that you are unlikely to get better unless you do. You need to come to terms with the fact that your weight and shape, based on a good diet, are normal for you. This is partly influenced by your genes and partly by what you eat and do.

- To start, help yourself find out what you are doing by keeping a detailed diary of all you eat and drink, when you vomit, when you take laxatives and how you feel at the time.
- Start trying to eat regular meals with other people. Plan a snack between the meals so you do not get too hungry. Always know when your next meal is coming and do your utmost not to graze between the meals. If you do, you are more likely to binge as you will feel you have broken the rules.
- Continue to keep a diary of what you are eating, drinking and when you are vomiting.
- Weigh yourself weekly. You will see that you do not really put on weight. Daily weighing is a bad idea as everyone's weight fluctuates a bit from day to day and it will only make you panic and start dieting again.
- Make a list of foods you think of as forbidden foods, such as cake or chocolate, and gradually try having a little of them in a planned way.

- Make a list of things to do as alternatives to bingeing. Go for a walk, ring a friend, clean a cupboard. When you do feel like a binge, try doing one of the things on it.

If you follow this plan you should gradually stop the bulimic cycle. But beware when you feel you are recovered as you will have unrealistic expectations that you will never binge again. When you are stressed or unhappy you may lapse. It is not the end of the world. Start the self-help plan before the pattern gets re-established. As you feel better you may also want to start dieting, but this will just set off the whole cycle again. Remember, it is normal to be greedy from time to time, to overeat at a party for example. That is not bingeing.

Coping after Recovery

> **Therese, 42:** *I was ... anorexic from eighteen to twenty-one and a half and then I started to binge and I couldn't stop all the way back up to that weight [180 pounds] ... I became a recluse ... I didn't want anybody to see me. I was very depressed ... I finally pulled myself together and gradually lost the weight but battled all through my twenties, hovering around 155, 160, then down to 130 ... so my poor body has taken a beating. My weight is about 130 now ... a marvellous woman, a nutritionist ... has helped me ... break the cycle of dieting and bingeing.*

Bulimics and anorexics usually continue to have a degree of struggle with food once they have recovered. Therese has maintained a healthy body weight for over a decade now. She takes her food philosophy from a nutritionist she consulted. It revolves around eating protein in the morning and at lunchtime which she says fuels her body for the afternoon's activities. She also snacks on fruits, vegetables and nuts such as plain almonds. For supper she tries to have carbohydrates which she finds calming, and sticks mainly to vegetable-based sauces. Therese tries not to go without food for too long – say more than three hours. If she does she gets hungry and finds she overeats for the rest of the day. Therese is doing well, but you can see she still works at it. We are not suggesting you follow Therese's diet, but if you have a problem with food try to work out a plan for yourself that will ensure you get the proper nutrition while allowing yourself to enjoy food.

> **Therese, 42:** *I'm not into penitential food. I love wine ... I definitely feel that I'll never go back to those days of being a huge, big mama, and at the same time I am always vigilant, I'm always fearful and I still don't trust myself completely ... If there is one consolation for getting older it is that ... I certainly feel better about myself.*

chapter 7

sex and the STI guide

Sally, 50: It's an amazing buzz. It's like a wave that spreads throughout my body starting in my clitoris. I'm left with a sense of intense well-being which sounds boring but it's beautiful. It's the feeling of just ... surrendering myself to a wave of pure pleasure.

> **Marge, 24:** *When I was a teenager sex was exciting just because you were taking off your clothes when you weren't supposed to.*

> **Janet, 40:** *I've never had any anxiety about being a lesbian ... it's just who I am.*

> **Emily, 48:** *I know perfectly well people fall in love with women in wheelchairs. I think there are all sorts of delightful possibilities.*

A sex life is anything but static, even though it might seem so in long periods of drought or if we sometimes lose interest. What sex we want, and how much, varies throughout our lives. We learn from experience, and try to make it better. Our sex drives wax and wane with our periods, with our age, with our partners, and the availability of a partner.

Since the sixties and the pill, and a shift to liberal attitudes towards sex, it has been possible for us to have sex if and when we want to — assuming it is available. Of course, religion, culture and morals influence women's freedom to choose to have sex. Two decades later sexually transmitted infections (STIs — see pages 178–93) such as Aids, herpes, chlamydia and genital warts made casual, unprotected sex unsafe. The latest British figures show transmission of STIs is still on the increase (see page 178).

In this chapter women talk about their sexual practices, what they like and what they do not like. We look at what can go wrong with sex and what to do when it does not work. And we offer a guide to your sexual health, to help you should you pick up something unwelcome along the way.

Myths and Misunderstandings

> **Dr Jenny Cozens, Psychologist and Agony Aunt for *Good Housekeeping*:** *My mailbag suggests that if anything goes wrong with sex it's always bound to be the woman ... the man is always perfect.*

> **Dr Paula Nicolson, Psychologist, Sheffield University:** *I think that most people believe that the erogenous zones are below the waist, but as a psychologist I know better and I can tell you they are actually above the neck.*

> **Charles Kingsland, Gynaecologist at Liverpool Women's Hospital:** *The difference between the G spot and a pub is a man can always find his way to the pub.*

> **Arlene McCarthy, MEP, Peak District:** *Personally I prefer a Jaffa Cake and a cup of tea.*

sex and the STI guide

149

The Kiss

Adrianne Blue, Author of *On Kissing* and London City University Lecturer: *First kisses when they really do have passion, the first erotic kiss anyone has, usually is remembered and can really knock you over. In fact Mohammed Ali, the boxer, fainted after his ... Many people think that a kiss is even more intimate than coitus. It's unprovable really but I was surprised how many men, especially young men, said that they were not really particular about how many women they went to bed with but they were very particular about which ones they kissed, which ones they kissed intimately.*

Hannah, 42: *It is true, it may be more intimate. It's not just him. His tongue is in your mouth and your tongue is in his mouth. It's the most equal thing. You're both giving so completely and you're both so open to each other. A part of my body is in him and a part of his body is in me. And you're also prolonging the inevitable.*

A sexy kiss can be a prelude to sexual intercourse. It can be a tease. It can be part of a snogging session which does not lead to consummation. A kiss – especially a first kiss – can be the biggest turn-on there is. It can also be a flop.

Kelly, 21: *It was gross. It was a big fat tongue in my mouth. It wasn't that unpleasant, it was just strange. I remember thinking it was rather funny.*

Adrianne Blue: *For many many decades a kiss was a metaphor of orgasm in the movies. There's no doubt about that, yet it also symbolized passion, intimacy, love.*

Arousal

It may only take a kiss, and sometimes just the mere thought of a kiss with someone who turns you on, to find yourself in a ready state for intercourse. In ongoing relationships, however, it usually takes more and sometimes considerably more. One of the common problems with sex is the way couples often skip the foreplay or do not prolong it enough to put maximum excitement into the sexual experience. Occasionally it is a thrill to 'get right to it' but more often we need the stimulation of foreplay.

Kissing is the obvious starting point – not just on the mouth but anywhere. Everyone has places they like to be kissed – on our neck or in our ear. Some of us like our partner's tongues, others do not. Hands are extremely useful in exploring our partner's and our own bodies during sex. We need to tell our partners what we like and where we like it. As shy as you may feel about talking about what you like, do speak up in this department. Good sex partners will want to please each other.

The main noticeable change in a woman's body as it prepares for sex is vaginal wetness. The transparent or milky white vaginal discharge we have, even when we are not contemplating intercourse, increases, giving us the slipperiness needed for comfortable sex. At the time of ovulation this discharge increases all on its own. Other parts of the body are involved too. When a woman is aroused her nipples stand up, her heartbeat quickens and her genital area becomes engorged with blood.

> **Hannah, 42:** *It's like electricity, almost literally. It's as if you're plugged in and there's an energy source and the energy – even though it might be focused on your nipples and your genitals it's in your fingers, it's in your toes, it's in every part of you.*

All the Way

The age at which we have our first sexual intercourse has changed dramatically over the years. Women born in the early 1930s usually remained virgins until the age of twenty-one. But the age has been steadily dropping ever since. This is one of the many discoveries made by the *National Survey of Sexual Attitudes and Lifestyles* which was published in 1994, the most comprehensive study of its kind ever carried out in Britain. It surveyed 18,876 men and women and was carried out by four women.

Baroness Castle of Blackburn – Barbara Castle – remembers the lack of sexual information in the 1930s during her days at Oxford:

> **Barbara:** *Oh it was absolutely absurd, the sexual darkness of those times ... I had a whip round in the JCR [junior common room] so that I could buy a book I'd seen advertised in the* New Statesman, *all about the facts of life. I passed it round the JCR. It was the best-read book in the whole of St Hugh's College. It was thumbed and ear-marked and all the rest of it because we none of us knew the facts of life.*

The 1994 survey found the modern median age of first sexual intercourse for girls is now seventeen. And nearly one in five girls loses her virginity when she is under the age of sixteen. The legal age of consent for sex between men and women is sixteen. At whatever age it may have happened, practically everyone can recall their first sexual intercourse. But there is always that one per cent who cannot quite remember:

> **Sally, 50:** *I'm not really sure when it was because I don't quite know when I lost my virginity. There was a lot of groping that went on when I was in my early twenties. It's awful isn't it, I don't even know which man was first, which man actually penetrated me first because there was so much sort of nearly screwing – do you remember? – in those days that you got close but you're not quite sure. So it's sort of a blur. I may have blocked it out actually.*

Who Wants What?

> **Sarah, 14:** *I'm looking forward to sex ... I'm curious about what it feels like and how I'll be feeling at the time and who it will be with. I think ... I'll feel closer to the person. I imagine it hurting, kind of maybe a sharp pain ... I'm nervous about what will happen and if I'll do it right.*

Sex is loaded with anticipation and expectation right from the beginning. When it is at its best it can be out of this world. When it is bad it can be embarrassing, painful, empty, regrettable, damaging to our emotions, and even to our bodies. But with practice and experience our sex lives can only get better.

> **Fiona, 36:** *I have a new man. I'm having sex all the time. I look back at years without sex. Years! I'm very fussy ... The drought is over. I walk down the street in the morning and I grin at strangers and I think, 'Ha, I'm getting it!'*

> **Joyce, 50:** *When I was first married I had sex every night with my husband but I don't think I can really actually remember a memorable occasion. My husband kind of forced me to do things I didn't want to do ... I enjoy doing those things now ... I have a friend and we make love together and it's wonderful, absolutely wonderful. It's just that feeling inside that makes you want to burst, makes you want to scream out ... it comes from deep down I suppose. I've got no inhibitions when I'm with him and he hasn't either.*

But frequently the sex we want and the sex we get do not match up.

> **Sally, 50:** *I love a cuddle but the trouble is I know what's coming next. It would be great if my husband just occasionally took me in his arms and gave me a lovely cuddle without it always being a prelude to sex. It's a shame because sometimes when he does try to cuddle me I find an excuse to get out of bed because I really don't feel like having sex.*

Other women would love to trade places with Sally, because the way they see it there seems to be a shortage of reliable men available for sex and relationships.

> **Jennifer, 44:** *I don't think the men are out there, at least the ones I want to be with. There's the kind of man who wants to have sex with you and they're usually married. And then there are the ones who are recently divorced and don't want to be alone. They just have problems to work out. My experience has been that men will often not take the time to work things out between relationships. They'll move on and carry their baggage with them. And the actual man who's single and has worked his stuff out and is on the same wavelength as you is hard to find.*

Statistically, there is no man shortage until we reach middle age. There are more boy babies born than girl babies, but the statistical odds do change as we age. By the time we reach the age of forty-five there is a switchover with women beginning to outnumber men. By the time we reach eighty-five there are twice as many women as men at that age.

Part of the reason for what appears to be a shortage of available men around middle age may be a trend towards older men choosing much younger women for their partners, passing by their contemporaries to be with women sometimes decades younger.

> **Jack, 53:** *My wife's ten years younger than I am and I think that when you're in a close relationship with someone younger it helps you to feel younger. I also think it's hard to deny that younger women are sexually and physically more attractive and that's why men trade in their wives for younger women.*

But what is going on before middle age? A recent survey in Britain found that four out of every ten women in their thirties are not having sex. Of course, some women do not want to have sex, although most young women certainly do. Aids and other STIs have made us more cautious about who we sleep with. Another factor in women either choosing not to have sex, or not being able to find the right partner for it, may be changes in the way we live our lives. It is now quite common for a woman to focus on her career first, delaying marriage and motherhood. Professional women endeavouring to work their way to the top may find themselves married to their jobs, with little time and energy left over for sexual pursuits. Working in the fast lane is tiring and can be all-consuming. Survival in the professional jungle takes skill and dedication.

> **Jennifer, 44:** *I think if you're a woman anywhere in your thirties and forties and really liking your job and dedicated to it, it's difficult to meet people outside the workplace. I think that's true for most people whether they're on their own or not and I think you definitely run out of energy. I also think once you're past a certain age and have had a number of disappointing experiences it takes a lot of emotional courage to try and set out again. And I think there are probably too all sorts of different people. People who like to date, who see it as a fun social thing to do and there are people like me who find it's largely hard work. You have to find a date in the first place and then you have to work at the date. So there's a lot of effort to put into it, when it could be easier to go home and read a good book.*

There are many reasons for not having sex, even when you do have a partner. You can be too tired, too busy, turned off, ill, depressed, repressed, angry or uninterested. There may be no partner or the partner may not be the right one. For many women the menopause (see Chapter 3) heralds a new stage of sexual liberation and therefore more sex. The fear of pregnancy is gone, and you may have more time for sex if your children have left home. The sexual drive is mysterious, however, and many women say just the opposite, and talk about a dwindling or even complete loss of interest in sex as they age. There may also be a problem of vaginal dryness during menopause (see page 57).

> **Sally, 50:** *My sex drive was much higher before I had children. I could go several times in one night. It's almost as if nature has some sort of built-in mechanism so that once you've procreated your libido drops.*
>
> **Linda, 50:** *My husband and I, luckily, don't have an awful lot of sex. We both feel the same. We're not making love every night. It might be three or four weeks but we're both that way inclined. I think to go to bed now and have a cuddle means more to me than perhaps making love. Not always. But we go to bed and we cuddle every night and kiss every night and that's lovely. It's relaxing.*

> **Margaret, 58:** *I'm not so interested in sex now I must admit ... it's still all right ... my husband's a very sexy man. People say 'Aren't you lucky!' He's always had a very strong sexual urge which I used to find a nuisance when we were younger but we've more or less evened out now and we're quite happy with the way things are ... but it helps when your husband is away all week, then he comes back and you're suddenly jolly pleased to see him and it sort of wakens up the interest.*

There is a great variation in women's desire and enjoyment of sex. In older age the death of a lifelong partner often leaves women without any interest in finding a new sexual partner. Of course this can change if a new partner is found, but when a woman does not want sex it does not mean anything is wrong. Some women lose interest after the menopause or after a hysterectomy. If you have had your ovaries removed at the same time as your uterus you may need to be on HRT, otherwise the acute menopause brought on by the oophorectomy may cause a sudden loss of libido. Sometimes the menopause comes on earlier even if the ovaries are left in. One large study found that most women had no sexual problems after having a hysterectomy and some even found that sex was better because the problem for which they had the hysterectomy had been cured.

> **Mary, 74:** *You sort of eventually reach the stage where you just totally forget about sex. I can't remember when or why. I haven't thought of anything related to sex since the hysterectomy, eight years ago ... I just maybe unconsciously thought that was the end of everything because they had taken out my uterus and just the thought of even anything penetrating me ... If I were a married person it would be different because I imagine something would have happened!*

The 1994 Sex Survey also found:

- Nine per cent of married women over the age of forty-five had not had vaginal intercourse in the previous year.
- More than one-third of all single women had no vaginal intercourse in the previous year.
- Half of single women had had no sex at all in the previous month.
- More than half of women in their late fifties had had no sex in the previous month.
- Cohabiting couples have more sex than married couples do.

Orgasm

Joyce, 50: *I would say it's the most wonderful thing that could ever happen to you ... it's like having a volcano erupt inside you. It just goes voom inside you! It's just a wonderful feeling. I always want to scream out at the top of my voice but I can't because the neighbours will hear!*

When a woman has an orgasm the walls of her vagina contract rapidly. The younger we are the more contractions we have – on average eight to twelve. After the age of fifty or so the number of contractions per orgasm falls off to about four or five so the orgasm may feel less intense. However, a woman can enjoy multiple orgasms at any age, unlike most men however young they are. It does, however, take longer for an older woman to become lubricated – say five minutes instead of mere seconds. Most women's orgasms are achieved by direct stimulation on her clitoris, and not just through sexual intercourse (see also pages 171–3). Stimulation can also be brought about through masturbation, oral sex, or a vibrator.

Hannah, 41: *When I have an orgasm it's such a full body experience – my eyes, my breasts, my knees, every single part of my body is affected ... it is unbelievable.*

Marge, 24: *I turn into a bowl of quivering red jello.*

This is an accurate physiological description because we really do quiver and turn red just before we climax. The labia – the lips surrounding the clitoris – swell a little and become deep red.

There are all kinds of reasons for not being able to have an orgasm easily or for not being able to have one at all, and this can be normal. Some younger women find they do not get an orgasm for several years after starting to have sex. You can be unhappy with your partner, unhappy with yourself or perhaps you feel guilty about sex. Often it is simply that you are not getting the right stimulation. See the section on masturbation (pages 158–9) and have a look at page 172 for more on this problem.

Oral Sex

For you: when you have oral sex your partner uses their mouth and tongue to stimulate your genital area. The formal name is cunnilingus. The Sex Survey found that more than two-thirds of women in Britain have oral sex. The study also found that oral sex is usually reciprocal but not always.

> **Lynn, 44:** *I find most guys want it for them but they don't think that you want it. I think any woman would be self-conscious having it. If I was anticipating oral sex for me, me being the recipient, then I'd want to have a bath because it's actually kind of a turn-off for me to think of what might be down there.*

Some women feel very self-conscious about the way they smell in the genital area. But in fact some men say our smell is part of the turn-on, and they enjoy knowing that oral sex gives immense pleasure to a woman. If you have trouble reaching an orgasm and you feel comfortable enough to try it with your partner, oral sex sometimes helps.

For him: when you perform oral sex on a man, using your mouth to suck his penis, it is called fellatio. Sometimes it is done as a prelude to vaginal sex. The man may climax in your mouth, or not. Some women swallow the ejaculate, others do not. There is nothing wrong with swallowing. But if your partner has or may have an STI (see pages 178–93) he must wear a condom during oral sex, or for any act involving the intermingling of bodily fluids.

> **Joyce, 50:** *The first time I had oral sex with my husband he said, 'I won't come' and he did and I was just horrified. I mean I was only twenty-one at the time and I was just appalled ... I couldn't wait to spit it out. But now I do swallow it because I enjoy what I've done. And I obviously love him more than I ever loved my husband ... when you're doing it to the man he's obviously enjoying it so much and I feel good about doing it and it's not only that. He'll touch me while I'm doing it to him so it's good!*

> **Sally, 50:** *I don't get any pleasure out of performing fellatio on my husband. I can't breathe! And when he comes, swallowing his semen is pretty unappetizing. I enjoy it when he does it to me but I actually prefer coming when his penis is inside me.*

Anal Sex

Anal sex is now legal between men and women over the age of eighteen in England and Wales. In Scotland it is legal at sixteen, and in Northern Ireland it is illegal. The anal muscles are much tighter than the vaginal muscles, so it is important that the woman always lets the man know if he is going too fast, particularly if it is the first time you are trying anal sex – physical damage and pain may result if it is done too roughly. Using a lubricant such as KY jelly will help, and the man should wear a strong condom to ensure that no STIs are transmitted. If you have anal sex it is also important for your partner to wash his penis before switching to vaginal intercourse otherwise bacterial infections may be transmitted. The same goes for anal stimulation using the fingers.

The Sex Survey also asked about anal sex and found that younger women have it more frequently than older women. Over 8.5 per cent of eighteen to twenty-four-year-old women had experienced it in the previous year. Cohabiting couples were found to have anal intercourse more frequently than married couples. Nearly 10 per cent of women cohabiting with men had had anal sex in the previous year, compared with 5.4 per cent of married women.

Masturbation

Masturbation, or self-stimulation, is little talked about but up to 75 per cent of women do it and enjoy it even though they may feel guilty about it. It was too sensitive a topic even for the Sex Survey which dropped questions about the practice when respondents reacted with 'distaste and embarrassment'.

Rachel, 44: *I don't have a man in my life so ... masturbation is my sex life. I have to say I often resist the impulse because there's still something in me that's a ten-year-old going, 'ooh that's bad and that's shameful'.*

Elizabeth, 30: *In my last months of pregnancy I couldn't get an orgasm if my life depended on it ... So right after, in the weeks following, I masturbated because it had been a long time ... sometimes I feel a little guilty because David's not around and I'm doing it behind his back. But I know I shouldn't feel that way.*

Betty, 74: *It's probably ten or fifteen years since I tried that ... it was only really a few times. I probably felt guilty and thought it was a dirty awful thing to do or something, knowing the mother I had who didn't tell me anything. Even now I think I can't imagine telling somebody this is what you do if you want to masturbate.*

Masturbation is the victim of a disinformation campaign, although this is less true today than it used to be. But even now some parents warn their children not to do it, telling them that masturbation can make them mentally deranged, or they may teach their children that touching themselves for pleasure is bad. In fact it is good for all kinds of things. It can help you reach a better understanding of your body. It can be very enjoyable and relaxing. If you do want to masturbate but you feel uneasy about it, take some time to explore and make sure you have privacy so you know you will not be disturbed.

> **Cheryl, 42:** *Normally I would start by massaging my nipples with some pressure. And then I ... stroke my clitoris with a lot of pressure, up and down. What happens is my hand becomes numb so you can't quite continue! I can't give myself multiple orgasm ... which is why I have often thought of buying myself a vibrator.*

> **Francesca, 42:** *I used to do it more than I do now. When I was a single woman and I would have sexual partners and then fallow periods I would definitely masturbate and like all kinds of rhythms you feel more sexual at times than others and it's a great way to relax. I might go through fallow periods where ... I felt as if my whole furnace had shut down. In fact nothing was really working so I didn't masturbate and then somehow the buds started stirring again and I felt more sexual and if I didn't have a man around I'd masturbate and even if I did have a man around I'd masturbate. Sometimes we'd even do it together and that's always nice when people feel comfortable enough to do that.*

> **Gertie, 42:** *I do it, regularly ... I like fantasizing. My fantasies are mainly lesbian sex because I think a woman's body is really nice. Although I don't think I could ever do it [with a woman] though. I suppose I'd like to just for the experience because I don't want to reach eighty, sort of a shrivelled old woman, and think, 'oh I'd like to have done that'.*

However, masturbation is not for everyone.

> **Vicki, 40:** *I just think it's the grossest thing I could imagine ... I would just feel like an ass lying there by myself. If there's not a man there what's the point?*

Fantasies

Having sexual fantasies is normal and may even help a flagging sex life. Or they can be an enjoyable pursuit in themselves.

> **Francesca, 42:** *I have very predictable fantasies. They're always domination fantasies which are very common I gather ... A rape, not pain, just domination. Several men, a man and a woman, a couple of women. I'll even say I've gotten as far as a German Shepherd! I like to take risks ... in my fantasies. I don't take big risks in my sexual life, but I take them all in my fantasies.*

Lots of women do report fantasies about being dominated by men and sometimes heterosexual women fantasize about sex with female partners as we saw in the masturbation section. One of the positive things about fantasies is that you get a chance to try things out in your head that might not work for you in reality. They are safe. They may make masturbation more fun and may even help perk up your sex life if your relationship is in a rut.

> **Hannah, 42:** *I have had sleeping dreams where I'm having sex with women. I've never consciously said, 'Let me have a fantasy about a woman,' but I've definitely had dreams about women and woken up aroused.*

Lesbian Love

> **Janet, 40:** *From the day that I discovered it or it discovered me, from the first touch that was it for me... I went home and I bragged to everybody that I'd just had this amazing discovery. It's just who I am.*

Lesbians arrive at an understanding of their sexual orientation in all sorts of ways. They may start out in heterosexual relationships and soon realize something is not right. Or they may clearly and early on know they prefer women. They may just feel they have a different orientation but not be clear what this is. Some women, often in later life, make a conscious decision to orient to women after a life of unhappiness in heterosexual relationships. Some 'natural-born lesbians' question whether these women are true lesbians. Some women are bisexual throughout life while others experiment with both sexes eventually settling on one or the other.

Lesbian love is out. Gay women are coming out on TV, in movies, and in politics, attracting both praise and ridicule. Women who love women are freer than ever before to be open about their relationships. This does not mean they are free from discrimination. Family members may shun them and at work they sometimes feel a need to keep their relationships private.

> **Susan, 35:** *There's still a lot of social stuff to get over. I've never felt any prejudice directly but I think indirectly you sometimes feel excluded from things ... in part Louise and I keep our private lives separate from work and that can make you feel very schizophrenic.*

The 1994 Sex Survey found that 3.4 per cent of women had had a homosexual experience some time in the past with 1.7 per cent having had genital contact. Less than 1 per cent (0.6 per cent) of women had had a homosexual partner in the previous two years. It is difficult to know how many lesbians there really are. Some women simply will not have had a partner, others may not have come out – either to themselves or to others. Ninety-five per cent of women said their sexual relations were exclusively heterosexual.

> **Janet, 40:** *It was a physical thing. It was like a chemical thing ... When you know, you know. I was twenty-one, twenty-two. That's fairly late but I was a farm kid. I was miserable before that as a sexual being. I was always happy as a child and then all of a sudden when I became an adolescent and started having sex I was miserable. I hated it.*

Susan has been living with her partner Louise for five years.

> **Susan, 35:** *I think all the pluses are emotional. It has to do with living with a woman and women can be much more supportive and much better partners to my mind. Every decision you make about your relationship is open to discussion because you don't have any of the usual baggage of conventionality which goes with a heterosexual relationship ... I think it's a popular misconception ... of same-sex relationships that we slip into male-female roles, that you're either butch or fem. Those roles are completely flexible in my experience. There are absolutely no assumptions about who you are in that partnership. In my relationship with Louise, Louise for the moment is very happy to be the breadwinner. But even though she's perhaps perceived by others as being the more male character in our partnership she's actually the one who wants to stay at home and raise the children if there are any.*

Infidelity

The 1994 National Sex Survey found that 80 per cent of people believe in being faithful to their partners, with women only slightly more disapproving of extramarital affairs than men. Of course having this view does not mean a person *is* faithful. Still, most married individuals reported they had been faithful to their spouses. Less than a third of married women said they had had a sexual partner outside of marriage, and only one woman in 500 said she had had more than one partner outside of her marriage.

> **Joyce, 50, and divorced:** *My lover now is married and I've been having this affair for fourteen years ... and I feel very guilty about it for her but I know that we do things that he's never ever done with his wife. I suppose he's getting the best of both worlds because he won't leave his wife ... I'm quite happy on my own ... I do get very lonely at weekends like on a Saturday evening ... and sometimes I think, 'Oh why isn't he'. I wish he was here with me and I know he feels the same. He'll phone me and he'll be phoning me from the loo on his mobile phone!*

Emily is a Yorkshire woman whose sex life has been thrown off track. She has a degenerative condition which means her body is gradually losing its flexibility. Emily, however, is not losing her sexual drive, but she needs to explore new ways of having sex. The problem seems to be her husband. He is having trouble adapting.

> **Emily, 48:** *You tentatively suggest things and when you feel you meet a brick wall you back off ... there's this huge potential for creativity in sex involving one or more disabled people and it's something I would really like to explore but [my husband] is probably regretting what is lost and past, more than he is thinking about any kind of future possibilities. I think I've taken steps to talk to him about it but I think I have also backed off ... I have very great self-respect but I'm not prepared to risk being insulted in that area ... If I have sex with my husband and I feel he's being impatient with me I feel deeply insulted. It's been a couple of months since we had sex.*

So Emily is contemplating having an affair.

> **Emily, 48:** *I've got plans but they don't involve him. I know enough to know that I'm still attractive, that men still fall in love with me and it's my belief that there are possibilities for exploring sex in the context of a love affair ... I am in love with somebody ... I don't know whether we will be able to get together ... but the point is that whether I have something I can act on or not doesn't matter. I know perfectly well people fall in love with women in wheelchairs. I think there are all sorts of delightful possibilities.*

Gertie was inspired by a modern movie, and she acted on it.

> **Gertie, 42:** *I had this whole fantasy, you know that movie with Alan Alda,* Same Time Next Year. *I just worked on this whole fantasy that this guy would be somebody I would meet once a year.*

Gertie, a happily married mother of twins, turned her fantasy into reality. She planned her own *Same Time Next Year*, and travelled to another country to see it through.

> **Gertie:** *I wanted real excitement. I wanted to do something that took me away from my family completely ... I just felt so free and liberated. When I got back I realized that something I needed to do once a year was go off, and sleep with somebody else. Just to remind me who I was. He's married as well. He's got children ... It was just truly wonderful. The journey from the restaurant to the hotel was electric. I just hadn't experienced excitement in that way for such a long time, just in anticipation of what was going to happen. It was really wild and really passionate and when he left my body just tingled for days.*

Gertie's *Same Time Next Year* man may turn into a *Same Time Next Season* man. When we last saw her she was planning a reunion just a few months after her first thrilling encounter. She said she felt no guilt about it and could not imagine why she should. Her affair, she says, reminds her of another side of her which needs 'tapping into'.

Affairs can damage your marriage, even if they seem fun at the time.

> **Barbara, 44:** *All through the affair I felt guilty and worried that John would find out ... in the end I couldn't cope any more and I jacked it in ... I still feel guilty and worry that he'll discover it. It's made the sexual side of our marriage more difficult. I still think about him when I have sex [with John].*

Affairs can make a woman feel attractive, loved, needed, wanted. They are thrilling – perhaps all the more so because of their forbidden nature – and they are more intense partly because you are not free to see the object of your ravenous desire whenever you want. This can also be very painful.

> **Valerie, 42:** *You know the first few months you didn't mind sharing him with somebody else and then after a while, when you weren't going to be able to spend your birthday with him or you were distressed and you knew you couldn't pick up the phone and call him because he was at home with his wife, it became an irritant and in fact it became an impediment to the growth of the relationship.*

When it is your partner who is the unfaithful one, the hurt is usually deep and the ensuing insecurity debilitating. We feel rejected and unattractive and preoccupied with the other woman's looks. Is she prettier, slimmer, smarter? What does she have that I do not, and so on. How could she? How do I get him back? We may take a lover to retaliate. We try to improve our own looks – very difficult when we feel unwanted and unloved. Even after the affair ends, assuming it does, it may take years before we can let go and forgive. We may never forgive and trust again.

Char, four years on, is still with her husband who had an affair, which she believes lasted for eight years.

> **Char, 47:** *I still feel angry inside from time to time. What gets me upset is he has never once really been able to apologize for having hurt me. He just goes on about how everyone has affairs and I'm old fashioned and stupid to be upset. He thinks we've talked about it and sorted it out but his way is not to really talk about it and just put it behind him. It hasn't been so easy for me.*

Gina is 50. Her marriage ended ten years ago leaving her with four children, aged three to seventeen.

> **Gina:** *Affairs sabotage everything you've ever tried to do in your adult life. They undermine your self-confidence entirely. I was consumed with questions in my grief and immediately looked to blame myself. I searched for horrendous deficiencies in myself which could have undermined my marriage. In the end I realized it was a pretty fruitless search. We're none of us perfect but I couldn't find any really monstrous qualities. I have taken ten years to recover ... my children are still scarred and fear they will not make long-term relationships. I still harbour murderous rage towards the younger woman who claimed my man. What is particularly galling is the way he appears amazingly cheerful at all times and has never once acknowledged the enormity of the pain we all suffered from his affair. He talks to me as if I were a neighbour or a customer, as though we share no common past.*

Jo, 47, found out she had cancer the same week she discovered by chance that her husband was having an affair.

> **Jo:** *I'm not sure what was worse the cancer or the affair, probably the affair. At least I felt I had some control over the decisions I was making about the cancer but one of the worse things about the affair was feeling so humiliated and powerless. Before that I thought our relationship was amongst equals. It's been a struggle but we're still together. The thing that made it easier for me was the fact that I did not tell him about my cancer until he had decided to dump the woman. I never wanted to be accused of playing the cancer card to stop the affair and I didn't. I'm sure the other woman thinks that's why he dumped her but he knows that's not true. It has helped me keep some self-esteem about the whole affair.*

When you are the adulterer your ego may get a boost. If you are in a marriage where your husband does not like to have sex with you, an affair can be reassuring, as Celia found.

> **Celia, 41:** *Having assumed that I would never have a sex life again it was an awakening ... to find that someone actually fancied you even though you had a nine-month-old baby under your arm was very uplifting. It was amazing how easy it was. Although it felt quite strange to be treated as a sexual being, after four years of not being, it made me feel great.*

The need for repeated affairs may mean something is missing in ourselves. Then we may be using affairs as part of a search for that good feeling we cannot seem to find and keep in one monogamous relationship.

> **Frances Campbell, Oxford Psychotherapist and Marital Counsellor:** *Some people can't cope with intimacy and they have to keep falling in love to maintain themselves. The best antidepressant in the world is to fall in love. So if somebody is very depressed or uncertain, one way they maintain their self-esteem is they can fall in love with one person after another and in that sense they can annihilate their partner.*

It sometimes seems our society is obsessed with affairs. It probably is. But very many of us have no first-hand experience of them whatsoever.

> **Sally, 50, and married for 22 years:** *I've never had an affair, isn't that amazing? I have no need for out-of-marriage sex. Our sex life is very good and more than frequent enough as far as I'm concerned.*

Sexual Intercourse and Pregnancy

> **Sally, 50:** *I wasn't keen on sexual intercourse during pregnancy because I kept thinking it was going to damage the baby. I knew that was ridiculous and we did make love while I was pregnant but I never really felt like letting myself go.*

There is controversy over whether orgasms can induce labour or even cause miscarriage. Prostaglandin hormones are released in the cervix during orgasm and we do know some prostaglandins are involved in the initiation of labour. But no direct link has been established between orgasms and premature labour or miscarriage. The foetus is well protected in your uterus with a bag of fluid and layers of muscle between it and anything that might be moving around near or next to it. Women who have had a previous miscarriage or miscarriages may prefer to avoid sex in the first few months. There is no definite link between sex and miscarriage. Some couples try having sex to stimulate labour when the baby is overdue. Once again we are not sure if this really works, although there is some evidence that nipple stimulation when the baby is due might help to initiate labour, presumably because it releases prostaglandin.

Lise, 38, due to have her baby in six days: *Funny enough you feel very good about everything. You feel very sexy, except not this week. The very end is not an attractive-feeling time but right up until about the ninth month you feel ... really healthy, invigorated and all those things make for good sex.*

Sex and Retirement

The story of Rose, 53, and Guy, 60, one year after Guy's retirement, may ring true for many retired couples who find sex becomes more enjoyable with the pressures of work behind them.

Rose: *It's a whole lot better now because we're more relaxed. When you're younger you have more responsibilities. We've shed those responsibilities. You're not fussed about the day-to-day worries now. So there is a big window of opportunity before you get old and decrepit.*

Guy: *It's better because you're not so tired ... I worked bloody hard and came home and slumped in front of the television.*

Rose: *I think it's made it more alive because we enjoy doing things together. Because working is stressful and he would come home exhausted and strained by what was happening at the office and he's more relaxed now. I think I'm more relaxed.*

Ideally, if you have a partner and you both live long enough, retirement should make time for enjoyment of each other and adventure too, in the bedroom and elsewhere. But this time of your life can also be an upset. Routines and patterns change when suddenly your mate is home after being away all day every day. It may make you feel claustrophobic to have your space invaded twenty-four hours a day. So it is important for you and your partner to make time for each of you to be alone. You do not need to wait for retirement to begin this pattern. Start on weekends while you are still working. It helps to prevent total dependency and to prepare yourselves for the time when one of you may be on your own.

But there is also great joy in finding you are home together again after all those years of being parted by work, and taxed by the children, to actually have time to do as you please.

Claire Rayner, Agony Aunt: *You might not be quite as passionate, quite as vigorous, but you're more skilful. And in my experience it's infinitely more satisfying. We've learned each other's little ways, the shorthand. You don't have to worry about what you look like, you can let yourself go and have fun.*

Sexual Dysfunction

All societies for all time have been fascinated with sex. Centuries of sexual explorers have experimented with a range of aphrodisiacs to enhance the sexual appetite. Ancient Arabs ate asparagus. The smell of asparagus, seeping out of our sweat glands, is supposed to be similar to our own natural sex smells called pheromones. The Greeks made fennel and nettle soup to enhance sexuality. The Aztec emperor Montezuma is supposed to have relied on chocolate for stamina (he had a harem of 600). The French like oysters and Champagne. A glass of wine might help to relax a nervous couple and create the start for a romantic evening, but it is unlikely to proceed much further if there are actual sexual dysfunctions to mend. There are many disorders related to sex and most of them can be helped.

In the 1970s Masters and Johnson, the leading American sex research team, shocked the world by claims that half of American marriages were troubled by sexual problems at some time. In 1988 a survey in the UK found that a third of women over the age of thirty-five with partners had problems with sex, as defined by experts. However only one in ten of these women felt they had a sexual problem and only half of these wanted help.

Both psychological and physical factors can lead to sexual problems and often it is a combination of the two. Some problems have their roots in childhood and young adulthood. Family attitudes to sexuality, sex education, religion, and bad sexual experiences, all play their part. If sex is treated by the family as a taboo topic, as something shameful and wrong, this can create guilt over sexual feelings. Poor and inadequate sex education and misinformation fuel sexual myths. Women who have trouble with sex are often found to have been sexually abused or raped.

Other experiences may interfere with sex too. Some women lose interest in sex around the time of childbirth and immediately after (see pages 289–90). Discovering that your partner has had an affair may act as a sexual turn-off and make a woman feel protective of her sexual feelings. Being involved in an affair yourself can lead to loss of sexual interest because of anxiety resulting from guilt. Our partner's sexual problems, such as premature ejaculation or impotence, affect us too.

Perhaps the most important cause of sexual difficulty is a more general problem in the relationship. Anxiety, poor communication, lack of foreplay and depression, can all be involved. Sometimes medical problems such as diabetes and heart disease decrease libido. If you are on medication and you have noticed you are losing interest in sex, the two could be linked. Tell your doctor. If this is the problem there is probably an alternative drug. Other conditions such as endometriosis (see pages 38–40) cause pain and discomfort during sex.

Some operations may cause trouble because they interfere directly with the parts of our bodies involved in sex. Sometimes with an episiotomy after childbirth there is a raw area around the episiotomy scar. This can easily be treated at your doctor's surgery by applying liquid nitrogen. Rubbing steroid cream into the affected area can also help. Occasionally you will need a small operation to get rid of the scar tissue, but often the problem goes away in time without treatment. Other operations have psychological effects. For example, it has been found that a third of women have a deterioration in their sexual relationship after a mastectomy. An oophorectomy – when your ovaries are removed – causes an acute menopause, often accompanied by loss of sexual interest. This is usually helped by having an oestrogen implant or taking HRT.

Many drugs are known to affect a man's ability to get an erection, his sexuality generally and his libido. Much less research has been done on the effects of drugs on women's sexuality, but antidepressants such as Prozac and beta-blockers (used to treat high blood pressure) can have negative effects on sexual interest. If you are on any medication at all and having trouble with sex, check it out with your doctor.

Loss of Sexual Desire

Frances Campbell, Oxford Psychotherapist: *One of the things sex therapists find most difficult is the gone-off-its. You can treat premature ejaculation or phobic anxiety more easily. Those are very treatable ... but the gone-off-its, and especially if they've been together since they were quite young, it usually means the relationship has become a brother/sister relationship ... it's partly a developmental problem. People often marry too early before they are a fully mature adult, out of insecurity or naïvety and those kinds of marriages are very painful to break up ... and it is very difficult to fix this kind of problem without completely restructuring a marriage and I don't mean candlelit dinners and stockings and suspender belts.*

sex and the STI guide

Loss of sexual desire is the number one sexual problem for women. It can strike without warning and leave the same way or gradually. The reason for it may or may not be found. It can be due to stress, tiredness, unhappiness in a relationship or a drop in hormonal levels.

> **Hillary, 43:** *I lost mine. I hated it. My doctor told me I might never know why ... I tried to analyse myself, my husband, my history. I was beginning to resign myself to the loss when it came back but it had lasted for a few years and it was depressing.*

> **Emma, 28:** *My affectionate life with my partner is excellent. I'm with a man who I am constantly kissing and cuddling. However, when either one of us becomes really embroiled with work to the point where we're working twelve-hour days we seem to lose interest in each other sexually ... it's probably both of us. I think it's equal but it's always to do with work. Then it becomes unbalanced because if he's working hard and I'm not then it just becomes a drag. It doesn't worry me because we are so affectionate with each other ... but I'm more worried that it worries him actually. It's very sexist. I think because he's a man he's more interested in that.*

You can wait it out or you can check it out. If you are in a relationship and you suspect the relationship is the problem, try talking about it. It might be you think he is having an affair and do not know how to bring up the subject. It might just be you and the way you are feeling now: overly tired, worried about something, depressed. It is quite normal not to feel desire for your partner all the time, especially when you have been together for a long time. As well as talking to your partner, try talking to a counsellor (see Useful Addresses on page 390) or your family doctor.

When things wane a bit, some of us have been known to plot to try to get that light turned on again. We might spend time apart, organize a bedroom picnic, plan a weekend away from home or use that old standby: try to make him jealous.

> **Emma, 28:** *Have lunch with an extremely handsome other man. And then the sparks fly again. I think there's a lot about sex which is conquest sex, you want to acquire that person so you are having conquest sex. That's why when you have your guy it starts to slow down. Once you've been living with him for two years you don't need to conquer him any longer and that's why it gets boring and in my experience the best sex we ever have is when the other person is threatening to stray. I think it is a time-honoured truth about relationships and I don't think my relationship is any different than anybody else's.*

Frances Campbell: *I think it really is just the way it is. If you're jealous you stop seeing your partner as just part of you. You feel 'My God, somebody else fancies him! I'm going to have a bit of that'. That's jealousy. That's why love affairs work so well because you are never sure of the other person in the way you are in marriage ... the brother/sister types of marriages are more likely to have affairs. Affairs are one of the things that bring them to an end.*

Vaginal Dryness

This can be a problem especially at the time of the menopause when a woman's falling oestrogen level can leave her dry (see Chapter 3). It may also be because of lack of foreplay and this can be sorted out, again by talking and then acting. Tell or show your partner what you would like. If this is difficult for you, try to think about why this is. Are you afraid of how your partner will respond, or not respond? The worst scenario is total rejection, or to be laughed off but this is not likely. On the practical side, you can try KY lubricating jelly or cream, available without prescription. Sometimes women who take the oral contraceptive pill complain of vaginal dryness. This can be remedied by swapping to another pill. The dryness which occurs at menopause may be remedied with some forms of HRT (see pages 60–71).

Orgasm

Some women cannot achieve an orgasm, or can only have them in limited circumstances. The loaded word 'achieve' is often used, as if an orgasm is something one should receive a prize for. The myth of the female orgasm was zapped by the American sex researcher, Shere Hite, in her 1977 *Hite Report on Women's Sexuality*. She was the first to grab the headlines about what it really takes for a woman to reach orgasm. Her apparently astonishing discovery was something most women privately already knew. Most of us cannot have an orgasm with sexual intercourse alone. Many men were shocked to learn that the in-and-out action of their penis during intercourse was not enough. The clitoris usually needs direct stimulation.

Sally, 50: *It's fairly rare for me to reach orgasm with just intercourse but sometimes if we're in a position where his penis is rubbing against my clitoris it's possible to reach orgasm but it helps if he's also touching my clitoris with his fingers.*

It may be you are simply not getting enough direct stimulation. Try having sex at different angles. If you are on top during intercourse it may be easier for him to stimulate your clitoris with his fingers. Or if you try kneeling and he enters you from behind, the same thing applies or you can even try stimulating yourself during intercourse. A lot of women do this. It is important to tell your partner what you like. Experiment. It may be difficult to speak up but if you can find your nerve the results may be spectacular. If you think the problem is with your relationship you must talk about it with each other and perhaps see a counsellor for help (see Useful Addresses on page 390). Reading one of the many sex manuals may help. Sometimes masturbation (see pages 158–9) can also help you to improve your orgasms.

> **Celia, 41:** *I was about twenty-nine or thirty. I think I found it was a bit like an exploration ... I didn't feel guilty. I felt I wouldn't particularly want to get hooked on this ... but I think it did actually help me to a sort of greater sexual confidence because it made me know my body a bit more rather than having some man just fumbling away at you.*

Vaginismus

This is when the muscles of the vagina do not co-operate for intercourse. They tighten and are resistant to it, making an attempt at intercourse painful. The problem often relates to a woman's fear of sexual intercourse. This could be because of a previous bad sexual experience, sexual abuse as a child, because your partner tries to penetrate before you are ready, or because sex was seen as something shameful and wrong by your family. Most women with this problem can be helped. Self-exploration and gradually getting to know your own genitals, helps. You should practise inserting a finger, then two, then three into your vagina. Then your partner can try this using a lubricant like KY jelly or cream until you feel comfortable. If this exercise induces anxiety, your partner needs to know about it so try to think positively about it, talk it through and fix it – together. Trying out an exercise like this represents progress and it might even be fun. Take it slowly and do not do anything you are not comfortable with. Sexual problems can become areas of total conflict so it often also helps to see a counsellor early on, to keep this problem from escalating out of control.

Dyspareunia

This is painful intercourse. It can mean pain at the opening of the vagina or deep inside. This may be caused by other conditions such as a vaginal infection or endometriosis (see pages 38–40). It may also happen after childbirth, especially along the scar of an episiotomy (see pages 283–4) or after other operations involving the vagina, womb or ovaries. It can also be linked to vaginismus and anxiety. If you feel very tense and think sex is going to hurt, then you are likely to tense up the muscles of your vagina, which means your partner may have to use more force than normal during sexual intercourse which itself leads to setting up a cycle of 'pain, vaginismus, more force, more pain'. Talking about it and trying different positions and using a vaginal lubricant may all help. But do seek help from your doctor if it continues.

Erectile Dysfunction

For men, the most common sexual problem is not getting or not being able to sustain an erection. It may be his problem but it swiftly becomes yours as well, since it affects your sex life too. Furthermore, he will need your help and understanding. There are many reasons for what is formally known as erectile dysfunction. It can be related to anxiety and other psychological problems. Medication may interfere with a man's erection, as well as medical conditions such as diabetes and multiple sclerosis. Beta-blockers, commonly used to treat high blood pressure, sometimes interfere with a man's ability to get an erection.

> **Roger Kirby, Consultant Urologist, St George's Hospital:** *Sexual function is so intertwined with emotion that it is very difficult to separate the two ... it isn't just simply a question of giving them, for example, an injection to give them an erection and sending them off because the whole thing is much more complicated than that.*

In the case of Paul and Linda the problem was guilt.

> **Paul, 56:** *I had a bit of a guilt thing about the fact that she was married and I said to Linda, 'Look, if you and your husband split up I want to be there the following day'. And eventually she and her husband did split up and I was there the following day and I found that I could not maintain an erection, sometimes I couldn't get an erection.*

So Paul went to a sex therapist on his own. She recommended he try a special vacuum pump designed to help give a man an erection.

> **Paul:** *The results were absolutely disastrous. Even on my own, completely on my own in the house, I felt embarrassed, I felt humiliated.*

After the disaster with the vacuum pump Paul and Linda went to see a sex and relationship counsellor, together.

> **Linda:** *The treatment ... was not centred on my partner. My needs were considered, what I wanted out of the physical relationship considered, in great detail and the idea I felt was to make it a mutually satisfying experience and I was so amazed to find that it really did help me as well as help him.*

The counsellor began by forbidding Paul and Linda to have sex, an approach pioneered by the renowned sex researchers, Masters and Johnson, in the United States in 1970. Paul and Linda felt silly at first. The counsellor asked them to make sure no one would disturb them. They had to be at home alone. Then the counsellor suggested they both take a hot relaxing bath and meet in a warm, comfortable candlelit room. Next they were to massage one another, slowly. Most importantly they were not to touch each other's intimate places.

> **Paul:** *It nearly drives you mad.*

Paul and Linda then endured a second session of restraint ...

> **Paul:** *And then hallelujah, the third time you are allowed to do whatever you wish – but the massage comes first – and all of a sudden your impotence is cured ... you're on the way.*
>
> **Linda:** *You feel that once you've been – if you can say cured – you want to sort of tell everybody, you want the whole world to have the same treatment ... The relationship has been enriched by it and the sexual side has become something that I never thought it could be.*

The slow, step-by-step, build-up to sex approach is much tested and reliable. Variations on it are used by therapists helping couples on both sides of the Atlantic. The same type of approach can be used for women too. As well as these techniques, injection therapy for erectile dysfunction is now commonplace and can be helpful.

Nearly all men experience impotence or premature ejaculation at some time in their lives. Impotence is when a man cannot get an erection and does not ejaculate. Premature ejaculation is when he ejaculates too soon after arousal – sometimes even before he has put his penis into your vagina. Try not to panic if this happens, even if it goes on for a few weeks. Within a good relationship it can usually be sorted out. If it does become a persistent problem, first try the not-having-sex approach that we have already talked about. Another technique is called the 'squeeze'. After the man has an erection and before he ejaculates, try squeezing his penis for about fifteen seconds which will stop him ejaculating. He might even lose the erection. Then start stimulating him again and repeat the squeeze twice more. Only on the fourth time allow him to ejaculate. There are various other things to try so check out the many sex guides. A good one is *The Relate Guide to Sex in Loving Relationships* by Sarah Litvinoff. Or contact Relate (see Useful Addresses on page 390), your GP or a family planning clinic for advice.

Sexual Abuse

Sexual abuse has been given huge attention in the UK and around the world in recent years. Yet children and adults continue to be abused. Social workers, doctors and teachers have a new awareness. There are procedures to comfort and counsel the abused and to report the abusers. Sexual abuse is not only news, it is now treated as entertainment. Made-for-TV movies, dramatic serials, detective shows and popular novels, all use sexual abuse as a theme. The popularization of sexual abuse has done nothing to stop it.

The first problem is that for all our knowledge and supposed openness about abuse statistics are not reliable. Many people still do not report it. Several 'recovered memory' scandals, where victims were shown to be fabricating the abuse story, have created problems for the many who have truly suffered. Recovered memory is when a victim supposedly suddenly recalls an alleged abuse many years after the fact. The nature of the relationship between the abuser and the abused adds tremendously to the complication because often the two love each other. Most abusers are known to their victims. They are frequently family members or neighbours. He is a father, uncle or brother, sometimes a teacher. Mothers and sisters are also abusers. But father/daughter or father/stepdaughter is a classic combination.

> **Anne Marie West:** *I didn't know any different. I didn't know that it was not normal. It was a life that I was brought up in. It was the only life that I knew.*

Anne Marie West, who told her story to *Woman's Hour*, is a victim in an extraordinary and extreme case. But her feelings and response to what happened are similar to others who have suffered what we might regard as far less torture. It is extremely difficult to measure the abuse of a child.

Anne Marie suffered a lifetime of sexual abuse at the hands of her father and stepmother, the serial killers Fred and Rosemary West. Fred West hanged himself in prison before his trial could take place. Rosemary West is now serving a life sentence for a string of murders of young girls and women. Anne Marie West's natural mother and two of her sisters were among her father's victims. Abusers are adept at covering their tracks and the Wests did so for two decades. The authorities – trained to spot abuse – often miss it. They may well suspect it, but have difficulty proving it when good cover stories are provided. Abused children are constantly under threat not to report the abuse.

> **Anne Marie:** *I remember an occasion when I was about nine. I was at a school in Gloucester, infant school, and I used to be given notes excusing me from PE. Or I'd have to make an excuse myself and this one occasion I was told that I had to do PE and I was changing and the teacher noticed marks on my body and sort of asked me 'what's the problem?' and we were always told to say that we'd fallen over or something ... and I carried on the day and when I got home it was a matter of, I should say, minutes and there was a knock at the door and a lady came in and I was told to get changed and to make a cup of tea. And Rosemary my stepmother and this lady were talking and as I come out to make a drink for them this lady was saying, 'oh well that's fine thank you very much, it's not a problem', and left, and I did get what I recall was the biggest hiding of my life for that and being young and not realizing I decided that, well, obviously the things that my father and stepmother had been telling me, that authorities and people like they are out to hurt you, to me, it seemed that that was the way it was.*

Such is the peculiar and tragic twist in abuse relationships that the victim is made to feel guilty, not the perpetrator. This helps to sustain the relationship. So the child co-operates in two ways. She or he may love the offender and feel protective towards that person. If the child speaks up, family life, as precarious as it is, may be shattered. If the child stays silent the family stays together and the abuser is rewarded. You may be afraid to report an offender to the police, but local police now often have special units designed to deal with sexual abuse. Ask for a trained officer and ask for a woman to talk to, if you prefer. You might save someone else the suffering you have endured by reporting an abuser.

> **Anne Marie:** *I was very much of a Daddy's girl. I loved my Dad. I did idolize him. He was everything to me and ... I never argued or fought back or objected to things and this is where I say I was very much of a coward.*

If you have been abused in the past and feel that it is interfering with your life today, sexually or in other ways, get help for yourself. Talking to someone such as a counsellor (see pages 103–7), The Samaritans, Women's Aid or Childline (see Useful Addresses on page 390) might be your first step to recovery.

Rape

Rape is being forced to have sexual intercourse against your will. Sometimes there are arguments about what 'against your will' actually means. If you voluntarily climb into bed naked with a man with an aroused penis, are you 'asking for it'? Do you forfeit your right to say 'no' before intercourse actually takes place? Cases where these questions arise are rare. Most rape is violent and clearly without the consent of a woman.

If you – or someone you know – is raped:

- Get help as soon as you feel able to – you may want to contact your local Rape Crisis Centre. If you do not know where it is, ring the London number (see Useful Addresses on page 390) to find out.
- Contact a friend to help see you through the next steps.
- Contact the police and ask to talk to their rape crisis unit. Police stations have special interview suites for women who have been raped. Non-uniformed female police officers are available to talk to you, offer advice and support. There is no obligation to press charges or even to have a medical examination, but you can have a medical examination by a specially trained doctor if you wish.
- If you decide to have a medical examination it is best not to wash or drink (if there has been any oral contact) until swabs have been taken.
- You will need to have swabs taken from your vagina, and any areas where there has been sexual contact. They may also want to comb your pubic hair for hairs and fibres.
- Specimens can be collected for evidence up to seven days after the rape has occurred.
- Alternatively, contact your GP. You should also consider getting yourself tested at a sexually transmitted infection clinic, even if you do not want to report the rape as a crime.

Domestic violence and marital rape are less likely to be reported than other crimes. Both of these, as well as being physically harmful, can lead to psychological problems, sleep disorders, depression and attempted suicide. See Useful Addresses on page 390 for details of organizations that help women who are suffering domestic violence.

Guide to Sexually Transmitted Infections

The problem with sex is that it often comes with trouble. Sexually transmitted infections –
STIs – are on the increase. They used to be called STDs – sexually transmitted diseases –
but health professionals are switching to the less stigmatizing sounding 'infection'. The 1994
National Sex Survey found that 5.6 per cent of women had visited an STI clinic some time in
the past. Many women also see their GP for STI treatment. According to the latest
Department of Health figures (1996) the number of new cases of STIs was 405, 000, an
increase of 6 per cent over the previous year. Out of the total number of new cases 228,215
were women, an increase of 8 per cent for women over 1995. These figures do not include
people with Aids (see pages 188–90).

New cases of STIs in women (at GUM clinics in England) in 1996
- Genital warts: 27,101
- Chlamydia: 18,163
- Herpes: 9,349
- Trichomonas: 5,302
- Gonorrhoea: 3,902

You can get an STI at any age and stage of your life if you have sex with someone who is
carrying an STI. It is also possible to get some of these infections without having sex,
although often there is a sexual connection. These infections are thrush, bacterial vaginosis,
and cystitis.

Sexually transmittable infections include HIV, Aids, chlamydia, trichomonas, gonorrhoea,
syphilis, genital warts and genital herpes. They come with a myriad of names and labels.
And they often hunt in packs, so if you get one you might get two or three along with it.

> **Erica, 40:** *All at once I got gardnerella [see page 180] and two or three other
> incomprehensible sounding things, plus herpes, after sleeping with someone
> once. I was in disbelief, sorry for myself and fairly disgusted with him. Where
> had he been? Who had he been with? Suddenly all the horror stories I'd ever
> heard were true.*

The best way to prevent a sexually transmitted infection from transmitting is to make sure
your partner wears a condom, whether it's for vaginal, anal or oral sex. Or you could try
having sexual intercouse without penetration by kissing, touching and masturbating, or
using sex toys such as vibrators. If neither you nor your partner have had sex with anyone
else there is no risk of an STI.

Remember STIs are everywhere. If you are planning to travel do not be lulled into imaginary safety because you are heading for a wonderful destination. If you think there is any chance you will be having sex on holiday go prepared. Take condoms with you. They are difficult to buy in a hurry in countries where you do not speak the language and can be impossible to find in others, even if you do.

If you suspect you have been infected, you must get help so go directly to the STI experts or see your GP. You can make an appointment yourself at a Genito Urinary Medicine (GUM) or STI Clinic. GUM and STI clinics are attached to hospitals and they are free and confidential. They specialize in sexually transmitted infections so they tend to be better if you are fairly certain you have an STI. It may be less embarrassing for you too because they are more anonymous than your local surgery. You can also visit a family planning clinic, who will also guarantee confidentiality. They do not even report your visit to your doctor (or anyone else) unless you ask them to.

> **Janice, 36:** *I went to one and they treated me just like a number which was perfect for the occasion. I was so relieved not have someone yell out my name in the waiting-room. It was confidential and the atmosphere completely trusting. And the woman doctor who examined me couldn't have been kinder.*

How Do You Know?

Sometimes our vaginal discharge tells us. All women have some discharge most of the time. It varies in consistency and amount, usually increasing at the time of ovulation and just before menstruation (see page 31). It may be heavier if you are on the pill or using an IUD (coil). The discharge often decreases at the time of the menopause. Normal vaginal discharge is white, but becomes yellow with a slight odour on contact with air because of a chemical interaction called oxidation.

When we get a sexually related infection our vaginal discharge may become thicker, and the smell and consistency can change. Infections that cause these changes are bacterial vaginosis, candida (thrush), chlamydia, trichomonas, gonorrhoea and herpes. Vaginal deodorants are heavily promoted to get rid of all our smells. But they are not necessary, and it is not good to put deodorants in the vagina. The lining is very sensitive and deodorants cause damage and irritation.

sex and the STI guide

STIs

(This guide also covers infectious gynaecological infections which may not necessarily be related to sex.)

Bacterial Vaginosis, or Gardnerella

Symptoms: Fishy-smelling grey watery discharge which is worse after sex. Sometimes no other symptoms.

Causes: Bacteria which normally live in the vagina (without showing symptoms) but which can multiply and cause trouble. The most common of these is *Gardnerella vaginalis*.

How it is Caught: It can be passed sexually between partners, but not necessarily as the bacteria is normally in the vagina anyway.

Tests: Swabs taken from the vagina and tested in a laboratory.

Treatment: Antibiotic tablets – metronidazole (Flagyl) or antibiotic cream (clindamycin) inserted into the vagina.

Treat Partner?: Only if it recurs in you.

Long-term Effects: The infection can recur. Can be a problem in pregnant women causing premature labour.

Candida, also Known as Yeast Infection, Thrush or Monilia

Symptoms: Itchy, white, curdy, cottage cheesey, vaginal discharge. Vagina and vulva may be red and sore and very itchy. Symptoms may be similar to cystitis (see pages 192–3).

Causes: Yeast infection called *Candida albicans*.

How it is Caught: Again, not strictly a sexually transmitted infection although it can be. The yeast lives on the skin especially in warm, moist places (such as armpits), in the intestines, and in the vagina of 20 per cent of women without them knowing. It is often associated with sex and sometimes it can be caught from a sexual partner who has thrush, though he might not have any symptoms. Some women get thrush after taking antibiotics or steroids, or when they are pregnant or diabetic, all of which probably cause a change in acidity in the vagina encouraging the yeast to multiply. Some women complain they are more susceptible to thrush when on the contraceptive pill. Men can get a red itchy rash on their penis, burning and itching under the foreskin, a curd cheese-like discharge under the foreskin or slight discomfort on urinating. But sometimes men have no symptoms.

Tests: A swab from the vagina and vulva is taken to sample the discharge. Microscopic analysis or laboratory culture confirms diagnosis. Once you have had it, you will recognize it the next time, and can treat future bouts without having a test.

Treatment: A variety of creams and pessaries, single or multiple dose, can be inserted into the vagina or applied to the vulva. One of these, clotrimazole (Canesten), can be bought without prescription. A pill called fluconazole (Diflucan One) is available with or without prescription. It is expensive but it is a one-pill treatment and some women prefer it over pessaries. However, it should not be used during pregnancy. Self-help remedies include vinegar in the bath, eating live yoghurt, and even putting live yoghurt on a tampon and inserting it into your vagina. Many women swear by these natural remedies; the medical evidence that they help is sketchy but there is no harm in trying them.

Treat Partner?: Only if he has symptoms of itching and/or soreness or you are getting recurrent thrush.

Long-term Effects: Usually none except the nuisance of recurrent thrush. Some women are repeatedly troubled by thrush. No sooner does one episode clear than another seems to start. That is why it is a good idea to get a swab taken to make sure it really is thrush.

Action on Recurrent Thrush
- Have a real blitz on treatment to rid the body of all the thrush yeasts lurking around. During the next attack use anti-thrush pessaries and cream and take an anti-thrush pill – all available over-the-counter or on prescription.
- Avoid all bubble baths.
- Look at your diet. Cut out the cakes, biscuits and sugary foods. Eat more live yoghurt.
- If it is linked to sex, use an anti-thrush pessary after sex.
- Get your partner to take anti-thrush treatment.
- Use an anti-thrush pessary once a week for a few months.
- Try not to take any antibiotics unless absolutely necessary.
- Don't wear underwear made from synthetic materials or trousers that are too tight.

Other Effects of Thrush: Candidiasis
Some people think that the yeast causing thrush, candida, can spread throughout the body and produce an illness called candidiasis. Fatigue, constipation, diarrhoea, wind, bloating, recurrent cystitis, catarrh, palpitations, recurrent thrush, poor memory, depression, irritability

have all been attributed to the disease. It is thought that the candida yeasts overgrow in the gut. Theories and some evidence link this to antibiotics taken both as medication and in our diet via the food chain as more antibiotics are now used in food growing and animal-rearing. It has also been linked to diets high in carbohydrate, refined sugars and yeast.

Candidiasis is especially diagnosed by therapists working in complementary medicine. Many conventional doctors question whether there is such a condition. Unfortunately this means there has been no good research to sort out the true nature of the problem. The treatments suggested include diet, nutritional supplements, antifungal drugs, desensitization and taking supplements of 'good' bacteria. Anti-candidiasis diets exclude refined sugars such as those found in cakes, biscuits and puddings, and eliminate yeast products such as bread. There may also be other food intolerances which should be eliminated on a trial and error basis. Various vitamin supplements, A, B, C, and minerals including selenium and magnesium, have all been recommended in varying amounts. Nystatin or other antifungal drugs can be tried. A special type of desensitization is offered by some therapists using extracts of candida. Taking doses of lactobacillus, a 'good' bacteria, is supposed to re-balance the bacteria in the gut. Although many doctors are sceptical about candidiasis, if you think this is your problem you can try some of the above and can find out more from the many books available on the subject. Check with your own doctor or seek help from one of the range of complementary therapists (see page 390).

Itching around the vulva and vagina need not, however, be caused by thrush.

> **Jenny:** *I have to say, the itching had been going on a very long time. I'd been to the doctor years before ... I'd been given things for thrush and cortisone cream to control the itching but [was told] not to use too much as it thins the skin. In the end they said there was no cause for the itching. But I still had this uncontrollable itching in my vulva which was worse once I got warm in bed and was just dropping off to sleep. I then noticed a raised area which I thought perhaps I'd caused by scratching. Then I began thinking there was something more to it. Maybe I've picked up an STD. It seemed unfair – there was only my ex-husband and one other man since I'd been divorced ... So I went back to the doctor as I was worried it was more than an itch. My doctor this time said it was lichen sclerosis after taking a biopsy. I was given a strong steroid and told for this condition to use it when needed ... Gradually it's got less and less.*

Lichen sclerosis affects the skin of the vulva, making it itchy and look white and thin. It is not related to sex. In many women the lichen sclerosis is easy to control with strong steroids, but for some it can be very uncomfortable with cracks and bleeding of the skin involved. Rarely, vulval cancer can develop in the lichen sclerosis so it should be checked every year. Unfortunately no one knows why it occurs.

Trichomonas, Trich or TV

Symptoms: A thin yellow or green frothy vaginal discharge which has an unpleasant fishy smell. Also soreness and itching around the vagina. Sometimes there are no signs at all but it is detected in a routine cervical smear. It is often found in association with another STI.

Causes: A tiny parasite called a protozoa named *Trichomonas vaginalis*.

How it is Caught: Unprotected sexual intercourse.

Tests: A vaginal swab to get a sample of the discharge which is checked in the laboratory.

Treatment: A short course of antibiotics usually with metronidazole (Flagyl).

Treat Partner?: Yes. Very important even if he has no symptoms.

Long-term Effects: Usually none, though there may be a link to pelvic inflammatory disease (PID).

Herpes (Herpes Simplex Virus or HSV)

Symptoms: Women who carry the genital herpes virus develop lesions like cold sores around the vagina or anus when the virus is active. They can be tiny itchy spots which last for a couple of days or they can come in groups – a little like a blistery rash – and be quite painful, lasting for weeks. The sores may crust over as they heal. The vagina and vulva may be very sore and red and glands in the groin may swell and cause pain. You may have difficulty peeing and have a general flu-like feeling which can last for a few days or for weeks. It takes up to a month for the symptoms to appear after you become infected and the first attack is often the worst. It may also be the only attack. You may notice subsequent attacks are preceded by a tingling or stinging sensations around the opening of your vagina or anus. If the virus is transmitted orally, sores may appear in your throat.

Causes: Herpes is caused by the herpes simplex virus. There are two types, 1 and 2. Both can cause genital herpes and cold sores. But Herpes type 2 (HSV2) usually causes the genital herpes and herpes type 1 (HSV1) is usually found in cold sores around the mouth. The swapping around of the two types of virus is probably linked to oral sex. The only way of knowing which one you have got is for a swab to be taken and examined under a microscope.

How it is Caught: Unprotected sexual intercourse or oral sex. Herpes can be transmitted skin-to-skin – for example, your mouth on his penis, if he has a sore or if you do on your mouth. The virus is most dangerous when it is active, but it may even be transmittable when it is dormant so use condoms. Whether you choose to use condoms for life or not depends on you and your relationship. If you are in a permanent relationship you may not be too concerned, especially if you let your partner know when you are having an attack. But as far as casual sex goes, insist on a condom and let your partner know of the risk.

Tests: Swabs from the lesions which are cultured in the laboratory. A swab test may produce a false negative, but not a false positive.

Treatment: An anti-virus drug, e.g. aciclovir (Zovirax) taken five times per day or famcyclovir (Famvir) taken three times per day, should be prescribed as soon as the diagnosis is made to reduce the length of the first attack, although it will not prevent future occurrences. Later on, these drugs may help prevent an attack if you take them as soon as you feel one coming on. There is also evidence to suggest that if it is taken for six months it may reduce the number of future attacks. If you get attacks more than five times a year, a lower dose taken every day may help. Tablets are expensive so some doctors are reluctant to prescribe them. If you want to try the drug, make sure you ask your doctor for it. The aciclovir cream is available without prescription but is useless for genital herpes. Even though there is no outright cure for herpes, there are several things you can do to prevent attacks, or shorten the length of their stay. Get plenty of rest, eat healthy foods, avoid too much alcohol. Some people claim taking vitamin C helps. Some women find that they get more recurrences when they are under emotional stress and trauma. When you have an attack, you can take paracetamol to reduce the discomfort, have a salt bath or use an ice pack for relief.

Treat Partner?: Only if he gets an attack. Men get sores on their penis or around the anus when they have a herpes outbreak and they have a discharge only if herpes is in the urethra in the penis.

Long-term Effects: 80 per cent of women infected with genital herpes do get recurrences, although many of these may be mild. Herpes can put your baby at risk if you develop it during pregnancy. If the virus is active during the baby's delivery, a caesarean birth may be recommended (see pages 284–5) as if the baby gets a herpes infection at birth it can cause an infection of the brain called encephalitis.

Comment: Herpes was hyped when it first came on the scene in the eighties. But it fast disappeared from the headlines when the news landed a far bigger and more serious story: Aids. But the stigma hangs over from early reports.

> **Rosemary:** *For a long time having genital herpes simplex wasn't a problem. I occasionally got a sore, it went away very quickly and that was it. When I saw (the) headlines ... I thought, oh my goodness it's not just a little cold sore virus. This is a fearsome, horrible, loathsome disease, yuck. And I started reading all about it and as a result I got more and more worried about it and terrified about it and started to think my goodness I should never have sex again ... and when I was worried about it I was getting lots of attacks. I mean for about a year and a half the attacks never seemed to go away.*

The virus need not be a big deal. You can make it into a bigger deal by not getting enough rest and by being stressed all the time. Remember, some people only get it once. If you have any doubt about your partner, use a condom. They are very effective in preventing transmission of this viral skin condition. Herpes is, however, on the increase. One reason for this is that more than half of the people who have it are thought not to show any symptoms, so they transmit it unwittingly.

Genital Warts, or Wart Virus

Symptoms: Small fleshy growths on the vulva, vagina, anus or cervix (or on a man's penis) which take about two months or much longer to appear after you have been in contact with the virus. Sometimes you can catch the wart virus but not have any obvious warts. They may itch, but usually they are neither itchy nor sore. You may not even know you have them unless you can see or feel them.

Causes: A virus called human papilloma virus (HPV). There are at least fifty different known types.

How it is Caught: The virus is passed by skin-to-skin contact, so it does not have to be through full sexual intercourse.

Tests: No tests are needed as they can be diagnosed just by looking at them. Sometimes you only know you have been exposed to the virus when it is seen on a cervical smear (see pages 374–9).

Treatment: Although there is treatment available to get rid of the warts, the virus may live on. There is not yet any treatment to eradicate it. Treatment of the wart(s) itself is simple but may need to be repeated several times as some take a long time to go away. A paint called podophyllin may be applied or the warts can be frozen or burnt off. Unfortunately they recur in 25 per cent of women after three months, though they may also disappear without treatment. You can help your treatment by wearing cotton underwear, avoiding tight clothes and taking salt baths.

Treat Partner?: Not necessary unless warts appear. The virus is still transmittable if warts are not visible. Use condoms to reduce the risk of spreading the virus.

Long-term Effects: Women who have certain types of the genital wart virus are more likely to have changes in the cervix which might turn into cancer later if it is not treated. The virus increases the risk but does not mean cancer will follow. Wart viruses 16 and 18 are the worrying strains. There are tests available to check for wart virus which are currently being assessed for reliability. If the wart virus is present in the cervix you may need more frequent cervical smears and possibly a colposcopy (see page 378). Unfortunately there is no way to treat the wart virus itself in the cervix.

Comment: The wart virus can linger for a long time and be passed on without anyone realizing or just go away. If you suddenly develop warts it may be because you have recently been exposed to them or the exposure may have been a long time ago and for some unknown reason they have suddenly developed. This can cause problems between partners who may suspect one of them has been unfaithful.

> **Pam, 39:** *I ... also felt resentful at being told that I'd probably come into contact with the wart virus. I didn't know who had infected me and the rational part of me knows it's not helpful to apportion blame – after all it takes two doesn't it. But I did think it statistically much more likely that the past sexual behaviour of my husband had been to blame ... To hear eminent male doctors hypothesizing on the increased incidence of cervical cancer among young women and laying it at the door of female promiscuity adds insult to injury.*

Chlamydia, or the Silent Disease

Symptoms: Vaginal discharge or just extra moisture from the vagina or perhaps no symptoms at all. Cystitis, due to inflammation of the lining of the urethra causing pain and stinging on urinating, can also be an indication. If your partner has non-specific urethritis (NSU) get yourself tested for chlamydia. NSU is an inflammation of a man's urethra usually caused by chlamydia. It may cause the man to have cystitis-like symptoms, a discharge from his penis, or he may not notice anything.

Causes: A bacteria called *Chlamydia trachomatis*.

How it is Caught: Vaginal or anal intercourse.

Tests: Special swab inserted into the cervix, or a blood or urine test. None of the tests is 100 per cent certain of identifying the infection even if it is present. GUM clinics are more likely to test for this routinely than a GP will, though there is talk of screening all young women for this infection.

Treatment: Antibiotic treatment as soon as possible after the diagnosis.

Treat Partner?: Vital to treat him to prevent reinfection. No sex until you have both completed the course of antibiotics.

Long-term Effects: If not treated or if there is delay in treatment, chlamydia can cause pelvic inflammatory disease (PID). PID can be caused in many ways but most commonly it is transmitted when a bacteria from the vagina is pushed up into the reproductive organs during sexual intercourse. Up to two-thirds of cases of PID are caused by the bacteria Chlamydia. It is common to get a low-grade, niggly abdominal pain which can be constant or come and go, a bit more discharge and trouble with periods – nothing dramatic. The local infection causes redness and swelling in the fallopian tubes. Two per cent of teenagers contract the disease and 1 per cent of twenty to thirty-four year olds. Older women can also be at risk. It is sometimes known as a silent disease as it can go undetected, but if left untreated, in the long term, it can cause chronic illness and infertility. The problem with PID is that it can block the fallopian tubes, a cause of infertility since the egg cannot travel through. Or it may lead to an ectopic pregnancy if the fertilized egg develops in the tube (see page 294). With a mild attack of PID, the risk of a blocked fallopian tube is 3 per cent whilst three bad attacks increase the risk to about 75 per cent. PID evades diagnosis because the symptoms are often vague or there may be no noticeable symptoms. Frightening estimates suggest that by the year 2000 PID could affect one in four women.

> **Celia, 21:** *I caught chlamydia from my boyfriend last year. He suddenly phoned and said I ought to go for a check-up as he'd been having trouble peeing but he wouldn't talk about it. We're both at college in different towns so communicating is a real hassle with neither of us having our own phone. I hadn't noticed anything except possibly a bit more discharge. I've had the treatment – we've finished and I'm terrified that my tubes are blocked. The awful thing is not knowing until you try to have a baby. If I can't I'll kill him.*

HIV and Aids

Elizabeth Glaser spent the last years of her life campaigning for Aids victims. In 1986 she and her husband, *Starsky and Hutch* star Paul Michael Glaser, discovered their daughter had Aids. Elizabeth acquired HIV through a blood transfusion she received during her ninth month of pregnancy. She was carrying her daughter Ariel. Ariel is believed to have contracted the virus through her mother's milk during breast-feeding, not when she was inside her mother's womb.

> **Elizabeth Glaser:** *I think that the sad part about this was that people listened to me because I wasn't gay, because I wasn't a drug abuser, and because I was white and because I looked like them and I was maybe the first, or one of the first people with Aids who looked like them and I was telling them a story that could have been their life.*

Aids took Elizabeth's life in 1994 when she was forty-seven. Her campaign had a huge impact in the United States and abroad.

Symptoms: HIV (Human Immunodeficiency Syndrome) is the virus which causes Aids (Acquired Immune Deficiency Syndrome). Once you have been infected with the HIV virus you are HIV positive, but your blood may not test positive for three months after getting the infection. Most people who are HIV positive do not have Aids and will be well for as long as ten to fifteen years, though nearly all HIV-positive people will eventually develop Aids. Whilst you are HIV positive you may be more susceptible to infections as your immune system is affected by the virus. You are infectious and able to pass on the HIV virus to other people throughout this time, even in the first three months after catching the HIV virus when you do not test positive. This is especially worrying if you are having unsafe sex – that is sex without a condom. HIV becomes Aids with the appearance of certain illnesses and changes in the immune cells of your blood. It can lead to recurrent infections, pneumonia, tiredness, weight loss, and skin cancer.

Causes: Human Immunodeficiency Virus (HIV)

How it is Caught: Vaginal intercourse, anal intercourse, sharing needles, blood transfusion or contaminated blood products and, rarely, oral sex. Women are more likely to get it by having intercourse with an infected man than a man is to get it from an infected woman. If other STIs are present and these cause open sores, this increases the likelihood of transmission.

Tests: Blood test which may not become positive for three months after exposure to the virus. It is available from your GP or anonymously at an STI clinic. There are concerns that if you have the test via your GP the results are in your notes which might affect your ability to get life insurance in the future. Ask that it is not recorded in your notes. In fact, although insurance companies regularly ask applicants about their sexual infection history, doctors are not yet obliged to answer these questions.

Treatment: There is no cure for Aids as yet. AZT in combination with other drugs given to people who are HIV positive may protect the immune system and delay the onset of symptoms and Aids itself. This is a fast-changing area and there have even been recent claims that aggressive treatment with a combination of drugs might provide a permanent cure for some Aids sufferers, but it is too early to make certain predictions. Many HIV-positive people believe exercise and diet play a role in fighting off the onset of full-blown Aids.

Treat Partner?: No treatment available, but the partner should be monitored to see if the disease has been contracted. Partners should always use condoms.

Long-term Effects: These vary enormously. Some HIV carriers are living longer, healthier lives than anyone expected a decade ago. Yet recent studies indicate new HIV strains can be more virulent.

Comments: HIV- or Aids-awareness has launched the 'safe sex' generation. Many teenagers now know about the risks even before they begin to experiment with sex.

> **Sarah, 14:** *I know a lot about sexually transmitted diseases from magazines and we learn about it in school so I am very aware that when I have my first sexual experience he should use a condom and I think a lot of people in my school take that view as well.*

Aids, however, is on the increase. At the time of writing, the total figure for Aids cases reported in the UK since 1982 was 13,720. Women accounted for 10 per cent or 1402 of these. The year 1996 saw an 18 per cent increase in new Aids cases over the previous year, and 8 per cent of these new cases were women. Most women in the UK get Aids through unprotected intercourse. In 1996 alone 224 women developed Aids through unprotected intercourse, while thirty-seven women contracted it through sharing needles. Between 1982 and 1997, 916 women died from Aids against 9584 men.

All blood products are now screened for the HIV virus. But if someone who has very recently been infected with HIV gives blood, the test will not show this, i.e. it will screen negative when in fact it is positive. Fortunately in this country relatively few people are infected with HIV. There is also no financial incentive to give blood so the risk of getting a blood transfusion which is infected with the HIV virus is very, very small. In countries where blood donors are paid and the incidence of HIV is higher, the risk is greater. Blood products like plasma and other vaccines made from blood can all be treated to destroy any infection with HIV so these will be 100 per cent safe from HIV.

HIV is transmitted via:
- Vaginal intercourse.
- Anal intercourse.
- Sharing needles and injecting drugs.
- Infected blood transfusions and blood products.
- Oral sex.

HIV is not transmitted via:
- Lavatory seats.
- Kissing.
- Masturbation.
- Swimming-pools.
- Drinking out of the same cup.
- Handshaking or hugging,

It was thought until recently that HIV could not be transmitted via oral sex. There have now been several reported cases, so it is possible but rare. If you have oral sex with a man when you have a sore or a cut in your mouth, it is possible for the HIV virus to be transmitted. Always use a condom.

Gonorrhoea, or 'the clap'

Symptoms: Women often do not know they have this until it has spread causing pelvic inflammatory disease (PID) or other symptoms. If you get gonorrhoea through vaginal intercourse you may notice a change in your discharge. There may be more of it, it may be thin and watery and the colour yellow/greenish. You may notice symptoms like a burning sensation when you urinate (as in cystitis – see pages 192–3) or develop a sore throat when gonorrhoea results from oral sex. Men are more likely to know when they have it since they will see a white or yellow discharge from the penis, four days to two weeks after catching it. They may also feel cystitis-like symptoms, have an anal discharge (if it was transmitted via anal sex) or a sore throat (if it was transmitted via oral sex).

Causes: Infection with a bacteria *Neisseria gonorrhoea* passed during sex. It can affect the vagina, cervix, urethra, rectum and occasionally the throat.

How it is Caught: Through sexual, oral or anal intercourse. It often accompanies another sexually transmitted infection.

Tests: Swabs need to be taken from the vagina, urethra, rectum and throat to get samples of the bacteria which are then cultured in the laboratory.

Treatment: Large doses of an antibiotic – usually amoxycillin.

Treat Partner?: Your partner must also be treated with antibiotics and use a condom.

Long-term Effects: It can cause pelvic inflammatory disease and infertility if not treated.

> **Joanne, 39:** *I had it and it was nothing. It's two shots of penicillin and you're cured. I don't even remember because at the time that I had it, it was so unbelievably treatable.*

Pubic Lice, or 'Crabs'

Symptoms: Intense itching in your pubic area because of the lice bites.

Causes: A parasitic insect called pediculosis.

How it is Caught: There are lots of myths about pubic lice. We usually get them from sex. But people also say you can get them from sheets, towels or even from sitting on a toilet seat, although if this happens it must be very rare. Having lice is not a big deal. Your pubic hair will feel very itchy and you will probably be able to spot the tiny lice. Their minute legs are claw-like – hence the nickname crabs – and cling to your hair.

Treatment: Shampoos with a special anti-lice concoction are available without prescription and after a couple of uses you should get rid of the pubic lice. They do not return on their own. You need to have contact with them again.

Treat Partner?: Yes or you will get re-infected.

Long-term Effects: None.

Cystitis

Symptoms: Needing to pee a lot, yet when you try to go little or nothing comes out. It stings and can be extremely painful. In mild cases it is a feeling of minor irritation. Sometimes the urine is cloudy or can be blood stained.

Causes: It is an inflammation of the lining of the bladder and urethra. This is most commonly caused by a bacteria, *Escherica coli*, which normally lives in the rectum but has crept up the urethra, often during or after sex. A woman's urethra is much shorter than a man's. His urethra has to travel the length of his penis to reach his bladder, ours has only a short trip, making it much easier to develop a bladder infection. (Men get cystitis too but less often and it is more likely to be STI related.) So although cystitis in women is not usually an STI it often pops up after sex, brought on by friction and travelling bacteria. It can also be caused by other bacteria, viruses and allergies to soaps and vaginal deodorants. Wiping yourself from front to back after going to the toilet will help to keep bacteria away from the urethra. Women who use a diaphragm for contraception are also more likely to get cystitis. One in two women get cystitis at some time in their lives.

Tests: A urine test using a special stick impregnated with chemicals which changes colour when dipped into urine infected by bacteria, although this test does not tell you exactly what is causing the infection. A urine sample needs to be cultured in a laboratory to identify the organism. Some women get symptoms of cystitis even though no bacteria can be cultured.

Treatment: Drink a lot. Just about anything will do but an alkaline solution is best to fight off any bacteria. A teaspoon of baking soda in a cup of water works to flush it out. Cranberry juice is excellent. Avoid coffee and alcohol. Take aspirin or paracetamol for the pain. If the condition does not improve after a day or two you will probably need a prescription for antibiotics so you need to see your doctor. A short course lasting one to three days should be enough. Some women get thrush (see pages 180–2) as a side effect of taking antibiotics and may need to take anti-thrush medication at the same time.

Cystitis Prevention Tips
If you are particularly prone to attacks of cystitis after sex:

- Try washing before and after intercourse and get your partner to do the same, particularly after anal intercourse if you are going on to have vaginal intercourse. This also applies to fingers and sex toys.
- Pee immediately before and after intercourse.
- Drink a glass of bicarbonate of soda after sex.
- Use a lubricant (e.g. KY jelly or cream) if your vagina is dry to cut down the friction.

Long-term Effects: Sometimes the infection causing the cystitis spreads and infects the kidneys, causing pain in the back. This infection is known as pyelonephritis and it is more likely to happen if there is some physical problem with the kidneys or during pregnancy. If this has occurred or you are getting very frequent attacks of cystitis, it is a good idea to have an ultrasound or special X-ray to check out the kidneys and bladder.

Syphilis

Symptoms: The infection lodges around the openings to the vagina and the urethra. The glands around the vulva may become swollen. There is a sore (chancre) at the point where the infection settles in but this may be so tiny it is not visible. It appears 3–90 days after catching the infection, and disappears within five weeks. A rash may also appear in other places on your body, such as hands, back and tummy, 2–8 weeks later. Other symptoms include aching bones and muscles, and fever.

Causes: Syphilis is caused by a small organism (similar to but not a bacteria) called a spirochaete passed during sex.

How it is Caught: Syphilis is transferred through an open wound or tear in the skin. Nowadays it is fairly rare for women in Britain to get it, but pregnant women are checked for it because of the potential danger it poses for the baby. Women with syphilis may miscarry.

Treatment: Syphilis is easy to treat – and cure completely – by penicillin injection.

Tests: Swabs from the sore and blood tests.

Treat Partner?: Needs treating with penicillin.

Long-term Effects: None if treated early. If left untreated it can have devastating effects on the brain twenty to thirty years later, causing dementia as well as damaging many other parts of the body.

chapter 8

contraception

Jane, 27, on the condom for women: I was aware of it but it didn't particularly interfere. The noise didn't bother me although there are a few little squeaks and things like that, but it's really out of earshot, isn't it?

Jenny, 23: *I've taken the morning-after pill ... I've taken it twice and neither time did I have any sort of bad reaction. I didn't have any qualms, I was more worried about getting pregnant. I didn't think to myself I am aborting a foetus. I was more scared of the possibility of actually becoming pregnant and just worrying that it wouldn't work, that I hadn't followed the instructions properly.*

Geraldine, 24, after her second abortion: *'I promise I won't come' must be the most unreliable method around. Don't believe it.*

Jean, on natural birth control: *I feel it has added to our relationship ... just because you can't have intercourse doesn't mean you can't make love ... it has enriched our relationship and it makes those days that I am infertile even more appreciated.*

Susan, 40: *I was a bit worried ... that the Norplant implant may hurt but I didn't feel a thing ... I'd tried all other forms of contraceptive and I've had bad side effects with them all and this seemed ideal.*

Contraception was revolutionized in the 1960s with the advent of the oral contraceptive pill. It gave women control over their fertility for the first time.

Ann, 50: *It was a great relief to go on the pill and forget about becoming pregnant. I was in my twenties when it became freely available and, to tell you the truth, I'm glad it wasn't around when I was in high school. The stigma of being an unwed mother was a powerful disincentive to have sex too early. If I had had access to the pill I'm sure I would have been quite promiscuous at a time when I was neither emotionally nor physically equipped for sex.*

The pill was a dramatic development, and it continues to be the most popular form of birth control for younger women. Although condoms have increased in popularity, over three million women in the UK use the contraceptive pill despite pill scares (see pages 199–202), because it is such an effective method. This may also be because many GPs do not offer an informed range of choices and prescribe the pill without discussing the options first. Over two-thirds of women see their GPs for contraceptive advice. Some women, especially those in their teens and twenties, prefer to go to family planning clinics because of the anonymity this gives them.

Women want contraception which is effective and without side effects and risks to their health. A survey by the Family Planning Association (FPA) in 1996 found women are critical

contraception

of some parts of the contraceptive service. Many women said there was insufficient discussion about choices of contraception. They want more information about the adverse effects and health risks of birth control. Unfortunately many clinics are closing because of financial constraints. Unplanned pregnancy is common, even with modern contraception methods. Over 170,000 abortions were performed in England and Wales in 1996. Sexually transmitted infections – a by-product of unprotected intercourse – are also on the increase (see pages 178–93).

In this chapter we look at the range of contraceptives available today. We report on their reliability, advantages and disadvantages, and cost. We also examine the sterilization option.

Contraception Fact File

- Under the age of forty, up to nine in ten women having regular sex without contraception will get pregnant within a year.
- You may ask any GP for contraceptive advice (you do *not* have to see your own) or visit a family planning clinic or Brook Advisory Clinic.
- Pills, coils, diaphragms, and spermicides are all free on the NHS.
- Condoms are free from family planning clinics and from some GPs and are easily available from chemists, supermarkets and petrol stations.
- Emergency contraceptive pills work even if you wait for up to seventy-two hours to start taking them after having unprotected intercourse. Having an emergency coil (see pages 213–14) inserted is effective even five days after intercourse. The Accident and Emergency Department of your local hospital will supply this or emergency contraceptive pills if you cannot make contact with your doctor or any other agency.
- Some GPs have done courses in family planning, so check if your doctor has. You are likely to get the best service at your local practice if there is a family-planning trained person.
- Many nurses working in general practice are family-planning trained and can give advice about contraception.
- If you want to see a woman doctor, always ask for one.
- If you are not satisfied with the service you get from your own GP, try a family-planning clinic where all the doctors and nurses will be family-planning trained.

Choosing the Best Method for You

There is no ideal method of contraception. There is a variety of methods to choose from, each with advantages and disadvantages. One method may suit you best at one stage of your life and another later on. The reliability of different contraceptive methods is calculated on how many pregnancies occur for each method if 100 women use it for a year.

Reliability of Contraceptive Methods

Methods That Have No 'User' Failure

Injectable contraception implant
over 99% effective in first year (over 98% per year over five years)

Intrauterine system (IUS)
over 99% effective

Intrauterine device (IUD)
98- over 99% effective (depending on IUD type)

Female sterilization
over 99% effective
failure rate 1–5 per 1000 depending on the method used

Male sterilization
over 99% effective
failure rate about 1 per 1000

Methods That Have 'User' Failure

Combined oral contraceptive *over 99% effective*

Progestogen-only oral contraceptive *up to 99% effective*

Male condom *up to 98% effective*

Female condom *up to 95% effective*

Diaphragm or cap + spermicide *up to 96% effective*

Natural family planning:

Rhythm method *up to 98% effective*

New technologies (Persona) *up to 94% effective*

(Reliability rates of methods with 'user' failure reflect success when used absolutely correctly and consistently. Where methods are used incorrectly, they will be less reliable.)

Reproduced with kind permission of the Family Planning Association.

Remember that 95 per cent reliability in a particular contraceptive means that five times out of 100 the method will fail or, put another way, one in seventeen women using the method for a year will get pregnant.

Which method you choose depends on:

- How old you are.
- What sort of relationship you are in.
- Whether you find one method rather than another interferes with sexual activity.
- How terrible it would be if contraception failed and you were to become pregnant.
- Your partner's attitude to contraception.
- Whether you have any medical problems that might prevent you using certain types of contraception.
- Whether you want to have any – or any more – children.
- How often you have sex.
- Whether you have sex with one partner or more than one.
- The current fashion in contraception.

Occasional Sex

Use condoms for occasional love-making and to avoid sexually transmitted infections, or combine the pill and the condom to stay safe. A condom is reliable against STIs if you always use one.

Regular Sex with a Regular Partner

There is less risk of picking up a sexually transmitted infection if you have only one partner, as long as you are his only partner, so the pill may be a good option as it allows for spontaneity. But consider the other methods too, particularly if you are a smoker. Barrier methods, including the diaphragm (see pages 205–6) are also a good method over the long term.

After Having a Baby

Exclusively breast-feeding your baby, especially on demand, makes pregnancy unlikely in the first six months after delivery since breast-feeding stops ovulation. However, once you go over to bottle feeding (partially or totally) and add solids to your baby's diet you will not be breast-feeding regularly enough to ensure that you do not ovulate, increasing the chance of conception. A barrier method or the progestogen-only pill (see pages 201–2) are good options. Progestogen injections can also be used. Although a small amount of the progestogen hormone is excreted in a mother's milk there is no evidence that it harms the baby in any way. The combined oral contraceptive pill may decrease your production of breast milk. An IUD (see pages 208–9) can be used after six weeks. If you do not breast-feed, ovulation can occur as early as twenty-eight days after delivery and just ten days after a miscarriage or an abortion.

Older Women

Choices become even more difficult for older women who have had their children and who want a break from the pill because of risks associated with staying on it for a long time, and risks linked to their age. You might consider an intrauterine device (IUD), an intrauterine system (IUS), a diaphragm, or sterilization (see pages 211–13). Over 50 per cent of couples where the woman is over the age of forty-five choose sterilization of one or other partner.

> **Tess, 45:** *I was worried about being on the pill for such a long time – but when it came to my daughters – I just told them they ought to be on it. I wasn't into being a grandmother yet!*

When to Stop Using Birth Control

There is no reliable test to indicate the end of fertility. The FSH (follicular stimulating hormone) blood test (see page 42) will give some indication but it is not absolute. Experts recommend waiting for two years after your last period if you are under fifty and one year if you are over fifty at the time of your last period.

The Methods

The Pill (Combined Oral Contraceptive)

How it Works

'The pill' usually refers to the combined oral contraceptive pill. It combines two hormones, oestrogen and progestogen, in varying proportions depending on which brand you take. It works by stopping ovulation (see page 30) each month.

The pill has to be prescribed by a doctor, although you can also see a specially trained family planning nurse. Your medical history and blood pressure should be checked before starting the pill to make sure there is no reason for you not to take it. Make sure you understand exactly how to take the brand you are given. The main problem with being on the pill is remembering to take it, but with the combined pill you do have a bit of leeway. Taking it as part of your morning ritual – when you clean your teeth for instance – should help if you find remembering difficult. You do have twelve hours to remember before needing to use condoms as a back-up and follow the seven-day rule: take the forgotten pill as soon as you remember, use condoms for seven days and, if there are fewer than seven pills left in the packet, start the next packet straight away, without having the usual break for your 'period'. When you need further supplies, every 3–6 months, your blood pressure should be checked again to make sure that it has not gone up. Again this can be done by a doctor or a family-planning nurse.

Advantages

This is the most commonly used method of contraception by young women because it is almost 100 per cent reliable in preventing pregnancy. It does not interfere with sex and it is not messy. An added bonus is that it regulates your periods, they are usually lighter and it often relieves painful periods and PMS. The risk of cancer of the uterus and ovaries is also reduced.

> **Joan, 34:** *I started on the pill as a cure for period pain so the two are linked for me ... It also meant I was the only woman I knew who didn't hide the packets from my mother! However, I still recall hiding my packet from boyfriends because I felt it left me no convenient excuse not to sleep with them.*

Disadvantages

> **Kate, 45:** *I worry about the side effects of the pill – it's not natural, all those hormones, but I really want my daughter to use it as it would be disastrous if she got pregnant now.*

For all the pill's reliability, many women have reservations about taking it. Scientific research into the pill is much publicized, especially when the results are worrying. This sends a shock wave through the community. The facts you need know are these:

STIs The pill offers no protection against sexually transmitted infections (STIs). To protect against STIs you or your partner need to use a condom with or instead of the pill.

'Minor' Side Effects The pill can cause some side effects. Doctors call them minor because they are not life-threatening. They may not seem minor to you, though. They include depression, headaches, nausea, light bleeding between periods, weight gain, tender breasts and loss of sex drive. Most side effects settle down within three months of starting the pill. They also go away when you stop taking the pill without causing any long-term damage. If the side effects do not settle down after three months and you want to continue on the pill you should ask to try an alternative brand which may better suit you.

Thromboses, Heart Attacks and Strokes You do have a greater chance of having one of these if you are on the pill, but it is still very, very rare. In 100,000 healthy women not on the pill, about five will get a venous thrombosis (a blood clot in a vein). If the same number of women were on the pill, fifteen to thirty of them would experience thrombosis – depending on the type of progestogen in the pill. Out of 100,000 pregnant women (obviously, not on the pill) the figure is nearer sixty. Newer pills such as marvelon, femodene and mercilon are thought to have a higher risk than the older pills such as microgynon and ovranette. This is related to the different type of progestogen content. However, some women develop other side effects with the older pills like breakthrough bleeding or nausea so they prefer the newer ones. There is also some evidence to suggest that the latest pills with the newer progestogens may produce fewer heart attacks as a side effect since they do not have such a harmful effect on the blood fats. There is still much to learn about which brand of pill is safest overall and which brand is best for each individual woman.

Venous thrombosis can usually be successfully treated and only a very small number of women die from it. There is now a blood test available which can help identify women who are at increased risk. If there is a history of blood clots in your family you might be at greater risk so do ask your doctor for the test. Clots can also block your arteries, for example in your heart when it causes a heart attack, or in your brain when it causes a stroke. The best way to prevent this is not to smoke. Smokers who are on the pill may increase their risk of an arterial blood clot by up to eleven times that of women not on the pill. The newer pills may be better for your arteries.

Cancer There is a small increased risk of developing breast cancer and cervical cancer if you are on the pill. The risk for young women appears to be very small and there does not appear to be any difference between the brands of pill. If you do develop breast cancer while on the pill, it seems that it is less likely to spread than in women not on the pill. The link with cervical cancer is less certain, although some studies show you are twice as likely to develop cervical cancer if you have been on the pill for ten years than women not on the pill. The risk is still small as cervical cancer is relatively uncommon. If you have regular cervical screening, any abnormality should be able to be checked and treated before it ever develops into a cancer (see pages 374–9).

Some women should definitely not use the combined oral contraceptive pill, including women with high blood pressure, a history of severe migraine, heart disease, liver disease and breast cancer. It is not a good method for women who are breast-feeding as it can decrease the milk supply.

Progestogen-only Pill (POP)

How it Works
The POP is also known as the mini-pill. It contains just one hormone, a progestogen, and, like all birth control pills, needs to be prescribed by a doctor. It works by changing the

mucus around the entrance to the uterus so that the sperm finds it more difficult to get in. The POP also alters the lining of the uterus so that if the sperm does get through the mucus to fertilize the egg, implantation in the uterus is unlikely to occur.

Advantages

POP is a good alternative to the combined pill if you are getting side effects or if there are medical reasons for not taking it. So far, research shows the POP is safe to take while you are breast-feeding. It has not been linked to heart disease or breast cancer.

Disadvantages

It is not quite as effective at preventing pregnancy as the combined oral contraceptive pill – one in 100 women on it for a year get pregnant with careful use, and four in 100 with less careful use. For maximum effectiveness this pill must be taken at the same time every day with only two hours leeway. A watch with an alarm might help here. It can cause irregular periods with some bleeding in between and some missed which can be a nuisance. It may also make your skin more greasy and spotty.

> **Sue, 35:** *I really liked the [combined] pill but ... my blood pressure went up and they said I had to come off it. I tried several other pills but they all caused trouble. In the end they put me on the progestogen-only pill and that suited me, but remembering to take it the same time every day was a real pain. Finally I put it next to the toothpaste and that seemed to help me remember.*

Condoms

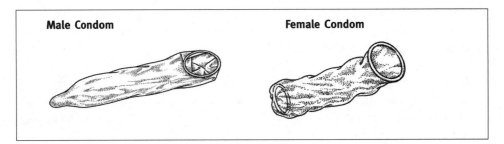

Male Condom   **Female Condom**

How They Work

Condoms are made of thin rubber and fit snugly over the man's erect penis. They work as a barrier to stop the sperm getting into the woman's vagina.

Advantages

Condoms protect you against pregnancy, with up to 98 per cent reliability when used properly and used every time. They also provide effective protection against sexually transmitted infections and diseases, including Aids and cancer of the cervix. Although cancer is not an STI, some STI viruses are linked with cervical cancer (see page 377).

Condoms are very convenient for last-minute, unplanned sex because they can be bought everywhere from garages to supermarkets and men's loos. You do not need a prescription, although you can get them free from family planning clinics and some GPs. They come in different colours, shapes (flared, contoured, ribbed and so on), flavours, sizes and strengths – a stronger one should be used for anal sex.

It can be fun to help a man put on a condom – although plenty of men are adept at getting them on by themselves and quickly – and need not be seen as a scientific procedure. All you need is an erect penis. The condom is placed over the head of the penis and gently unrolled down the shaft to the base of the penis. They are made of remarkably stretchy material and they should fit snugly on any size of penis, large or small.

Disadvantages

Condoms have an image problem, although less so now than in the past. Many people shun them, believing they are unreliable or inconvenient, and many men feel they reduce sensitivity.

> **Rita:** *Not being in a long-term relationship, condoms have to be the main contraception as nothing else gives me the same protection against the dreaded diseases. I'd be happier with condoms if it weren't such a struggle to convince the men. It is not the putting on of a condom that spoils the spontaneity of sex so much as the persuading of recalcitrant males to employ it.*

Some men say they prefer not to use a condom because, as thin as the material is, it is still between him and you, interfering with the sensation. There is probably a psychological element to this too. You want to be close and a condom is between you. Do not feel intimidated by a man's reluctance though. You should not feel bad about insisting that he wears one if you want him to. Many men, however, do not mind at all.

Some couples feel uncomfortable and get an irritation from the condom itself. Condoms are made from latex (rubber) and more recently silicone condoms are available. Most of the latex varieties are now made from low-allergy latex so allergies are less of a problem. If you do find one brand makes you feel itchy and uncomfortable, try another or one without a spermicide. There are lots to choose from.

contraception

There are some creams and pessaries that should not be used with condoms. Vegetable- and mineral-based lubricants like baby oil or vaseline can damage rubber and destroy 95 per cent of the condom's strength in just fifteen minutes, so if you are using a lubricant, make sure it is a water-based one such as KY jelly. All spermicides and Canesten, the commonest anti-thrush treatment, are fine but other treatments for thrush can cause damage.

Although condoms can expand 600 per cent they do sometimes split, usually in the putting on stage and often by a fingernail getting caught in them. They pollute, too, so do not flush them down the toilet. They float and there are already enough of them in the North Sea.

Female Condom

How it Works
The female condom is a thin polyurethane sheath. The material is very soft and comfortable. At the closed end of the sheath there is a small flexible ring, also made of polyurethane which is one and a half times the size of a fifty-pence piece. This is bent in and inserted rather like you would insert a tampon without an applicator. There is a larger soft outer ring that lies external to the body once the condom is inserted.

> **Marjorie, 35:** *Of course I had to show it to everybody in the office ... everybody's reaction was 'Ugh, it looks awful, it's so big, it's like a plastic bag, it's sticky' and of course there was this terrible giggly negativeness towards it ... OK, it doesn't look brilliant when you see it but ... it might be absolutely perfect for you and then it's a fantastic form of contraception as I know I'm protected against STIs and he doesn't lose it when he gets an erection like with the condom which he seems to have a problem with.*

Advantages
The female condom does not require fitting by a doctor or nurse and is available in chemists and supermarkets as well as some family-planning clinics. It is probably about as effective as the condom for men. Studies have shown that the polyurethane sheath provides a very effective barrier to all kinds of organisms including HIV (see pages 188–90) and some other viruses that are responsible for sexually transmitted infections like the herpes virus (see pages 183–5) for example. It is a barrier contraception and has to be used properly in order to be effective. It can be inserted a few hours before intercourse and it should be removed soon afterwards. It is particularly useful for women who are allergic to the spermicide or the latex of the male condom, since the female condom is made of very low-

irritant and low-allergenic material and the lubricant used is non-spermicidal. Older women around the time of the menopause may find it helps with lubrication if they have problems with dryness (see Chapter 3).

Disadvantages

It is expensive with a cost of about £4.50 for a pack of three. No large-number studies have been carried out to examine the effectiveness of the female condom. It has been difficult to find enough women to take part.

The Cap or Diaphragm

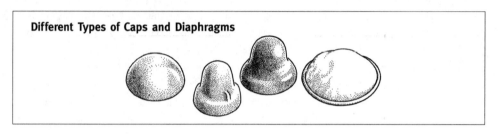

Different Types of Caps and Diaphragms

How They Work

There are various types of diaphragms and caps. They are made of rubber and come in different shapes and sizes. They all work by acting as a sperm barrier at the entrance of the womb. Vaginal diaphragms are circular domes which keep their shape because there is a pliable metal ring covered in rubber around the edge. Cervical caps are smaller and thicker and fit neatly over the cervix. These devices go inside your vagina, covering the area around your cervix, at the opening of your uterus. They are quite easily put in place once you have practised. Most women have no problem putting the diaphragm in. It is a bit like inserting a tampon. Usually you do not need an applicator but some women find it easier to use one. The diaphragm is stretched over the end of the applicator and just pops into place quite naturally once you learn how to insert it. You need to learn how to feel for your cervix to check that the diaphragm or cap is in the right place and is actually covering the cervix. Your doctor or nurse will show you. You know when the cervical cap is in the right place because it sort of snaps around the cervix with a fairly tight but not at all uncomfortable feeling. It is as if suction is holding it in place. If you feel too embarrassed to accept help in inserting it, try it at home alone but you do need to get over any fear of touching yourself. You will soon get the idea – and be reassured that the device is in the right place.

Both caps and diaphragms should be used with spermicide. This is a gel which comes in a tube and is squeezed around the rim of the device. It also helps make the insertion of the cap or diaphragm even easier.

Advantages

You do not need to stop in the middle of love-making to insert your cap. It can be put in place well ahead of time, up to three hours in advance – unlike the male condom. You can increase the advance time by adding more spermicide just before sex. The cap is easy to learn to use. Another plus is that it is 'natural'. It gives control to the woman and it also offers some, but not 100 per cent, protection against sexually transmitted infections, including the virus STIs which can, albeit rarely, lead to cervical cancer.

Disadvantages

You need to see a doctor or nurse to be fitted but this should be a good chance to talk about any other contraceptive options you may not have discussed before. You also need to get it checked every year and after having a baby as your size may change. You may also need a different size if you lose or put on more than 8 lb in weight. Some forward planning is needed as you have to insert it before intercourse and leave it in for at least six hours afterwards. It is a little messy since you need to use spermicide with it for extra contraceptive protection. Some women have trouble with cystitis (see pages 192–3) when they use the vaginal diaphragm. It is not as reliable as the pill. For every 100 women who use it carefully for a year four may get pregnant. It seems to have a higher failure rate when you first start using it and in younger women.

> **Sylvia, 48:** *I used the cap. I had no problems with poking around inside me – but it didn't exactly make for spontaneity. "Scuse me, could you just stay in that position while I pop to the bathroom?"*

Spermicides

How They Work

Spermicides are chemicals which come in cream, jelly, foam or pessary form. They operate by killing sperm. Spermicide on its own is not a reliable method of contraception although it is better than using nothing. Spermicides should be used with all barrier methods, although most condoms come pre-treated with spermicide.

Advantages

They are available without prescription and when used in conjunction with a condom or cap are effective 96–98 per cent of the time. They are more reliable in older women in their forties who are less fertile. For example, a woman of forty-five who uses no contraception for a year, has a 10–20 per cent risk of getting pregnant, compared to an 80–90 per cent risk in a woman younger than forty. They also add some lubrication which may be helpful to older women experiencing dryness.

Disadvantages

They are less effective in young women, simply because they are more fertile than older women. They are messy, sometimes sticky, and can be unpleasant tasting so they interfere with oral sex. It is rare to be truly allergic to spermicides but quite common to get some irritation. If this is so, try a different brand which, though it will usually contain the same spermicide, may be made up in a different way and have a different acidity, so hopefully will be less of an irritant.

Natural Methods (Rhythm or Safe Period)

How it Works

A woman ovulates fourteen to sixteen days prior to the first day of her next period, her temperature goes up slightly and her vaginal mucus changes in character at ovulation. By taking your temperature and testing your vaginal mucus, and charting the timing of your periods over several months, you can learn which times are most risky to have intercourse. For training in natural family planning, contact the Family Planning Association (see Useful Addresses on page 390).

> **Jean:** *My husband didn't want to use a condom and so for us it was that freedom of intercourse and the sensitivity and no side effects on either side ... if you think of it as learning to drive a car we put that time and effort into a skill that we'll have for the rest of our lives.*

Advantages

For Roman Catholics, natural family planning is the only method of birth control permitted by the Pope but it is also gaining currency in medical circles. The *British Medical Journal* recently compared it with barrier and chemical methods and concluded that if you do it properly and are highly motivated, it can be reliable with only two failures per 100 women. With less expertise the failure rate can be as high as twenty. You learn an enormous amount about your own body since you need to monitor it closely. You will become much more familiar with when your period is due because you will be very in tune with your body's changes such as breast tenderness and premenstrual syndrome (PMS: see pages 45–51). There are no side effects.

There are a variety of test kits available to help you monitor your hormone levels and therefore your ovulation days. You may find they help make practising natural birth control a little easier. They are available without prescription from chemists. A start-up kit may cost you around £50. The makers of these kits claim they are 93 to 95 per cent reliable, but this is no guarantee against pregnancy.

Disadvantages

You need dedication. The method relies on regular checks and monitoring of your body, following your vaginal secretions, and taking note of your body temperature. It is very difficult if you do not have regular periods even if you use a test kit. It restricts the times when you can have sex. But it can be used in combination with other methods like the condom. This method offers no protection against STIs.

The Intrauterine Device (IUD) and Intrauterine System (IUS)

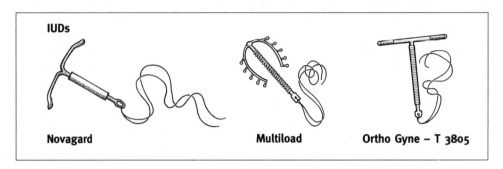

IUDs

Novagard   Multiload   Ortho Gyne – T 3805

How They Work

These are small devices inserted into your uterus through your vagina. They are usually T-shaped. The IUD, or 'the coil', is made of plastic and copper. It prevents pregnancy in several ways. It interferes with the egg and sperm getting together and stops any eggs that do get fertilized from settling in your womb. No one knows exactly how or why this happens. It can also be used for emergency contraception (see pages 213–14). Gynefix is a new type of IUD made of six small copper beads threaded on to a length of nylon. A tiny knot in the thread helps fix it into the top of the womb. It works like other IUDs, lasts for five years after insertion and has a failure rate of 1 per cent.

The IUS is another type of intrauterine device which gives off a progestogen hormone. This changes the mucus around the cervix making it more difficult for sperm to swim through the cervix into the uterus. If the sperm do get there it hampers their swim toward the eggs. It also makes the lining of the womb (the endometrium) thinner so that any eggs that do get fertilized cannot start to grow. The IUS is not good for emergency contraception.

IUDs and IUSs are both available on the NHS. Both have to be fitted by a doctor who has been especially trained to fit coils. IUDs are most commonly used, especially in younger women. The IUS is more often used in older women, especially if heavy periods are a problem – it tends to make periods lighter, shorter and they may even stop altogether. However, for the first few months after the coil is inserted, many women get a little bleeding or spotting of blood every day or every few days. The IUS coil is a little bit thicker so it can be more difficult to insert. It is more expensive so some doctors may be reluctant to prescribe it on the NHS.

Advantages
The good thing about these methods is that once the device is in you do not have to worry about contraception again until it needs changing, every three to five years depending on which type you use. Both types are fairly reliable with a failure rate of about one or two in 100. Another advantage is that fertility returns immediately after the device is removed.

Disadvantages
IUDs and IUSs are not usually recommended for young women who have not had children, or women at risk of contracting a sexually transmitted infection, as they increase the possibility of infection in the fallopian tubes. This may affect future chances of getting pregnant. It is a good idea to have a swab to check for chlamydia infection (see pages 186–7) before having a device inserted. The IUD tends to make your periods heavier and more painful. Both insertion and removal, especially the latter, can be painful. Both devices may cause a bit of bleeding between periods, but this is especially problematic with the IUS where light bleeding may go on for several months (see above). If you do get pregnant with an IUD in place, which happens rarely, it is more likely to be an ectopic (in the fallopian tube) pregnancy (see page 294).

Hormone Implants

How They Work
Contraceptive hormone implants (such as Norplant) consist of soft, small rods filled with progestogen under the skin. The rods are about two inches long. They contain a white powder encased in a soft covering which allows gradual release of the hormone over five years. The rods are put in a fan shape on the inner side of the arm. They are inserted (and removed) under local anaesthetic by a specially trained doctor. Sometimes removal can be difficult. They usually cannot be seen but you can feel them. There is initial bruising but it should not hurt. At first, the amounts of progestogen released are the same as two mini-pills. After a year to eighteen months the amount is reduced to about the same per day as the progestogen-only pill. The implants are available on the NHS.

Advantages
There are no fluctuations of hormone during the day so it is very effective. It is one of the most effective forms of contraception. From the studies done in the US, fewer than one in 200 women will get pregnant each year using this form of contraception. Within the first

couple of days after removal, the normal fertility rate will return. The rods can be removed at any time.

Disadvantages
Between 50 per cent and 60 per cent of women who use Norplant will get some irregular cycles initially. This can be occasional spotting or missed periods or you might have a brownish loss for ten to twelve days each month. Other reported side effects are very similar to the progestogen-only pill – slightly greasier skin, more spots, some breast tenderness and an increase in appetite. There is no protection against sexually transmitted infections.

Hormone Injections

How They Work
The hormone progestogen is injected into your arm or bottom. Over two to three months it very slowly and steadily releases small amounts into your bloodstream, stopping ovulation. The injections are available on the NHS and can be given at a GP's surgery or family-planning clinic by a doctor or nurse.

Advantages
An injection lasts for about two or three months, depending on the type of progestogen, and you do not need to think about contraception for that time. It might also protect you from uterine cancer as it makes the lining of the uterus thinner and less active. Similar hormones are used in the treatment of this cancer.

Disadvantages
If you suffer from negative side effects you have to wait it out – the injection cannot be removed. Periods often become irregular or stop and some women gain weight. When you stop having the injections, regular periods and fertility can return immediately or they may not return for up to a year. Injections offer no protection against sexually transmitted infections.

Withdrawal (Coitus Interruptus)

How it Works
This method involves the man withdrawing his penis from inside the vagina before he ejaculates. This is probably used more often than people admit. Couples probably do not plan to use it as a regular method, but do so when they do not have a condom handy or just get carried away.

Advantages

It is free. It may work if he is well controlled at doing this, but even so there is sometimes a leak of seminal fluid (come) before his orgasm actually happens. But it is certainly better than not using any method at all.

Disadvantages

It offers no protection against STIs. It can cause anxiety and frustration for both partners. It is a risky business and a dangerous method to use if you really do not want to get pregnant.

Female Sterilization (Tubal Ligation)

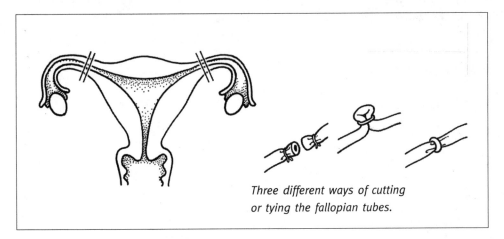

Three different ways of cutting or tying the fallopian tubes.

How it Works

The fallopian tubes are cut or blocked so that eggs cannot travel from the ovary to meet up with the sperm (for a full description of the operation see page 358). The eggs go down the tube and, as they are not fertilized, they just disintegrate and get absorbed.

Advantages

It is permanent in all but one to five out of 1000 women who have the operation. It is more likely to fail if carried out immediately after childbirth or termination of pregnancy, or on a younger woman. The reliability of this method means peace of mind for a woman who is certain she never wants to become pregnant again. It also means an end to all the caps and pills, rhythm method and withdrawal. And, unless STIs are a worry, it means the end for the condom too. You can get it free on the NHS, although how long you have to wait varies according to where you live.

Karen: *I just knew I didn't want any more children whatever happened. It made me feel a bit worried that he might go off and have some more children with a younger woman but I knew I'd done the pregnancy thing. It did make my periods heavier as I'd been on the pill for years but it was great not to worry about side effects or remembering to take it.*

Disadvantages

Since it is permanent you should only have it done if you are certain you do not want to have children in the future. The procedure usually involves a general anaesthetic but can be done under a local anaesthetic in some units. It is not as simple as a vasectomy (see below). You may need to stay overnight in hospital. As in vasectomy, reversal is expensive and not guaranteed. Undoing a tubal ligation costs upwards from £3500 which includes three nights in hospital. According to the Surgical Advisory Service there is a 40 per cent success rate for reversal. The success rate is lower the longer you wait after having your tubes tied in the first place. It does not protect against STIs.

Male Sterilization (Vasectomy)

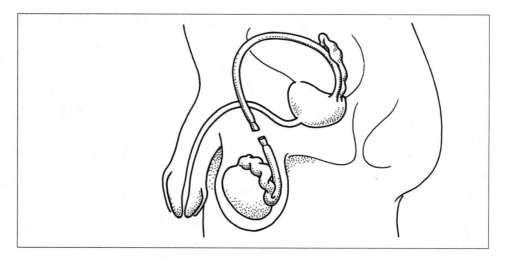

How it Works

The tubes carrying the sperm are cut so that when the man ejaculates there are no sperm present in his semen. Sperm are made in the testes which are in the scrotum. During sex and ejaculation sperm are swept to the penis via small tubes called the *vasa deferentia*. When a man is sterilized these tubes are cut and a small length of tube removed so that when he ejaculates there is semen but no sperm.

> **Liz, 40:** *He took a bit of persuading ... Although he wouldn't admit it, I think he thought he would become impotent, which he certainly didn't! Having reached forty I was fed up with being on the pill, and even if something had happened to one of the kids, we didn't want another pregnancy thank you. I'd been the one looking after contraception up to now and now it was his turn. I didn't see why I should have to go through the sterilization operation as well.*

Advantages

The operation only takes about fifteen minutes and it is done under local anaesthetic. There may be a bit of bruising and some discomfort for a short time after the operation, but this is minor. This procedure is about as close as he can get to a guarantee that he will not make a woman pregnant. The failure rate is less than one in 2000 and happens because the tubes rejoin. You can have sex without worrying about pregnancy.

Disadvantages

The availability of vasectomies on the NHS depends on where you live. Vasectomies are usually done privately and cost about £250. Your doctor will tell you who does it locally.

A man cannot have a vasectomy one day and depend on it as contraception the next. It can be three months or longer after the operation before all the sperm have disappeared. He must have two semen specimens checked before he can rely on it for contraception. A vasectomy does not offer protection against STIs. There have been anxieties about possible long-term side effects such as increased risk of heart disease, testicular and prostate cancer. Recent studies have found no evidence to support this.

Undoing a vasectomy costs about £2500 which includes a one-day stay in hospital. Successful reversal is not guaranteed. The Surgical Advisory Service in London told us the success rate is 80 per cent.

Emergency Contraception

How it Works

There are two usual methods – a pill or an IUD. With the first method, you take four pills, two to start with, and two after twelve hours. They are taken by mouth and contain oestrogen and progestogen at higher doses than the ordinary contraceptive pill. They work by stopping implantation of the fertilized egg. Alternatively you can have an intrauterine device put in. This also works by stopping implantation of the fertilized egg. Another alternative for women who cannot take oestrogen is a progestogen-only pill.

contraception

An estimated 100,000 abortions in the UK could be avoided each year if everyone who was at risk, because of split condoms or because they got 'carried away', used emergency contraception.

Advantages

This method is often misleadingly called the morning-after pill. In fact, following unprotected intercourse, you have three days to start taking the pill and five days for the IUD method, within which time these methods will effectively prevent pregnancy. It is a myth that you can only use the emergency pill method once in your life. You can take it many times and even, if necessary, more than once in a month. But if this is happening to you, you are avoiding dealing with the need for reliable contraception. With the IUD method, you can leave it in and then you have proper contraception in place.

Although you cannot yet buy emergency contraception pills over the counter in the UK, they are available from quite a few different places. You can get emergency contraception from any GP (not just your own), a family planning clinic or Accident and Emergency Department at any hospital, and it is free. It is highly effective – 96 per cent for the pills and virtually 100 per cent for the IUD.

Disadvantages

About 50 per cent of women taking emergency contraception pills feel nauseated and roughly 10 per cent will actually vomit, but taking an anti-travel sickness tablet can help stop this. If you vomit you should take two more pills to replace the two you have lost. You may be given two extra pills just in case – otherwise you need to get back to the doctor. The IUD has to be inserted by a specially trained doctor.

The Future

Major advances in contraception have been made, but many of us still feel there is a long way to go before we can truly relax and rely on our chosen device.

one in three: abortion

Francesca, 42: I want a child so desperately now, I think how could I have had something so precious growing inside of me and have destroyed it consciously, but at the time . . . I knew I could neither support the child myself nor bring it up properly.

One in three women in Britain will have an abortion.

> **Ella, 22:** *I found out that I was pregnant in my first year of university, aged nineteen. For some reason I didn't really think I could be pregnant. I was convinced that the reason why I was feeling so nauseous early in the morning was a recurrence of a bug I'd had in Nepal ... to anyone else it seemed blindingly obvious what was wrong ... after I'd recovered from the shock I knew exactly what I had to do.*
>
> **Celia, 41:** *I was waiting for some emotion to hit me and it hasn't yet. Maybe it never will. I had a momentary sort of slight wobble when I saw, in the room of the doctor who was going to do it, a board with pictures of babies he'd delivered, but not one bit of me could imagine thinking that could be me. All I could think was this is very sad ... but the relief ... was just enormous.*

The vast majority of women who have abortions do not regret their decision, difficult as it can sometimes feel to choose to go through with one.

In England and Wales in 1996, 177,495 abortions were performed, showing an increase of 13,857 over the previous year. The jump (in 1995 abortions were down over 1994) is blamed on a contraceptive pill scare. Late in 1995 thousands of women hastily went off the pill upon hearing reports that it was a serious health hazard. The result was thousands of unwanted pregnancies. (We address the pill scare on pages 200–1.)

It is impossible to calculate the number of unwanted pregnancies and how many of these pregnancies are actually followed through to delivery. In one study, over 25 per cent of women in their third pregnancy and almost 40 per cent of women in their fourth, said they regretted their pregnancy. But having regrets does not necessarily mean a child will be unwanted or unloved once it is born.

Abortion was legalized in Britain in 1967 with the introduction of the Abortion Act. Until that time it had been illegal except when a woman's life was in danger. Abortion law had begun to liberalize a little in 1938 when a judge decided that there could be a legal termination of a pregnancy not only to save a woman's life but also if her doctor believed continuing with the pregnancy would turn her into 'a physical or mental wreck'. In the intervening years women who could afford to pay did manage to get safe abortions for other reasons, while women without means often suffered terrible infections and loss of fertility from unsafe abortions, and some even died after having a backstreet abortion.

one in three: abortion

May, 71: *There'd been one or two that tried it and died ... She was the same age as me, Mary would be. She was my friend in school with me. She had that and she died. Oh it was a dreadful thing.*

Rose, 56: *I was young. It was very difficult to get at the time. It was somebody I knew did it. Gosh, this is bringing back awful memories. Years ago someone always knew somebody who would do that sort of thing. I went to her house several times. She used soapy water and they just actually pump it up inside you. And I can remember I went several times ... but the baby didn't abort ... I was having terrible clots, and I was thinking ... it was gone ... I had the most dreadful pains. It worked in the end and I passed a tiny little foetus.*

A decade later, women like Rose would be spared her horror. On 27 October 1967, Britain passed the Abortion Act. Joyce had her abortion in November after the act was passed but before the law came into effect.

Joyce, 50: *It was just very undercover. It was like a covert operation. Everything was done in whispers and I just went along with it ... it's kind of frightening you know, being there and having it done, the whole shebang ... I went to a clinic at the top of Harley Street ... there was this guy with some kind of Polish-sounding name ... and there was another guy there as well and he held my hand ... and the guy performed the abortion. I couldn't have been more than ten weeks pregnant ... and my husband, well my boyfriend at the time, was waiting outside and we came out and went straight to the cinema ... We saw* Thoroughly Modern Millie, *can you believe it?*

Over 90 per cent of abortions now are performed on the grounds that the risk of injury to the physical or mental health of the woman is greater if she continues the pregnancy than if she had the pregnancy terminated. Having an abortion and having a baby are both safe today, but, in statistical terms, an abortion is slightly safer than continuing with a pregnancy. Ninety per cent of abortions are carried out early, in the first twelve weeks of the pregnancy. Many of these could be done even earlier if there were no delays in the system. Some hospitals do not have sufficient resources, creating further delays of two or three weeks before the operation can be done. Women also sometimes delay before seeking an abortion because they need time to consider whether this is what they really want. Many abortions could be avoided altogether if more women considered using emergency contraception after having unprotected sex (see pages 213–4).

218

In later abortions, the risk of abortion may become greater than carrying through with a pregnancy. But there are still occasions when women choose to have an abortion after the twelve-week period. Three per cent of abortions are carried out after sixteen weeks. Many of these are because a foetal abnormality is detected in antenatal screening, or because the pregnant women is very young, mentally ill or mentally disabled. In these cases the woman often does not realize she is pregnant until late in the pregnancy.

- Fewer than one in 100 of all abortions is carried out because of a risk to a woman's life.
- One in 100 of all abortions is carried out because of a risk of the baby being born seriously handicapped.
- Just over two in 100 of all abortions are done to prevent serious harm to a woman's physical or mental health.

The Unwanted Pregnancy

Even though your period is late it does not mean you are pregnant, but it is important to check out whether you are or not right away. You can buy a do-it-yourself pregnancy test from any chemist for under £10. They are the same tests used by doctors. You can use it within two days of the expected beginning of your missed period. If you do not know when your period is due, and think you might be pregnant, try the test anyway. If the result is negative, repeat it one week later just to be sure. The tests are usually reliable but sometimes they give a false negative which means it says you are not pregnant when you are. If you want to double-check try the test again in a few days. If you are still worried, or if you miss another period, you can also see your GP or visit a family-planning clinic to have a pregnancy test without paying a fee.

Some anti-abortion organizations offer free pregnancy testing and what they call non-judgemental counselling, but they obviously will have some bias towards adoption or you keeping the baby yourself if you are pregnant. If this is, in fact, what you feel you would do, they can be helpful by offering material support as well.

There are various other agencies which will help you too. Start by asking your GP for a referral. Talk, too, to your family and friends. Ask for their support. You may well get it and find that this helps you to make the best decisions for you and the baby.

Adoption of the baby was standard procedure for countless girls who got pregnant before abortion was legalized. But while adoption may still seem to be the best choice for some women, twenty or thirty years later one may regret the decision.

Patsy, 45: *I was seventeen at the time … and I felt like my heart had been ripped out. There is still a big tear in it today. I remember having to sign papers … I remember kissing her goodbye with a lump in my throat the size of a golf ball. But I couldn't hold back the tears. When I left I turned at the door to look at her one more time and the tears started to flow … She was born on Valentine's Day. That's a hard day for me … I want and need to find her. I need to know she's well and happy. Or even if she isn't. I need to see her, to touch her, to hold her, to talk and talk. To apologize for giving her away … to tell her I've never stopped loving her. I need to heal and I don't know if I ever will. I would love for her to know her full brother and two half-sisters … I feel so helpless when I think that I possibly will live out my lifespan on this planet and never have known her … Looking back, was it the right thing? Yes and no. Yes it was right that she went to a mature couple whom I know wanted a baby so much it hurt. There is no doubt in my mind that they loved her as their very own and still do. I don't know if I could have provided her with what every child deserves. I'll never know now. But no it wasn't the right thing either. To sever all ties, blood ties. It is wrong.*

Most women who get pregnant by mistake and do not want to have a child, choose abortion over adoption. The choice you make may depend on your personal morality, your religion, the stage of your pregnancy, the nature of the relationship with your partner, your age, your financial situation, and your family's attitude, if you decide to tell your family at all. In coming to a decision, it may be helpful to think about:

• Why the pregnancy is unwanted.
• What your feelings were when you first knew you were pregnant.
• What is the worst aspect of your present situation.
• Is there a positive side to the present situation.
• Is this a crisis out of the blue or is it linked to other problems.

If you have a friend to talk to, see if this framework of questions helps in decision-making as you talk them through. Once you have decided what to do, reflect on why you became pregnant and how you can prevent a future unwanted pregnancy.

Ella, 22: *A terrible image of myself, heavily pregnant struggling to get to the next lecture, flashed across my mind, and I definitely wasn't ready for it. The actual abortion was not as traumatic as I thought it might be – just uncomfortable. It also made me feel embarrassed about being there in the first place … contraception was explained to me, several times, much to my chagrin.*

one in three: abortion

When you cannot decide what to do, go for counselling. If you feel comfortable with your GP, start there. The aims of pregnancy counselling are to help you reach an informed decision that you will not regret, to reduce the risk of depression and to help sort out emotional problems once your decision is made. Whatever you do, do not delay the talking it through process. See also page 390 for the details of organizations which will offer help.

> **Sandra, 42:** *I got pregnant a month or less after [my first abortion] ... I was using a diaphragm ... I was irritated at myself and at my body and I was also a little humiliated. I was going back to the same clinic and I thought they're going to look at me with such disdain ... I don't have any ethical problems with it but the second time was more difficult and I resolved I was never going to have an unwanted pregnancy again and I ran out and got an IUD.*

Whatever you decide, you may feel sad afterwards. This does not mean that you have made the wrong decision. It is not an easy decision for most women to make, even though you may be certain that it is right. You may believe that abortion is acceptable but find it is hard to go through with one. You may not believe in abortion but find yourself wanting one.

> **Maggie:** *My youngest child was ten. I had had three children ... I just couldn't face ... starting again and it wouldn't have been fair on the other children. I'd just started back at my career in teaching. They say having a baby is good for a marriage but I think another baby then would have finished ours off.*

Getting an Abortion: The Options

If You Find Out Early:

You discover you are pregnant by doing your own pregnancy test up to eight weeks from your last period. You do not want to be pregnant, and decide you want an abortion.
- You arrange an immediate appointment with your family doctor who agrees with you.
- The doctor signs a special form, and makes an appointment for you on the NHS to see a gynaecologist who your doctor thinks will help.
- You see the gynaecologist who agrees to do the abortion for you. He or she also signs the form and an appointment is made for the abortion to be done at a hospital before you are twelve weeks from your last period (it will need to be earlier for a medically induced abortion – see page 224). Counselling will be available if you want it.
- After the abortion, you decide on the best future contraceptive plan for you.

one in three: abortion

221

If You've Delayed:

You discover you are pregnant but you are past the twelve-week mark.
- See your doctor as soon as possible anyway. It is still possible in some circumstances to have an abortion up to twenty-four weeks after your last period.
- Your doctor says 'yes' but there is a long delay before you can be seen at the hospital, putting you past the twelve-week mark.
- Either ask your doctor to put pressure on the hospital for an earlier appointment, or consider having your abortion at one of the private charity abortion clinics such as British Pregnancy Advisory Service or Marie Stopes (Useful Addresses on page 390).
- Ask your GP to write a referral letter for you.

If Your Doctor Says 'No':

- Ask to see another GP in the same surgery or visit a GP at another practice. You do *not* have to see your own GP to get an abortion if you do not feel comfortable with him or her. You can also go directly to a family-planning clinic or Brook Advisory Centre (Useful Addresses on page 390) who will refer you to a hospital or tell you of other doctors in the area who are sympathetic to women in need of an abortion.
- Contact one of the charitable or private abortion clinics directly. The BPAS (British Pregnancy Advisory Service) or Marie Stopes will arrange appointments for you to see a doctor and a gynaecologist who will arrange an abortion. They also set up counselling if you feel the need to discuss it further.

The NHS Abortion

Whether and how quickly you can get a free abortion on the NHS depends on where you live. In 1995, 70 per cent of abortions were carried out under the NHS. In Scotland the figure was 98 per cent. In the West Midlands it is much lower. Doctors and nurses can refuse to be involved with abortions on ethical grounds. The law is interpreted in different ways so that some clinics or hospitals provide a better abortion service than others. Some NHS hospitals now contract out their abortions to private charitable agencies such as the BPAS (see above).

The Private Abortion

Private abortion clinics are staffed by people who accept and understand abortion, virtually guaranteeing positive support. They also usually provide a quicker service. If you are under fourteen weeks pregnant and your own GP is informed, the cost is £315, including the consultation. However, if you want an abortion without your GP's involvement the cost is £355. The extra fee allows for an overnight stay in hospital, necessary because you are not being delivered back into the care of your doctor.

Marie Stopes International launched six 'walk-in-walk-out' clinics in England in the summer of 1997. These daycare centres provide abortion using a procedure which usually takes ten minutes or less. It is only available to women in their first twelve weeks of pregnancy. The procedure is done using a manual vacuum aspirator and is carried out with local anaesthetic. As quick and uncomplicated as this may sound, you still require the written consent of two doctors to have the abortion. If you feel you need counselling and time, a quick visit to a day clinic may not be for you – unless you have planned ahead and sought counselling elsewhere. Even with this quick abortion service, many women will still want to take time off and rest for a day or two.

Methods of Abortion

There are two main types of abortion: surgical and medical. A surgical abortion usually involves using suction to remove the contents of the uterus and does not involve any cutting. It is usually done while you are under general anaesthetic, although sometimes it can be done under local anaesthetic which is injected into the cervix. Medical abortions use drugs to induce labour. Whether you have a medical or surgical abortion depends on how far the pregnancy has advanced and also, in the first nine weeks, on a woman's preference and what facilities are available in your area.

The Surgical Abortion

This method is preferred for early abortions or first trimester abortions. First trimester means the first three months of a pregnancy. You usually have a general anaesthetic. A thin plastic tube, 6–10 millimetres wide, is then slipped into the uterus through the cervix. Sometimes the cervix needs to be stretched a little to get the tube in by using a thin metal dilator. The foetal tissue is removed by suction with a device called a vacuum aspirator. You usually stay in hospital for a few hours. You will need to see your own doctor, or visit the clinic, or hospital where you were treated about one week after your abortion to check that everything is all right.

It is a very quick and safe operation. Occasionally some of the pregnancy tissue is left behind and you will need to have the procedure repeated or have a D and C (see pages 356–7). Very rarely the womb gets perforated during the operation, but if it does it usually heals by itself. Persistent pain or heavy bleeding would alert you to a worry that this might not be so.

Celia, 41: *You're knocked out for ten minutes. You feel very woozy. I went home after lunch. I was bleeding for about six or seven days. A bit crampy. I found two enormous bruises on my legs which I couldn't attribute to anything but it turns out to be the stirrups that they put you on. You do then feel a bit vulnerable thinking what else did they do but it seems to have been straightforward.*

Celia's experience is fairly typical, although most women do not complain of bruising. A little light bleeding is sometimes associated with slight cramps and can continue for up to two weeks. If you have heavy bleeding, a fever or more than a fleeting pain, you should get this checked quickly in case something has gone wrong. An infection can cause heavy bleeding or continuous pain. This should be treated right away with antibiotics to prevent complications such as those arising from pelvic inflammatory disease.

The Medical Abortion

A medical abortion involves taking a drug which blocks the hormone progesterone which makes the lining of the uterus hold on to the fertilized egg. The drug is called RU 486 and it contains an anti–progestogen called mifepristone. This may be used for abortions up to nine weeks into the pregnancy. The drug also has the potential to work as an emergency contraceptive after unprotected intercourse (see pages 213–14). By law, the tablets must be administered at an approved hospital or clinic.

Two days after you first take them you return to the clinic or hospital to have a pessary containing prostaglandin hormones inserted into your vagina, or you may be given tablets to be taken orally. Both methods relax your cervix and make your uterus contract. Most women will abort within four to six hours of this step. The pessary often causes nausea or sickness and some diarrhoea. Most women will also need to take strong painkillers as the contractions may be very painful. For 95 per cent of women the abortion will be complete after this procedure, and for around 4 per cent it will not. For one in 100 women it will not work at all. In this case it is not advisable to carry on with the pregnancy because of possible damage to the foetus, so a surgical abortion is recommended.

So, about five per cent of women who have a medical abortion may need a further minor operation (usually an aspiration curettage – see pages 357–8) because the abortion is incomplete and some tissue has been left behind which may cause bleeding. Some bleeding may continue for two weeks after the abortion. An advantage of medical abortion is that it is less likely to cause any damage to the cervix or uterus. Some women may also prefer it because there is no need for general anaesthetic.

Late Abortions

Late abortions may legally be carried out up to twenty-four weeks into a pregnancy. The prostaglandins and mifepristone drugs are used for abortions from thirteen to twenty-four weeks, inducing a mini-labour. You are awake for the procedure. Prostaglandins are either inserted into the cervix or injected into the uterus which starts to contract within a few hours. The foetus is then expelled. Mifepristone, an anti-progestogen (see page 224), is sometimes also used to make the process shorter. In 50 per cent of cases the abortion may be incomplete so an operation under anaesthetic is needed to completely empty the uterus (see page 224). Late abortion is more traumatic because the foetus is more developed.

Sian, 22: *I was fifteen when I had an abortion ... I was on the pill but not taking it properly. I didn't realize I was pregnant and I just didn't want to admit to myself that I was. I wrote something in a letter, my mum read it and that's how she found out ... I was nearly four months pregnant. I was booked into the hospital the next day, my mum's birthday. They put things into my vagina to make me go into labour. Once the labour started it was terribly painful. At the time I just wanted it to be over and done with and to get out of hospital. I didn't think about the baby. Then it happened, the waters went, I wet myself. I felt this big thing fall out from my stomach. I was on a bedpan at the time. I thought there was another one coming and I screamed but it was the afterbirth. They gave me the choice whether I wanted to see it. I looked at it. It was a little boy. I felt like I was a murderer when I saw it – before that I could just ignore it. Now if I think about it I wonder what would have happened. But I have no regrets. I know it was the right thing.*

Sometimes our breasts produce milk after a late abortion. This can be very upsetting and women having a later abortion, for whatever reason, usually need a lot of emotional support. Most hospitals will let you take a friend with you and there should also be a nurse with you for much of the time. You will also be given strong painkillers to help with the pain.

Dilatation and Evacuation

Some doctors think that from thirteen to sixteen weeks, dilatation and evacuation is the safest method of abortion but it is more widely available in private or charitable clinics than on the NHS. It is carried out under general anaesthetic, the cervix is dilated and the foetus removed in fragments.

Foetal Reduction

This is the euphemistic term for selective abortion, the removal of one or more foetuses to prevent or reduce a multiple birth. The problem has arisen because of fertility drugs and in vitro fertilization (see pages 310–12). The best chance a woman has of becoming pregnant with this treatment is to start with, say, three embryos. This increases her chances of one surviving. However, it also increases the chances of a multiple birth because sometimes two or more do survive. Many prospective parents do not want twins, triplets, or more, so the practice of selectively aborting one or more foetuses is now possible. Multiple births are also riskier, so women may choose to abort selectively in order to increase their chance of safe delivery of one baby.

However, foetal reduction is not without its risks. It may cause the other foetus(es) to miscarry on their own. The decision about what to do can be very difficult and you will need to discuss it carefully with the doctors involved and your partner. The procedure worries some people who approve of abortion generally. And it has certainly angered the opponents of abortion.

> **Joanna Bogle, *Catholic Times* columnist:** *It is tragic. Imagine growing up knowing that your mother [chose] to abort either you or your brother or sister and it was just an arbitrary thing ... I think there is a great need for a debate ... all civilized societies have sought to control it. It's time Britain did the same.*

The Risks and Effects of Abortion

Abortion is a safe procedure whichever method is used but there can be complications. The earlier it is carried out the fewer these will be. Minor problems such as infection and bleeding occur in up to 10 per cent of women. Serious problems are very rare. The risk of dying from an abortion is one in 100,000 while eight in 100,000 women die during childbirth or in the month after.

One worry is how abortion affects future fertility. Early vacuum aspiration abortions, the most common method for early abortion, have not been shown to be associated with any subsequent adverse consequences on fertility and pregnancy, nor have they been shown to increase the risk of future ectopic pregnancy (see page 294). Later abortions may be linked to an increased risk of miscarriage in future pregnancies, but the studies are not recent and relate to old-fashioned methods of abortion which were more likely to damage the cervix and cause problems.

The anti-abortion lobby sometimes claims that most women get seriously depressed and psychologically disturbed after abortion. However, studies following up thousands of women who have had abortions show that, although many women experience feelings of sadness and guilt immediately after an abortion, these feelings are often transient and are also frequently accompanied by a marked feeling of relief. Women are likely to feel worse if they are made to feel guilty about having an abortion. Not surprisingly, depression is more likely in women who wanted to have the baby but decided to abort because there was something wrong with the foetus. And worries about having had an abortion sometimes return to women who have trouble getting pregnant later, when they are ready to have a baby (see Chapter 12).

> **Francesca, 42:** *I was pregnant when I was twenty-two and I had an abortion and there is a part of me that feels irrationally that I am being punished for having had that abortion. I suppose because I want a child so desperately now I think how could I have had something so precious growing inside of me and have destroyed it consciously, but at the time that I did have the abortion I didn't feel that way. I was very practical about it. I felt emotional about the idea that I had a baby growing inside me but I knew that I could neither support the child myself nor bring it up properly.*

Making the decision to have an abortion can be difficult enough without having to think about the effect it will have on you twenty years later. It is impossible to predict where you will be and what you will want. Women who do go on to have children later may deal with their emotions differently from women who do not.

> **Margie, 44:** *Most of my closest friends know about it. It's a long time ago now. But it still will come back to me as something really awful that I feel guilty about and have a lot of pain over ... Looking back, I made my choices because of the circumstances involved. I still don't understand it, why I chose the way I did and maybe that's why it's not resolved for me. I had two – two years apart – and I can't believe that it happened twice to me. That was extremely difficult. The first time you can say, 'OK I was stupid and sort of made a mistake', but the second time you think, 'how could I be so stupid a second time?' But there it was. On some levels I never could accept the argument – even though I've made it myself – that it was not a life and so, even though I really have moved on from it, from time to time if I'm feeling bad about myself that's one of the things that I'll beat myself up with.*

one in three: abortion

> **Sandra, 42:** *The third time ... ten years later and ... that one was difficult for every reason. The father that time was a married man with whom I'd been having an affair and with whom I was completely and totally in love who had been promising me that he was going to leave his wife for me. Realistically he never was going to. And so the abortion was emotionally difficult because it was killing something that was his ... I was killing a promise.*

For some women an abortion is like a bereavement. Initially you may feel disbelief, followed by sadness, then anger – perhaps at your partner or yourself or both. Eventually you come to terms with your decision and accept that it was the right thing to do. Or you may continue to feel you have made the wrong decision and have regrets. Consider going for counselling which may help you sort out your feelings and cope better now and later too when you look back. Other women more easily put it behind them.

> **Ella, 22:** *I had never, at any point, felt maternal instincts or thought of my pregnancy as anything other than a massive stumbling block to the rest of my life. Right or wrong, this was my first impulse, proving without a doubt that I was too young to take on the responsibility of being a mum.*

The Abortion Debate

Abortion continues to be a contentious issue and a deeply personal matter.

> **Ann Furedi, Director of the Birth Control Trust:** *An abortion's designed to end a pregnancy. It's inevitably designed to destroy a foetus but I don't think it's appropriate to weigh up the potential life of the foetus ... with the existing quality of life of the conscious woman ... It's easy to exaggerate the amount of repugnance that there is to abortion issues. Survey after survey shows that the vast majority of people agree with abortion as it's provided under the current law.*

However, the more we know the more difficult it may be to proceed. For some women abortion is made more difficult now that ultrasound technology (see pages 273–5) lets us watch the foetus and know its sex. We can hear its heartbeat and watch it move. An eleven-week-old foetus looks recognizably human. Research which tells us a foetus can feel pain is also extremely unsettling.

If you decide to terminate your pregnancy because there is something wrong with the baby, dealing with your emotions can be very difficult. You may have planned for this child, and really wanted it. You have felt pleased to be pregnant, planning the birth and becoming a mother. Learning there is a serious problem with the baby will be a shock and many women will feel confused over what is right to do. Deciding not to have the baby you badly want can be tortuous. Various people and groups may put pressure on you and make you feel guilty. The important thing is to sort out what is best for you.

Abortion for a pregnancy resulting from rape is often linked to enormous anger associated with the rape itself and can seem like a further violation of your body. But terminating a pregnancy conceived under such circumstances can also bring enormous relief. Counselling can help, as can having a trusted person help you manage the practicalities.

As well as the pros and cons of abortion there are other concerns about a father's rights when his partner becomes pregnant. Some men believe abortion is a woman's right, but others may try to prevent their partner from going ahead with an abortion.

The debate over abortion in the United States has erupted into violence. Women seeking abortion, and those supporting them, have been murdered in attacks on abortion clinics. Some members of the pro-life movement have brought tactics of violence to Britain too.

In the Republic of Ireland, abortion remains illegal – unless the woman's life is at risk. The struggle for women wanting abortion was highlighted in 1992 by the plight of a fourteen-year-old girl who was raped and made pregnant by a neighbour. The courts forbade her to travel to the UK for an abortion. But the Irish Supreme Court overturned the decision and she was eventually allowed to go abroad. It appeared that her foetus had more rights than she did. In the UK the law does not recognize the rights of the foetus.

However, campaigners against abortion continue to make an important point.

Joanna Bogle, *Catholic Times* **columnist:** *All the things we were promised that abortion would deliver it hasn't delivered. We have more illegitimate births now, more than a quarter of all births, and I remember being told repeatedly in the seventies that that was going to be a problem that would vanish with abortion on demand... so there's an overdue debate ... and it is honestly not going to go away.*

With proper use of contraception and more use of emergency contraception after unprotected intercourse the number of abortions would fall dramatically. No contraception is 100 per cent effective, however, and there will always be some need for abortion.

one in three: abortion

chapter 10

breasts

Valma, 50: I think mine are quite lovely … They're not hanging down to the south which someone of my age might be expecting. They're quite firm and round and nice to hold.

Breasts go in and out of style. How society regards breasts is constantly changing. Art history documents this well. In Rubens's 'Bathsheba' breasts are erotic, but St Agatha the Martyr's breasts are cut off – punishment of the female body for tempting men into sexual misbehaviour. In the twentieth century, Hollywood often decides how they should look. Post-World War Two, the ideal woman's body was the precursor of the Barbie doll. She was supposed to have enormous breasts, tiny waist, and broad hips: Marilyn Monroe, Jayne Mansfield, Rita Hayworth. In the sixties we burned our bras, in the eighties we celebrated them. Madonna wore hers as an outer garment. Vivienne Westwood designed big bras with pointed cones. The message became, 'Be proud of your breasts'.

The development of our breasts in adolescence confirms to ourselves and to others that womanhood is truly on the way. Even when covered up and neatly contained in a bra our friends monitor their progress. We are sometimes so anxious that we acquire our first bra before our breasts arrive.

> **Janine, 20:** *I can remember being mortified. I didn't actually need a bra but the embarrassment of having vest and knickers in the girls' changing-room was my main motivation. My mum was saying, 'You don't need one', but ... the next day there was a bra in a Marks & Spencer's bag on the dining-room table.*

Yet once we have them, we often complain that they are too small or too big.

> **Margo, 40:** *I've always thought of them as things that get in the way. They've never been really functional to me. They're either straining out of my shirt – and I don't have big breasts – but they're usually too big for what I'm wearing or they're not big enough for what I'm wearing.*

Most men of course enjoy holding breasts. They like to look at them and touch them. They can be fascinated with them, too, as objects they do not have.

> **Marc, 42:** *People think of them as symbols. But personally I think of them as part of a woman's anatomy. It's what differentiates men from women. For men they're a fascination with something you can't have ... That's part of the turn-on.*

> **Fred, 48:** *I look at women and I notice their breasts. It's not a power or dominance thing, just straight pleasure of looking at something attractive. I think it would be sad if I didn't. It's funny because page three girls are a complete turn-off, too blatant.*

breasts

Our breasts are unique to each of us and it is clear that women vary enormously on how they feel about them. Some women feel good about their breasts, others want to change them. In Britain, more than 5000 women a year have silicone breast implants (see pages 237–8). It is difficult to get exact statistics for cosmetic surgery since accurate numbers for operations carried out privately are not available.

In this chapter we look at how we feel about our breasts. We review periods and painful breasts, how to check your breasts and how to decide when a lump should worry you. We have a guide to the treatments available for breast cancer and tips on how to cope with breast cancer. Too many women have it, but more women than ever are surviving it.

The Bra

The bra is both functional and sexy. We have support bras for jogging, nursing bras for breast-feeding, lacy bras for seduction (or just to treat ourselves), strapless bras, push-up bras and ordinary everyday bras. Bras are a source of irritation when they do not fit, a source of power, control and comfort when they do. The fitters who work at the Royal bra makers, Rigby & Peller, emphasize the importance of wearing the right size. They also say the average British bra size is 34 DD and that many women wear the wrong size without realizing. Commonly, women wear bras which are too small in the cup but too big around, so our breasts spill out and the back strap rides up. Most major department stores have specially trained fitters, so ask if you are not comfortable with your bra. If you have any fear of revealing yourself to a stranger in a fitting room you will soon lose it when you see the company you keep. Fitters and patrons alike represent the full range of the female bosom.

There is no evidence that wearing a bra benefits our breasts, although women who run or play any vigorous sport almost always wear a bra for comfort. Swimmers, too, make sure they have swimsuits that hold their breasts comfortably in the water.

Breasts and Breast-feeding

Our ideas about breasts and breast-feeding are set when we are young. One study found that while 70 per cent of sixteen year olds thought that breast-feeding was best for babies, only 40 per cent said they would want to breast-feed their babies when they had them. Education appears to make a difference. A Department of Health Survey of infant feeding found 93 per cent of women who continue in full-time education until the age of nineteen breast-feed their first baby, but of women who left school by the age of sixteen the proportion dropped to 57 per cent. (For more on breast-feeding see pages 288–9.)

> **Margo, 40:** *I first saw them as something other than a hindrance when I had my daughter and I had to breast-feed her. I had terrible problems breast-feeding so I had to have this breast-feeding specialist come and help and she sort of man-handled or woman-handled my breasts into position and my daughter into position ... and my breasts became this public object and for the first time I thought about them in terms of what they should be doing and I no longer saw them as a sexual organ. I saw them as a functional thing. And from then on I've been much less self-conscious of them. I've seen them more as something that's part of me.*

The 'Normal' Breast

> **Marc, 42:** *I don't have a multitude of experience but they come in many shapes and many sizes. No two are the same, even two that come on the same body.*

There is no such thing as a perfect breast. There is endless variation. How you view your breasts and how happy you are with your own body generally is in part due to self-esteem.

> **Jenny, 23:** *I like them. Sometimes I get annoyed because they are a bit big and it can be difficult finding shirts that don't make you look so top heavy. But I like them because they're nice, a nice round shape, a good size ...*

There is no evidence that doing exercises of any kind helps keep your breasts in shape or makes them bigger, smaller, higher, lower, more rounded or whatever. If you are very overweight, losing weight may help reduce your breast size.

Breasts are made up of fat (even in thin women), muscle, milk ducts and glands. Normal breast tissue feels like lumpy porridge and it tends to get even lumpier before a period as the glands are influenced by the hormonal changes that take place in the body every month (see pages 30–2). The nipple and areola – the darker circle around the nipple – are especially sensitive. The size of our nipples and areola varies from person to person. When you get pregnant, your breasts double in weight, and the areolae darken and stay darker after pregnancy.

Breasts change as we age. Fibrous tissue is the biggest component in our breasts and from about the age of thirty this tissue starts to get replaced by fat making our breasts softer and more droopy. There is no way of preventing this. Breasts sag after having a baby and after breast-feeding because the ligaments in the breast tissue get stretched and do not spring back into shape. But the most dramatic change happens at the time of menopause when the tissue thins even more.

Breast Problems

Jenny, 23: *The one thing that does bother me about my breasts is the fact that they are starting to sag already ... especially around the time of my period when they swell up. They get quite flabby and painful too, just because they are so heavy.*

Rachel: *My breasts get really painful especially before my periods. Sometimes it's too painful to wear a bra and as for sex, forget it. I can't bear him to touch me let alone anything else. Sometimes it even hurts to lie on my front in bed.*

Mastalgia or Painful Breasts

Many women get tender breasts before their periods (see pages 45–50) and this is normal. This can last for a day or for a week or more and nearly always disappears once the period starts.

For a few women the pain is severe and lasts much longer and may not be related to periods. This is mastalgia, which means painful breasts. Usually no cause can be found, but explanations range from water retention to neurosis. None of these has been substantiated. It is probably due to an abnormality of the secretion of the gonadotrophin and/or prolactin hormones. But the blood tests available are rarely helpful in sorting out the problem. The tests may not be sensitive enough. There has not been enough research perhaps because it is seen just as a nuisance rather than life threatening.

In 50 per cent of women who suffer badly, breast pain eventually settles down but it may take months or years. In the meantime if you suffer painful breasts try wearing a support bra. Some medicines may also help, but some of the drugs have side effects which may be worse than the pain itself. The drugs most commonly suggested are diuretics (pills which help to reduce water retention), progestogens, and vitamin B6. But studies have failed to show their usefulness. However, there is evidence that gamolenic acid found in oil of evening primrose or starflower oil sometimes helps to alleviate breast pain. The recommended dose is 300 milligrams daily.

The oral contraceptive pill (see pages 199–202) can both cause breast tenderness and cure the problem. Other helpful drugs are bromocriptine, danazol, and tamoxifen – all of which are available on prescription only. One difficulty in treating mastalgia is that the condition itself varies from day to day and month to month. Keep a diary so you know how it varies with or without treatment.

Leaky Nipples

Breast-feeding is usually the cause of leaky nipples. Leaking often starts even before the baby is born. It can also happen after an abortion or a miscarriage, especially those occurring after twelve weeks of pregnancy.

But nipples leak for all kinds of other reasons. The discharge may be milky, clear, or even a bit bloody. If you have discharge, get it checked. Usually no cause is found and doctors say it has to do with your hormones. Occasionally it can be caused by a non-cancerous tumour (a papilloma) in your milk duct or inflammation of the ducts (duct ectasia). It can also be a side effect of a medicine, such as some phenothiazine anti-depressants. Leaky nipples are occasionally linked to breast cancer (see page 239).

Itchy Breasts

Breasts may be itchy because of the cold, when you are pregnant, if your skin is very dry, if you have eczema, if your bra is too tight or made of a scratchy material. Nipples can get sore rather than itchy in women who jog a lot. This is known as jogger's nipple and it is caused by friction. If this affects you, put on some vaseline or try a different bra. Breast cancer does not cause itchy breasts.

Uneven-sized Breasts

Many women have one breast bigger than the other, but it is nothing to worry about unless one gets bigger because of the appearance of a lump and then it is the lump that is the problem. One breast often droops more than the other, and this is normal too.

In a few women there is a big difference. One breast may be hardly there while the other is a size C. This can be very distressing and embarrassing. Cosmetic surgery may help and in such cases could be and should be available on the NHS.

Stretch Marks and Sagging

Stretch marks frequently develop on our breasts during pregnancy and fade afterwards. They often start as purplish in colour and then become silvery whitish lines, running like rivulets down our breasts. But they can also be found in all kinds of places on our bodies, such as thighs and tummies, whether or not we have had babies. They can also occur if you gain weight. They are not fully understood but they are probably related to the type of skin you have. Breasts sag, pull on the skin and, over time, stretch it. This makes marks. Once you have them there is nothing you can do about them, although expensive lotions might make you feel better. Sue believes her oils prevented her from getting stretch marks during her pregnancies.

> **Sue, 42:** *The oil I used for my pregnancies I really believe in and should have shares in. There are different oils for the body. I had long, long talks with sales girls and bought the oil for me and diligently rubbed it in and never suffered one stretch mark.*

Some women say rubbing in oils or creams helps to 'tone' their breasts, although there is no scientific evidence to support this. It *may* be that the massage itself helps – rather than the particular product – since we know that massaging skin helps to disperse water which collects and creates cellulite. There is nothing we know of that will stop sagging. There is also no evidence that wearing a bra helps or hurts, but definitive studies are yet to be done.

Inverted Nipples

Some women are born with one or both nipples inverted – when the nipple pokes inward instead of out. In practical terms this does not matter. You should still be able to breast-feed though you may need extra help initially in getting the baby latched on to your nipple. However, if one nipple suddenly becomes inverted, this needs checking since this can be a sign of breast cancer (see page 239).

Sore Nipples from Breast-feeding

Breasts prepare themselves for breast-feeding during pregnancy. There is no need to scrub them – which might make them sore – nor any need to anoint them with lotions unless you enjoy it. Many women suffer sore nipples when starting breast-feeding. You need to make sure, when nursing, that your baby is 'fully on', with your nipple (including some of the areola) right in the back of his or her mouth. This is the best way to prevent soreness. There is a multitude of creams available, but many midwives recommend nature's way of easing sore nipples: rubbing some of your own milk on the area.

Cosmetic Surgery and Breasts

Breast Enlargement

Women sometimes have breast implants after surgery, when breast tissue has been removed for breast cancer (see page 250). Implants are also inserted for cosmetic reasons if we are dissatisfied with our breast size or shape. Before you decide on changing shape, remember that the way we feel about our breasts often changes with age, and for the better.

> **Ann, 50:** *I love my big boobs but when I was a teenager I was really embarrassed about them because they were very large. There were a lot of envious girls at school who used to ... look jealously at me and one flat-chested hussy said to me, 'At least when I fall in love I'll know my love is true love – you'll always be wondering if it's just your boobs that are attracting the men.'*

If, however, you are very unhappy with your breasts – suffering from physical pain or psychological distress – you may want to proceed. Do some research first. There are good surgeons and bad ones. Most surgeons who do cosmetic breast surgery work privately and are obviously going to give a very positive opinion about it. Surgeons who work in breast clinics in the NHS rarely do cosmetic surgery on healthy breasts and tend to be more cynical about its benefits. Talk to your GP and talk to women who have had the procedure. Read whatever you can find on the subject. Take plenty of time before going ahead as there is no going back.

> **Bob, 35:** *There's lots of other nice curvy bits and soft bits. I don't know why people like Pamela Anderson are held up. I certainly don't find her massive breasts attractive.*

Silicone breast implants have been used by over 2 million women in the USA. However, the American Food and Drug Administration (FDA) banned silicone breast implants because of reports that if they leak, which they sometimes do, they may be associated with cancer and damage to the body's immune system. Symptoms include fatigue and joint and muscle pain. Other studies refute these claims. Court cases are pending, but so far no one definitively knows what side effects are or are not caused by silicone implants. There is no ban in the UK, but to try to get a clearer picture of what is happening in this country a register has been developed for all women having breast implants whether for cosmetic reasons or because she is having her breast reconstructed after cancer. Saline breast implants are available as alternatives to silicone, but they are not so popular as they do not have the

breasts

same authentic feel of breast tissue offered by silicone implants. Breast implants are now being made from other materials such as soya which are meant to be safer since they are natural substances. But even though soya is a natural substance we have no idea of its effect on our bodies since it is not natural to have a lump of soya under our skin.

There is also no such thing as a 100 per cent safe operation, and breast implant procedures are not without complications. An incision is usually made in the crease under each breast. The smaller your breast is to begin with the more noticeable the scar will be. Some women get very lumpy, thick scar tissue (keloids) which can be painful and which can make you unable to breast-feed. Fibrous tissue forms around the breast implant. In some cases this can compress the implant making it hard and uncomfortable.

The NHS pays for implants associated with treatment for breast cancer and might pay in the case of a deformity, for instance if one breast is missing or very small. If you want implants just for the sake of having bigger breasts you will need to pay between £3000 and £3500 to have the procedure done privately. This involves an overnight stay in hospital.

Breast Reduction

This is not generally available on the NHS unless there are very powerful medical or psychological reasons for the operation. You may want it done if you have psychological problems about your size, if one breast is very much larger than the other, or if they are so uncomfortable and painful that they interfere with your life.

An incision is made under your breast and some skin, fat and breast tissue is removed. Your nipples are left in place but the procedure will leave you with scars under your breasts. The milk ducts are cut during the operation so this usually prevents breast-feeding in the future. The wound can also get infected or bleed.

> **Sheila, 56:** *I'm too big at the top and ... if I had the money I'd have them reduced. Because I think if you've got smaller boobs you look thinner all the way down. I think I'm all right everywhere else, just these. I just find they get in the way and I think I'd feel better if they were smaller.*

Becoming Breast Aware

Experts disagree on how often we should check our breasts. But whatever the opinion, and whatever the method, it *is* very important to be aware of our breasts and any out-of-the-ordinary changes that occur in them. It may mean getting a head start on a lump. The earlier a lump is detected the more successful the treatment if you do have cancer.

Check for the following:

• Change in the shape or size of the breast.
• Dimpling or pulling in of the skin.
• A new lump which is not in the other breast and does not disappear after your period.
• Unusual pain which does not go away.
• Discharge from one nipple.
• Retraction or change in the nipple.
• Any other change in the breast which is different from usual monthly changes.

We discover most breast lumps ourselves, informally, when we touch our breasts in the shower or the bath for instance. More formal checking is called breast self-examination. If you want to do this, do it monthly and at the same time of the month. If you are still having periods your breasts will vary with your cycle, feeling lumpier and fuller before your period and less so afterwards so it is important to know what part of your cycle you are in. If you are past the menopause, get familiar with the new shape and feel of your breasts. To examine your breasts you gently press down, circling around your breast – in small circular motions – starting from the outer edges, working towards the nipple in decreasing circles. Whether you want to formalize your checking in this way or simply be 'breast-aware' by noting changes through informal touching, do get to know your own breasts and check out any changes that concern you with your GP.

If You Find a Lump

Women worry about getting breast cancer more than they worry about any other illness. Finding a lump or bump sends most of us into panic, even though only one in nine lumps found by women who then see a doctor turns out to be cancer.

> **Marion:** *It was because my breast felt uncomfortable that I found a lump. If you've had children and you've had the sensation of milk coming in – that's the feeling I had and then when I had a bath I put my hand to where the pain was and discovered the lump. I just panicked.*

The way a lump feels gives clues to what it is but this does not provide a 100 per cent accurate diagnosis. A lump is much less likely to be cancer if you are young, for instance under thirty-five, and more likely to be cancer if you are over sixty. If it feels the same in both breasts or the whole breast is lumpy then it is unlikely to be cancer. When you have generally lumpy breasts it is especially difficult to tell what is going on, just by feeling. The most common causes of breast lumps are fibroadenomas and breast cysts. These are benign, which means non-cancerous.

Fibroadenomas

These cause about 15 per cent of the lumps women find. They are most common if you are young (aged fifteen to thirty). They feel rubbery, they are smooth and rarely hurt. They also feel very mobile when you try to locate them. They just slip away under your fingers. They do not change size during your menstrual cycle. They are bits of breast tissue which have become separated from the rest of the breast. Twenty per cent disappear, 5 per cent get bigger, and the rest – the majority – stay about the same size.

Breast Cysts

These are more common in women aged forty to fifty. They are just bags of fluid or jelly. Fifty per cent of women who have them have more than one. They can be quite big and painful. They are thought to be related to a hormone imbalance but we do not really know. They are treated by draining off the fluid through a fine needle.

Cancerous Lumps

These are more likely to be firm, be there all the time and may or may not hurt. They can be pea-sized or bigger. If you do find a lump you should see your doctor who will probably send you for a mammogram and perhaps to see a breast specialist to try to establish what it is. If you feel your doctor is brushing you off, get another opinion. Make sure you are seeing someone you trust and never be afraid to seek another view. A GP can never be sure just by feeling. Whether a lump is benign or cancerous can also be discovered by inserting a needle into the lump to extract a few cells (fine needle aspiration). These are then analysed in a laboratory. This is usually done at the hospital and you may even have the results while you wait. With increased awareness of breast cancer, more women are checking their breasts and finding small lumps and thickenings. As a result, operations to remove these lumps (lumpectomies) are on the increase even though the procedure may not always be necessary. There is a backlash against too much surgery. But many women just want the lump out, no matter what it is. Although most fine needle aspirations do establish a correct diagnosis, a lumpectomy offers the most reliable and definitive diagnosis.

The Facts About Breast Cancer

Breast cancer is the most common cancer in women in the UK, although lung cancer is catching up. On average, one in twelve women in the UK will develop the disease. The risk is greater the older we are. Every year in the UK about 35,000 women are found to have breast cancer. Annually, 15,000 women die from it. Britain has the highest mortality rate from breast cancer in the world. It accounts for 19 per cent of all deaths from cancer among women but only 5 per cent of all deaths among women. (Heart disease is the biggest killer.) Eighty per cent of breast cancers develop in women over the age of fifty, and 88 per cent of the deaths are in this age group. If the cancer is found early and treated before it has spread, about 85 per cent of women will be alive five years later. The average survival at five years is 62 per cent.

We are still very ignorant about why breast cancer happens and how best to treat it. Scientists do not even fully understand how a normal breast develops. However, we have some clues as to what may influence it. New treatments are being developed and we have better ways of finding breast cancers early through screening. This should mean we have a better chance of being cured if we do develop it.

Breast cancer usually develops in cells of the milk-secreting glands in our breasts or the ducts that carry the milk to the nipple. If the cancer is caught very, very early and is still only in the cells of the glands or ducts and has not spread at all, this is described as the 'non-invasive stage' (sometimes called in situ) and it is good news. If it has spread outside these cells it is called 'invasive'. Breast cancers are graded according to the type of cells and how far they have spread in the breast and to other parts of the body. The less it has spread the better the cure rates and survival chances.

breasts

Priscilla Welch, Marathon Runner, reflecting on the day she learned she had breast cancer: *I had arranged to meet my husband in a store ... and he just walked through the door with his thumb down and it was like being hit in the stomach, a low punch you know, and then immediately afterwards I looked at him and said, 'I'm not ready to go to the big blue sky yet, Dave, what can we do?' And he said, 'I've already made an appointment with the general surgeon for you this afternoon and we'll go together', and that's how we started the ball rolling.*

Three years later, in October 1997, Priscilla Welch was one of the top three finishers in 'The Survivors' Race' which was run in Denver, Colorado, to raise money for cancer research.

Breast Cancer Treatments

Gill: *It did worry me a lot because we'd only just got married and we were really enjoying a full sex life and obviously this was going to throw it. That side of it I felt very sad about.*

There are four main treatments: surgery, radiotherapy, hormone therapy and chemotherapy. There is no evidence that psychological or complementary therapies cure breast cancer, but they may be important to our general well-being and confidence during treatment.

Each case of breast cancer has factors which may help decide which treatment will be the most effective:

- The size: the smaller the tumour the better the outlook. (If it is less than 2 cm when first found, 85–90 per cent of women will still be alive after five years.)
- The nodes under the arm: the lymph nodes under the arm should always be tested for cancer cells and if none is found the outlook is better than if they are present.
- The type of cells: the tumour cells can be more or less active and the less active they are the better.
- Receptors: the tumour can be tested for special chemicals and receptors. One of these is the oestrogen receptor test (called ER status) which is a chemical test done to see if the tumour cells are sensitive to hormones or not. Women who have had the menopause are more likely to have a tumour which is ER positive and these tumours are more likely to respond well to the anti-oestrogen drug tamoxifen. There is a host of other receptors under review to try to help tailor individual treatments.

Surgery

Jane: *When I went in for the operation – for the lumpectomy – I was not aware at that time how much of my breast would be removed. What I was particularly concerned about was that if a mastectomy were to be necessary that I would want to come out of the operation to discuss it with my husband and if necessary have another operation because there was no way I wanted to go under general anaesthetic feeling that I was having one situation and come out of it and have a complete and absolute shock.*

Surgery is usually recommended once cancer has been found. In the past ten to fifteen years breast-conserving surgery and lumpectomy have been available, where the breast lump itself and underarm lymph nodes are removed rather than the whole breast. This is followed by five to six weeks of radiotherapy (see pages 246–7). The survival rate from this treatment is as good as mastectomy, though sometimes the tumour recurs locally and more surgery is needed.

Mastectomy – having the entire breast removed – is usually recommended when tumours are greater than four centimetres in diameter. The surrounding lymph nodes are also removed at this time to check for cancer cells. The prognosis is better if cancer has not spread to the lymph nodes in the armpit.

Phyllis: *When the nurse took the dressing off the wound the first time I remember her saying to me, 'Would you like to actually see the wound?' and I said, 'Well, next time'. The following day I felt I was ready to actually see the wound and I asked her to get my mirror and I was very pleasantly surprised believe it or not. It wasn't anything like I expected. It was just one long scar.*

Some women get severe swelling of the arm after surgery and this is called lymphoedema. This condition is linked to the removal of the lymph nodes under the arm and can occur after lumpectomy or mastectomy. Massage, gentle arm exercises and swimming can help.

Chemotherapy

Jo: *I was so frightened about chemotherapy. I immediately thought I was going to lose my hair and I thought of the dreadful sickness and things that you do read about with chemotherapy.*

breasts

243

Chemotherapy is a taxing process. Treatment regimes vary according to the type of tumour, your age and which cocktail of drugs you get. The most common regime is to have a combination of three drugs every three weeks. This involves going to the hospital as an outpatient and having a slow injection of drugs into the vein of your arm. You will need to have blood tests before each dose of chemotherapy to check that the chemotherapy is not reducing your white cells too much or making you too anaemic. If it is, you may have to delay treatment until your blood count improves.

> **Phyllis:** *I was pleasantly surprised. I'd heard so much about the chemotherapy and how people can feel but I was lucky enough that I could near enough carry on with my normal way of life.*

Chemotherapy drugs help to kill the cancer cells but they also affect some healthy cells, which is a drawback. Treatment is given over several months. A variety of chemotherapy drugs – cyclophosphamide, methotrexate, 5-fluorouracil and adriamycin – is used in combination or singly, depending on the type and stage of the cancer. It is administered by pill, intravenous drip and injection. The drugs enter the bloodstream and affect the whole body. The treatment also reduces oestrogen production in the ovaries and in some women this may induce the menopause if they have not already reached it. Chemotherapy is now nearly always recommended for women under the age of fifty, especially if they have not reached the menopause (when their breast cancer may be oestrogen-related). Recent evidence indicates that women with bigger tumours should have chemotherapy before any surgery is carried out because it helps to shrink the tumour.

> **Anna:** *Every time I brushed or combed my hair, my hair seemed to fall out but a lot of people didn't notice it because I had fairly thick hair to start off with. So it just got thinner and thinner but I didn't go bald and I didn't need a wig but I felt particularly ill, a bit depressed and sick and then it started to get better and I was just beginning to feel better again when it was time for the next session.*

Some drugs always cause hair loss, while others are less likely to. Other common side effects are tiredness, nausea, diarrhoea, weight gain and a general lowering of our immunity to disease. More drugs can be prescribed to counteract these side effects, including a cannabis-related drug which is very effective in stopping nausea. Young women may also experience menopausal symptoms (see Chapter 3).

Jeannette Matthey kept a diary during her battle with breast cancer. She was thirty-six years old and full of hope and pain, but did not lose her sense of humour, even when treatment made her lose her hair:

Jeannette: *How do bald people prepare for work in the morning? What do they have to work with? Men in particular of course. They don't have make-up ... they must learn to be very happy with themselves.*

And Julie, forty-seven, in the midst of her chemotherapy for breast cancer, told us:

Julie: *It was worse in the prospect than once it's lost. My fear about it going to happen was that I'd look like a cancer victim. You don't think about having hair but the idea of losing it makes you feel like a victim. I didn't want to be a victim. I wanted to be a survivor. Once it's off, you just get on with it. The actual reality has not been such a big deal. But for my daughter it's a big deal. I have to respect her feelings. I never let her see me bald as she doesn't want to. It would frighten her, so at night I wear a turban thing. Sometimes I wear a wig, sometimes a scarf. Mo Mowlam has been a terrific inspiration to me. The way she takes her wig off in the midst of talks on Northern Ireland. She's leading the way.*

Hormone Treatment

The hormone drug, tamoxifen, is usually given to women with breast cancer who have reached the menopause, especially if the tumour is oestrogen receptor positive (see page 242). Tamoxifen is an anti-oestrogen taken once a day in pill form. As in chemotherapy, it enters the bloodstream and affects the whole body. It is one of the most important advances in terms of breast cancer treatment in recent years as it increases a woman's length of trouble-free life after the initial breast surgery. Some women will have chemotherapy (see above) as well as tamoxifen. Most women tolerate tamoxifen reasonably well with only 3 per cent of women who take it for breast cancer giving up because of side effects. Weight gain is common and hot flushes occur in 50 per cent of women. Some women also experience depression, nausea and dizziness, vaginal dryness and loss of interest in sex.

Sian: *I took the drug and the first thing that I noticed was that I had a vaginal discharge, it wasn't particularly unpleasant but it was very noticeable. I had a dry vagina as well and that slightly bothered me but I didn't actually mention it. It's not the sort of thing you do mention, especially if you're only seeing the oncologist for two minutes for a check-up. I did have increased hot flushes but I found that relaxation could deal with hot flushes. I was able to control a lot of the symptoms myself.*

It has recently been noticed that women who take tamoxifen have a slightly increased risk of endometrial cancer. The endometrium lines the uterus. But this risk is very small and is far outweighed by the protection tamoxifen gives against developing breast cancer in the other breast or having a recurrence in the original one. Taking tamoxifen reduces the chance of having one of these second cancers by 40 per cent. Professor Richard Peto of Oxford University calculates that for every 1000 women with ER-positive breast cancer treated with tamoxifen for five years, approximately 160 breast cancer recurrences are prevented. He also calculates there will be eighty fewer deaths. Five to ten of these 1000 women will develop endometrial cancer, and one of these will be fatal.

There are concerns about other long-term side effects. Ovarian cancer (see pages 382–4), colonic cancer, and thrombosis may be associated with tamoxifen, but more research needs to be done. Tamoxifen has problems but overall the benefits far outweigh these risks. New hormone drugs are being developed all the time. Other drugs used in various combinations and doses are mitomycin, mitozantrone, taxol and lantron. They all have slightly different side effects and which one is most suitable for you will depend on the nature of the breast cancer and how much it has spread.

Surgery to remove the ovaries is being offered to some women, especially those who are oestrogen receptor positive (see page 242), as a way of reducing the body's oestrogen production. But the trouble with this procedure is that it immediately brings on a severe menopause.

Radiotherapy

Radiotherapy is usually given after surgery. Its main use is to prevent local recurrence of a tumour, especially if it was large or appeared under the microscope to be an aggressive type. It is nearly always recommended if a lumpectomy rather than mastectomy is performed, although if the cancer is at a very early stage radiotherapy may not be needed. It is also used after mastectomy if the glands under the arm are affected. Radiotherapy is done with a device like an X-ray machine which shoots out radioactive particles targeted at the cancer cells. Calculations are made as to how much radiation should be given and exactly where on the breast it should be targeted depending on the site of the original tumour. Tiny tattoos the size of a pin head are put on the skin of your chest to help the radiotherapist know where to direct the rays. The tattoos do not wash off – ever – so that if any further treatment is needed there should be no risk of giving too much to the same area even if your weight or shape changes in the future. Some women will have low dose daily treatment, whilst others will have a higher dose three or four times per week depending on the hospital they attend.

> **Margaret:** *I went for assessment for them to decide on how much radiotherapy I needed ... they had an accurate marker when they actually did the radiotherapy. Although they are tiny, I'd rather it wasn't still there or at least was brown like a freckle rather than blue/black.*
>
> **Christina:** *The first two weeks of radiotherapy for me were extraordinarily uneventful. Then I certainly had the effects of a very bad case of sunburn. I have great sympathy now for a chicken in a microwave ... the feeling of a spikiness that emanates from the nipple area and manages to spread itself almost like a spider's web over the breast area and the stabbing and the pulsating effect. Quite traumatizing actually and often quite unexpected.*

Most women have some problems with radiotherapy, though these vary and most will improve in time. Tiredness, depression and skin irritations such as soreness and swelling are the most common. The fatigue tends to increase as the treatment progresses. Your skin may take six months to return to normal. A few women have more severe reactions. If you are given too much radiation – and this happened more frequently a decade ago – inflamed nerves (neuropathy) sometimes causes pain in your arms. Women have formed a pressure group called RAGE (Radiotherapy Action Group Exposure) to draw attention to the problem and provide telephone support, organize care and to pressure the government to provide no-fault compensation to women who have suffered in this way.

Complementary Therapies

Many women feel they lose control of their bodies during breast cancer treatment. And they sometimes feel that while their breast is being treated, the rest of their body is ignored. Complementary therapies make some women feel they have more control, although there is no evidence that these therapies alone are successful in treating breast cancer. (Studies on aromatherapy and cancer are now underway, see page 350.) There needs to be much more research in this whole area as there is no doubt that complementary therapies may have an

breasts

important role to play. We know that feeling positive about things affects the immune system which in turn could affect how cancers progress. Most doctors see complementary therapies just as they are labelled: complementary. They do not regard them as a viable alternative to conventional medicine.

> **Flora:** *The next decision I made was to book into the Bristol Cancer Help Centre. They've got a whole range of complementary therapies. I chose visualization and relaxation which involves my using a tape. I'm encouraged to imagine my body defences attacking my cancer. At this point I override the tape slightly mentally and sort of visualize laser beams zapping my cancer, you know like Star Wars.*
>
> **Betty:** *The other therapy I went on was a wholefood diet. For me I decided to be quite rigorous because I didn't have any other treatment. Quite a lot of raw food, fresh fruit and vegetables, wholefood. I eliminate dairy products which don't agree with my cancer. This suits me very well in fact.*

You do need to be wary. Well-meaning friends, relatives and colleagues may bombard you with a variety of information. Or you, in your desire for a cure, may respond to offers of alternative remedies advertised in health magazines or newspapers, for instance. Some of these may have an appeal because they are sold as natural cures. In many cases very little is known about how successful they are or even what effect they will have on you, and they may cost a lot of money. Sometimes patients are made to feel that not to accept these alternatives will jeopardize their chances of recovery.

Which Treatment to Choose

If you find out you have breast cancer it will take time to get over the shock of it. But when you do grasp it, it may help you to be well informed on what is available in terms of treatment and support. Knowing too many details might make you feel afraid at first or you may be someone who wants no details at all. But knowledge can boost your confidence in the treatment you choose and how you cope with it.

The best treatment for you depends on how old you are, whether you have reached the menopause, the size of the tumour, how far it has spread and which type of cancer you have. Some cancers are more aggressive than others, some are made of different cell types and some, on special testing, are found to be influenced by oestrogen (see page 242). These oestrogen receptor positive cancers are the ones more likely to respond to anti-oestrogen therapy drugs like tamoxifen (see pages 245–6). Which surgery women want varies from woman to woman. Some want to have a mastectomy because it makes them feel safer about the cancer, even though a lumpectomy would do the job. Others want a lumpectomy because they are more anxious about the psychological effects of losing a breast.

Women with breast cancer are living longer now than ever before probably because of the increased use of chemotherapy drugs and tamoxifen. For some women the decision about chemotherapy is clear cut, for others it is not. Seventy to 80 per cent of women with breast cancer which has not spread (i.e. the lymph nodes are clear) will not have a recurrence after five years even if they do not have chemotherapy. In other words, chemotherapy will be of no use to them. For the remaining 20–30 per cent of women in this group, chemotherapy will stop or reduce the likelihood of a recurrence. The trouble is we do not know which of us is in which group and therefore it is impossible to tell which individual woman will actually gain from the treatment. So it is offered to everybody.

The effects of different treatments on the future quality of one's life also need to be considered in the calculations, something which the medical profession has been slow to acknowledge.

> **Kate:** *When they told me after the lumpectomy, I ought to have chemotherapy as well as radiotherapy, I wanted more information. Not just about the short-term effects to do with sickness, losing my hair and feeling awful. I felt I could cope with those. They did not seem to know whether long term these drugs could be a problem and that's what I wanted to know so I could make a better informed decision. I don't think they've done enough to find out how women really feel ten years after all the treatment.*

Making decisions is often very difficult. Weighing the risks and benefits can feel impossible when you are still trying to adjust to having breast cancer. And we are all different as to how we assess a risk or benefit. There seems to be little difference in survival whether you choose to have a lumpectomy or a mastectomy if the tumour is small, yet some women will feel safer with one method as opposed to the other. Similarly with reconstruction, some women definitely want it while others do not. Some of us want the choice made for us, while others want to be actively involved in the process. The important thing is to be able to get the information you want, in the way you want it, to allow you to make the best choices. Ask the doctors and nurses treating you and contact BACUP and Breast Cancer Care for more information and counselling if you want it (see Useful Addresses on page 390).

breasts

Prosthesis and Reconstruction

Antonella: *Sometimes it squelches, it makes a squelching noise but apart from that it's soft, it's movable, as your real breast would be. I don't have a sensation in the nipple as I did with my real one but I am aware when it's being touched. You wouldn't know the actual breast was fake.*

Susanna: *After the mastectomy, I felt very down in the dumps, very low and I felt I'd lost a bit of my womanhood quite honestly. I had to go and be measured for a prosthesis to pop inside my bra. I felt absolutely awful. It felt heavy, it wasn't part of me.*

After mastectomy there are many types of prostheses available to put in a bra or swimming costume, so make sure you end up with one you feel comfortable with. The NHS has a range or you can buy one privately (see Useful Addresses on page 390). You do not need reconstruction after lumpectomy, unless it is a very big lumpectomy in which case it is really a partial mastectomy. Some breast reconstructions are done at the same time as the mastectomy, so discuss this possibility with your surgeon. The cancerous tissue is removed, but the skin and nipple are saved and a silicon implant is placed beneath the skin. The most common style of reconstruction is an implant placed beneath the remaining skin and muscle.

Marcia: *The thought that I could be put back together, or reconstructed, that gave me the hope. It made living with it a little bit easier for me. It was a major operation – I felt a little poorly afterwards but the discomfort was well worth it. I would say it was a good month before I could really see what it was like and it was absolutely fantastic. I had a pair of matching breasts.*

There are also ways of reconstructing our breasts which do not involve any implants but use the skin and tissue from other parts of our bodies, usually from our back or lower abdomen. The option most suitable for you needs to be discussed.

Barbara: *My husband was keen for me to have it done. I knew that he would love me whatever. When he came to see me after the original operation he looked at the scar and tried to get me to look which I wouldn't and he kissed me there which I think was absolutely smashing. He was happy either way but he knew it would make me feel a lot better so he was 100 per cent behind me to go for it.*

If the Cancer Has Spread

About 30 per cent of women who have had primary breast cancer subsequently develop secondaries known as metastases in other parts of the body. Secondaries occur when cells from the original breast cancer break off and migrate through the bloodstream. They can settle in many sites, particularly in bones, but also in our lungs, liver and brain.

There are various options for treatment. The type of treatment you get depends on where the secondaries are located. Therapies can suppress the disease – putting it into remission – but the cancer may return. For localized secondaries, a localized treatment, such as radiotherapy (see pages 246–7), is given. But when the area is more generalized, throughout your body, a more generalized treatment is given – either hormonal therapy or chemotherapy (see pages 244–5). If one treatment fails another one can be tried.

> **Eliza:** *At the time I was totally shell-shocked. I had had a general check-up from my surgeon. When I went back to see him he said I had a couple of shadows on my lung X-rays and they were definitely secondaries. I had been given a good prognosis. I'd had a mastectomy and radiotherapy and I was led to believe that I was well covered and that I shouldn't have any more problems so it did come as an awful shock.*

New very intensive treatment using high-dose chemotherapy and 'stem cell rescue' is being used in trials with women who have relapsed or are found to have cancer which has already spread when it is first detected. The treatment involves having drugs by injection to stimulate cells in the bone marrow to reproduce very quickly. These stem cells then spill out into your blood and some of them are removed from the blood and stored. You are then given very large doses of chemotherapy which aim to kill off any cancer cells. However, the treatment also kills the normal developing cells in the bone marrow which is where your white blood cells are formed. White cells fight infection, so while you are having this treatment you are particularly susceptible to infection. The bone marrow cells previously rescued from your blood are then given back to you and gradually you start to make white blood cells again. You will need to be in hospital for about three weeks but this will vary. Although these treatments look promising, side effects are much worse than for the usual chemotherapy. Women often feel depressed, have nausea and sickness and diarrhoea and generally feel awful during the treatment. Some get chest infections or other infections because they have so few white blood cells which would normally get rid of such infections quickly.

breasts

Coping with Breast Cancer

Louisa on being in a breast cancer support group: *There's a lot of tears to start with but there's also a lot of laughter. We just support each other. Even if we have a down day we can ring one person in the group at least and say how we're feeling. We just talk openly about ourselves now. After a time your family get fed up listening to you, and your friends, they don't want to hear about all these things and so when you go to the group you let it out. That knocks the stress out of the illness.*

If you need help you can turn to your family doctor, your local breast care nurse, psychological counselling services, or local breast cancer support group. Ask about all of these at your GP's surgery or at the hospital. If there is no breast care nurse where you are being treated, you can ask to move to a clinic which has one.

Mary: *I knew I would need help caring for the children ... My sister-in-law got on to social services and we ... were pushed about and were told we weren't able to have any help and eventually we got the help. I've got home help twice a week and I have money to pay for a childminder to look after my two children when I have the treatment.*

Natalie: *It's very difficult to talk about it. I obviously did to a few close friends and to my family. I didn't want people's pity – I didn't want people feeling sorry for me and I didn't want people, every time I met them, asking me how I was. There's nothing more irritating.*

Alice: *I was just absolutely shattered. There was no one to talk to. I felt I was losing my mind actually. I thought I've seen this before, I've known people last a year, maybe eighteen months if they were lucky. I went home and tidied everything up and went and sought a solicitor and made preparations to die.*

Dusty Springfield: *The only time I had a bad fit was when I looked at the cat and thought, 'Who's going to look after you? And no way am I going to die.' And I never entertained the thought of dying after that and that's supposed to be very good. It is the people who just say, 'No way!' It has a lot to do with getting well and I'm fine ... I've got a check-up at the end of this month and you're supposed to be awfully scared about it and I'm not remotely.*

Risks of Breast Cancer – Facts and Myths

Inheritance

Some women are at higher risk of breast cancer because of genetic factors. We have long known that women with a strong family history of breast cancer are at higher risk than others. If your mother developed breast cancer under the age of forty, or if several close family members have had it, these are clues that it could be genetic. It is now possible to find out who is at higher risk and who is not by testing for the breast cancer genes, although these tests are not yet routinely available. Two breast cancer genes have recently been identified: the BRCA1 gene on chromosome 17 and, more recently, the BRCA2 gene located on chromosome 13. Less than 5 to 10 per cent of breast cancer cases appear to be genetically transmitted by these genes, but 80 to 90 per cent of women who carry the gene will develop breast cancer. If you have a strong family history of breast cancer, with two or more relatives having had it at a young age, your GP can try to arrange a test for you at a regional genetic unit.

If you do not have the gene, you may not have a higher risk even though you have a family history of breast cancer. There is uncertainty because more breast cancer genes may yet be discovered. Many of us will want the test in the hope of being reassured that we do not have the gene. Others will not want to be tested. If the test does show a breast cancer gene is present, it may cause severe anxiety and depression.

Heather's grandmother, aunt and first cousin have all had breast cancer so Heather assumes that it is 'in the family'. She has not yet had the gene test and she has mixed feelings about it.

Heather, 44: *My initial reaction is that I wouldn't want to know, then my next question would be, 'What happens if I actually have the gene?' If there are things you can do like diet, all this information that's coming out now that would actually have an impact on reducing your risk for genetic breast cancer, I would probably have it. It actually strikes me as one of those things I almost wish they hadn't invented because we have so many technological issues we have to deal with now around our health and we have so many unknowns.*

Earlier mammograms might help early diagnosis, but as yet there is no good way of preventing future breast cancer in women who know they are at high risk. A big study is underway now to see if tamoxifen (see pages 245–6) helps prevent women in the high-risk category from developing breast cancer. There is some evidence for this. Although it is known that tamoxifen is good for women who have breast cancer, it is not yet known what all the risks and benefits are of giving it to women who might develop the disease.

Some women at high risk decide to have a preventive mastectomy – having both breasts removed – even before there is any sign of disease. For some women with a very high risk this is available on the NHS. It is still possible to get breast cancer after the procedure because it is difficult to get rid of every breast cell, particularly as women often keep the nipple. In 1995 Denise, whose mother and three aunts all died of breast cancer, had a double mastectomy:

> **Denise, 25:** *I was very scared. Every spot and pimple that I found, I worried myself sick ... I was very worried more than anything for my children as I wanted to be there for them to grow up ... eventually I went to see the specialist and he was very good. He told me about the operation. I made my mind up there and then really ... it wasn't very nice and it was painful and it was nasty but I mean now, three months on from the operation I feel wonderful, the worry's gone. Now I can look at life in a whole different way. I can be here to see my children grow up and hopefully I'll be here to see their children grow up ... a lot of people do think that it is drastic but after losing nearly all of your female relatives I'm sure that anybody else in my situation would consider doing the same.*

The Hormone Connection

The hormone oestrogen which governs our menstrual cycles is linked to breast cancer. The earlier your periods start the higher your risk. If your periods begin before the age of eleven your risk doubles. The earlier you have children the lower your risk. Women who have children over the age of thirty-five are 50 per cent more likely to get breast cancer than women who have their first child under the age of twenty. And women who do not have any children also have a higher chance of getting breast cancer. Having a late menopause will increase your risk. Research suggests you have a 30 per cent greater risk for every three years' delay from the average age of the onset of menopause which is fifty.

The Pill and Breast Cancer

The combined oral contraceptive pill is made from two hormones: oestrogen and progestogen (see page 199). A comprehensive worldwide study has found that taking the pill increases your risk of breast cancer, but in young women the increased risk is very small. For women on the pill who stop taking it at twenty-five, by the age of thirty-five there will be one extra case of breast cancer for every 7000 pill users. For women who stop the pill at age thirty-five, by the age of forty-five, there will be one extra case of breast cancer for every 1000 pill users. For women who stop the pill at forty-five, there will be one extra case of breast cancer for every 300 pill users. The risk appears to disappear gradually once you stop taking the pill. After ten years the increased risk has disappeared altogether. We do not know whether women should take the pill if they have an increased risk of breast cancer already because of a strong family history. Common sense suggests you should think of alternatives, especially as you get older (see Chapter 8).

HRT and Breast Cancer

Hormone replacement therapy or HRT involves taking oestrogen and progestogen, or just oestrogen on its own (see Chapter 3). HRT makes breast tissue denser, and therefore mammograms (see pages 379–81) are more difficult to interpret. Some radiologists recommend cessation of HRT for two months prior to having your mammogram.

A 1997 a UK report has helped to clarify the link between breast cancer and HRT. It looked at almost all the studies that have been published before coming to its conclusion that the link between HRT and breast cancer depends on how long you take it. Women who use HRT for a short time around the menopause are hardly affected and do not have anything to worry about. For women aged fifty who do not use HRT ever, about forty-five in every 1000 will have a breast cancer diagnosed over the next twenty years. For those women who take HRT for five years, there will be an extra two cancers in every 1000 women over the next twenty years. For those women who take HRT for ten years this figure will be six, and for those of us who are on it for fifteen years the extra cancers over the next twenty years is twelve. The good news is once you have stopped HRT, the increased cancer risk returns to normal after five years. The breast cancers found in women on HRT do seem to be easier to treat successfully.

In 1997 two cancer charities, the Imperial Cancer Research Fund and the Cancer Research Fund, announced 'One Million Women', a research project which aims to ask all women having mammograms about their use of HRT. The results of the study should add further to our knowledge of the risks and benefits of HRT.

Diet and Breast Cancer

Breast cancer is highest in North America and Northern Europe, and lowest in China, India and Africa. This is probably due to differences in diet. Some researchers think that over 50 per cent of breast cancers in the UK are preventable because they are thought to be related to environmental or nutritional factors – for instance the Western high-fat diet. Limiting the amount of fat we eat may be beneficial in the prevention of breast cancer but it will not stop all cancers. Heavy alcohol consumption does appear to be linked with an increased risk of breast cancer. Results of studies on the link between caffeine and breast cancer are conflicting.

Age and Breast Cancer

Age is probably the biggest factor. Women under thirty can get breast cancer but it is rare. As we noted on page 241, 80 per cent of breast cancers occur after the age of fifty. In the debate over HRT and breast cancer, proponents of HRT point out what may be a paradox: HRT is thought to make us live longer, but living longer increases our chance of getting breast cancer. Breast cancers in younger women, as rare as they are, appear to be more frequently aggressive and have a worse prognosis. This may be because they are not diagnosed until a later stage, whereas older women are now being invited to participate in routine breast cancer screening (see page 379).

Accidents and Breast Cancer

If you fall, or accidentally knock your breasts, this does not cause breast cancer.

Breast-feeding and Cancer

There is a debate about whether (and if so how much) breast-feeding protects women against breast cancer, with a protective effect being reported in some studies. However, even if it does not offer protection, it is still good for the baby (see page 288).

Reducing Your Risk of Breast Cancer

Many of the risk factors are out of our control. There is little you can do to stop early menstruation and late menopause. When to have a baby is sometimes within our control but most of us plan this according to our relationship, job and other life factors rather than planning to have a baby early to reduce our breast cancer risk. We can try to keep fit through exercise and eating a low-fat diet, which should help reduce our risk of breast cancer. Women over fifty should have regular mammograms but of course this does not actually prevent cancer. Rather it aims to pick up any cancers early so treatment can be more effective. Twenty per cent of the so-called cancers found this way are not actually cancers. However, if left, some would develop into cancer over the next ten or fifteen years or even longer. They are called 'pre-cancerous' and this means they can be more easily treated and there is a better chance of recovery.

The Right Treatment

Not all women with breast cancer get the best treatment, although of course we all deserve it. Women referred to hospital should be seen in a proper breast unit which would ensure you see a specialist breast surgeon, with access to full pathological facilities for diagnosis. A breast care nurse should also be available. However, not all hospitals are equipped like this. Once you have been referred and if a cancer is found it can be difficult to change doctors. Research shows that women do better in specialist units than if they are left to a general surgeon who does occasional breast surgery.

Studies show that some women feel they are informed in a casual, off-hand manner, others that their concerns are trivialized and given little attention. They do not feel they are given enough information about the treatments available. Remember you can always ask for a second opinion.

> **Marianne:** *I had the misfortune to have my results over the phone – a voice saying, 'That lump, it must be removed sooner rather than later,' and he said, 'I've told your GP. Perhaps you'd get in touch with me tomorrow and make an appointment' and that was it. I was left at five o'clock cooking the dinner wondering what the hell to do next. I was just very confused. I didn't really know what was happening. He booked me in for surgery and I very meekly agreed at that stage. I felt very vulnerable and when I left there I came out and couldn't think of anything else but cancer and dying.*

If you (or a friend or relative) is diagnosed with breast cancer make sure you:

- See a breast cancer specialist. If you have trouble getting to see one ask your GP or phone BACUP/Cancer Link or Breast Cancer Care (see pages 392–3) who will guide you.
- Go to a centre accustomed to managing patients with breast cancer and which has good, modern equipment, to deliver the relevant therapy.

- Make sure you understand, do not be afraid to ask questions to make sure you get all the information you want.
- See a breast care nurse support service.
- Go back to your GP and discuss alternatives if you think your local hospital is not up to the job. Ask to see a different surgeon or ask for a second opinion if you are not happy with your treatment. Make a fuss until you feel good about the care you are getting.
- Contact the breast cancer help lines of BACUP or Breast Cancer Care who should be able to give you information about what else is available and where.
- Make a list of your concerns to discuss at your appointment.
- Take your partner or a friend with you for support, if you feel it helps.

One Woman's Fight

Lesley Elliott was thirty-five, married to a farmer in Dorset, and the mother of three children – Jack, Nancy and Eve – when she talked with Jenni Murray on BBC Radio 4's *Woman's Hour*. She knew her breast cancer was terminal.

Lesley: *The first time I found the lump I was breast-feeding my youngest child Eve who was then seven months. I went immediately to the doctor who found nothing that worried her, but I talked to friends and we decided the best thing would be to give up breast-feeding and note the changes in the breast and then return to the doctor in six weeks' time which is what I did.*

Jenni: *And still reassurance from the doctor?*

Lesley: *I saw a different doctor on this occasion. He reassured me that the breasts were normal which left me feeling happy and I was extremely pleased that it wasn't going to be breast cancer.*

Jenni: *So when you finally were diagnosed, when you found the lump under your armpit, how did you then view your chances of recovery?*

Lesley: *To start with I thought if lymph nodes were involved then it's got to be curtains and then I found out two out of twelve lymph nodes were involved and that was good news, the first good news I'd had. I could then develop a positive attitude which was what I did, followed by radiotherapy, and chemotherapy and the full works. Tamoxifen. I just really went for it and thought we're going to beat this.*

Jenni: *Now a close friend of yours had had the disease earlier, how much then were you prepared for the kind of treatment you would go through?*

Lesley: *I was very prepared and I was also very well informed about breast cancer because it was a close friend and I'd been very much there with her. The mastectomy was something I came to terms with fairly early on, but the chemotherapy I found terribly difficult. When you're going to the hospital they inject into the vein intravenously this burning substance which smells like bleach. I couldn't even clean the loos afterwards because the smell of bleach took me back to those hospital rooms. The only way I coped with that was thinking if this was happening to my child, if I was taking my child in for doses of chemotherapy I would wish it was happening to me ... so I told myself I ... was going in for them and that is how I got in each week.*

Jenni: *Now you have three young children, how have you approached telling them about your illness and about the operation?*

Lesley: *We've told them all about it. They saw the mastectomy very early on, they saw the scar and were terribly impressed by it as children are. I had a big plaster so I was a bit of a hero, but things changed a year later when I discovered I had secondary cancer: distant metastases of the lungs. I knew I was coping with a terminal illness and then what do you tell the children? We waited then very much for it to come from them and, after a lot of treatment going into hospital every two weeks for chest drains, my son asked me if I was going to die and I said I probably was.*

Jenni: *And how did he deal with that?*

Lesley: *He asked what would happen if Daddy died as well and I said that Grandma and Granddad would look after him and he said, 'Don't be silly they're so old they haven't got long to go'. So then I pointed out there were lots of friends and aunts and uncles that would help out and he seemed fairly happy with that.*

Jenni: *What have you done to prepare them for the future?*

Lesley: *I've written three books, one for each of them, which ranges from diary to fiction. This is partly written to them now as one would write to a child and partly written ... as ... one would write to an adult. So they chop and change quite a bit, they fill in all the details that I know my husband John will never* remember, like when they first learned to crawl and when they first learned to walk and when they lost their first teeth and that sort of thing. Apart from that it goes on into a fictional world of a family with no mother.

Jenni: *Now you've also thrown yourself into a lot of hard work for a charity called Breakthrough. In fact you did very soon after you'd had the mastectomy. Why did you push yourself into a public life?*

Lesley: *Because there was an awful lot of anger deep inside and it was either going to destroy me and I was going to go under or I had to get it out and direct it and focus it. When I was first diagnosed with breast cancer, my friends were more horrified by my mastectomy than they ever were by the fact I had cancer. The loss of a breast – although one would have preferred to have kept it – at the expense of my life was nothing and I really feel all the time we're so concerned with the mastectomy and the modification in surgery and I know this has certain psycho-sexual implications but it's mortality rates that concern me and how many women are dying.*

Jenni: *Your husband John, what about you and he, how have you been able to prepare for your death?*

Lesley: *We've always been terribly open about it and it's a very difficult thing … it's taking every day as it comes, making time for ourselves because that's terribly important … giving him the freedom to live a life after my death. This terrible lack of control after dying is something I find terribly difficult. I like to think I'll be there somewhere just giving people a bit of advice – so I write all that down and instructions for my funeral and instructions for life ever after and what to do about the children's schooling and how to tell the girls about having periods and how to explain sex to the children, and even to the extent of filling the freezer so that if it happened suddenly they'd have something to eat for a few months afterwards.*

Jenni: *Of all the things we've talked about, you're working extremely hard to spread the word about breast cancer. What is the message you most want people to hear?*

Lesley: *Women do survive breast cancer but a lot of women die from it … I want people to work towards finding a cure.*

chapter 11

nine months: pregnancy & childbirth

Lise, 38: The most amazing moment of the whole nine months is the first time you hear the heartbeat. It is astounding. The second was the time I heard a hiccup.

Martha, 31: *You could see a heartbeat, it was like a pulse of light in the scan and that was pretty amazing ... it sort of makes life real ... it's one of those things you can't believe has happened to you. It's like winning the lottery.*

Anna, 27: *The first feeling, I was in the kitchen washing up the plates and ... this whole sort of fluttering took over inside my tummy. The kicks came later.*

Amy, 30: *All goes well on the baby front, but each week is totally unpredictable. This week for the first time I have been famished all the time. And the baby must be sitting right on my bladder because I'm peeing every half hour practically. The things women put their bodies through!*

Lise, 38: *My husband and I haven't had a fight in nine months. The hormones have done me wonders. Never lost my cool over nine months.*

Pregnancy ought to be a happy and positive experience. It is not an illness, yet over the last few decades childbirth has been treated like one. After the war, women were told the only safe delivery is a hospital delivery. Having a baby became more like having an operation. Natural childbirths fell and caesareans went up. Midwives lost their skills and status and doctors took over. Many antenatal clinics turned into impersonal factories and some still are.

Sarah, 28, is seven months pregnant with her first baby: *I had a scan a couple of weeks ago and you're lying on the table and this lady just pulled back the curtain, made a few notes and went away. She didn't even say hello.*

The last fifty years, however, have also seen childbirth become safer for both mother and baby. One hundred years ago 150 babies died for every 1000 births, now it is down to about six per 1000 live births. Women, of course, want to retain low-risk childbirth, but they also want the personal care of midwives and to avoid unnecessary technological intervention. A debate continues to rage over how best to do this. In support of this campaign, the Department of Health launched 'Changing Childbirth' in 1995, an initiative to increase women's involvement in decisions about their own pregnancies and deliveries. It has led to a more midwife-led service, more choice in antenatal care and delivery and a move towards all women being in charge of their own notes during pregnancy.

nine months: pregnancy & childbirth

UK Baby Statistics

- In 1996, 35 per cent of babies were born outside of marriage. In 1961, just 6 per cent of babies were born to unmarried women.
- In 1994, 37,100 women had their fourth – or more – child, while in 1961 more than three times as many women – 124,800 – were having four, five or six children.
- In 1997, for the first time, the average age of the first-time mum topped thirty.
- The average number for a family in the sixties was 2.4 children. Now it is 1.88 children.
- At birth, according to 1996 UK figures, a baby girl is expected to live eighty years. In 1961 her life expectancy was just 73.8 years. Women are expected to live five years longer than men.

XX or XY?

Menstruating women usually produce one egg per cycle (see Chapter 2). Eggs only carry the X chromosome. Each sperm carries either an X chromosome or a Y chromosome. So the sperm decides the sex. When the egg and the sperm meet the resulting fertilized egg contains either XY chromosomes which develop into a boy baby or XX chromosomes which produce a girl. Fraternal twins may develop if a woman produces two eggs in one cycle. Identical twins develop when the fertilized egg splits into two.

There are more boy babies born than girl babies. In 1996 in the UK there were 376,000 boys compared to 357,000 girls. But by the time we reach forty-five there is a switch over with women becoming the greater number. By the time we reach eighty-five there are twice as many women as men.

In this chapter we examine the main features of pregnancy and childbirth. We review the tests on offer, women's feelings about them, the thrills of impending motherhood, and the range of deliveries women choose. We also look at the gloom of postnatal depression and the trauma of miscarriage.

Getting Ready for Pregnancy

If you are planning a pregnancy, and most women do plan, there are things you can do to try to prepare your body and mind, and to reduce the risk of complications.

- Check your immunity to rubella infection (German measles). You were probably immunized as a child or teenager, but it is a good idea to have a blood test before you get pregnant to find out for sure. Many rashes thought to be rubella are, in fact, other infections so knowing you have immunity will bring peace of mind. Having rubella in the first four

Best Time to Conceive

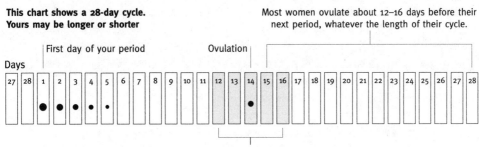

**This chart shows a 28-day cycle.
Yours may be longer or shorter**

Most women ovulate about 12–16 days before their
next period, whatever the length of their cycle.

First day of your period

Ovulation

Days

| 27 | 28 | 1 | 2 | 3 | 4 | 5 | 6 | 7 | 8 | 9 | 10 | 11 | 12 | 13 | 14 | 15 | 16 | 17 | 18 | 19 | 20 | 21 | 22 | 23 | 24 | 25 | 26 | 27 | 28 |

You are most likely to conceive if you have intercourse around this time

months of pregnancy may seriously damage the foetus causing cataracts, mental retardation and deafness. You are routinely tested for rubella immunity once your pregnancy is confirmed but it is then too late, as the immunization could damage the foetus.

- Avoid drugs and medicines where possible even before you try to get pregnant. If you must take medicine check out the possible effects on the foetus should you become pregnant. If you are on long-term treatment for depression, epilepsy, diabetes or any other medical condition, ask your doctor whether you should change drugs.

- Stop or reduce smoking (see pages 21–3). Thirty per cent of all women smoke, even though they know the long-term risks. Smoking also affects the developing baby. Babies born to smoking mothers are more likely to be underweight, premature, and prone to infections. The best time to quit is before you become pregnant. That way you avoid the added stress of struggling with nicotine withdrawal as you adjust to being pregnant. You will also enjoy the benefits of your healthier body while you try to conceive.

- Make sure you eat enough folic acid either through your diet or by taking folic acid supplements. You can buy folic acid at the chemist or get it on prescription from your doctor. Folic acid deficiency is linked to spina bifida – when the spine and nerves in the baby's back do not develop properly. You should take 400 micrograms (or 0.4 milligrams) of folic acid each day once you start trying to get pregnant, and continue until you are twelve weeks pregnant. It might be easier to take the supplements, though you can get enough by eating plenty of leafy green vegetables such as Brussels sprouts or spinach every day. If you have already had a baby with spina bifida or are taking treatment for epilepsy you will need to take even more folic acid and you should discuss this with your doctor.

- It is safe to drink a small amount of alcohol during pregnancy, though the exact safe upper limit is unknown. It is recommended to drink no more than four units per week (see page 24 for guidance on units of alcohol) and avoid alcoholic binges as the developing foetus can be seriously damaged by large amounts of alcohol.

nine months: pregnancy & childbirth

- Toxoplasmosis is a relatively rare infection in this country, which if caught during pregnancy can damage the developing baby. It is found in some cats' faeces which then get into the garden soil. Avoid emptying cat litter trays when pregnant and use rubber gloves when gardening. At present, pregnant women in the UK are not automatically screened for it. If you are particularly worried about it ask your doctor for a blood test or contact the Toxoplasmosis Trust (see Useful Addresses on page 390).
- If you are worried about an illness in your family which might be inherited talk to your doctor and get referred to a geneticist for further advice.

But even with all the best-laid plans, you still cannot dictate when you will get pregnant.

> **Lynn, 37:** *I'm used to controlling every aspect of my life so I thought I could control when I had a baby as well and postpone it until I got settled in my career. I decided the best time to have babies was when I was thirty-two or thirty-three. Unfortunately it didn't happen as early as I'd planned.*

Disabled Mum-to-be

> **Michele Wates, Author of** *Disabled Parents, Dispelling the Myths.* **Michele is a mum and she has multiple sclerosis:** *The interesting thing is I've been at every stage of it from a very slight disability to being in a wheelchair and I've had the whole range of being a mother in these stages. When I considered having a child I had to take into account that I had a progressive condition, I had to look ahead at all of that in deciding on whether or not to have a second child.*

Michele did go ahead. She triumphed with the discovery that the best kind of motherhood is one that asks for help. Collaboration makes it not only do-able but richer:

> **Michele:** *The truth of parenting is the more you share it the better it is for the adults and the children which is what you see in many more tribal societies. Another important part of all this is there has to be a sense of reciprocity and for some disabled parents that can be difficult because you feel you're not in a position strictly speaking to reciprocate the favours that are done for you.*

Disabled and able women alike report that pregnancy and motherhood are made easier when we accept help. If you cannot reciprocate in kind, try to think of what else you have to offer. And when you meet a disabled mum-to-be, keep in mind what Michele told us: The first thing a pregnant disabled woman often hears when she announces her news is, 'are you sure you can cope?' People may be well meaning but this question is undermining, especially when we hear it over and over again.

How Do You Know You Are Pregnant?

Martha, 31, mother of nine-month-old Madeleine: *My periods are down to the minute practically so a couple of hours after I missed that period I knew, and we were trying too, but I didn't really believe it and on the Sunday my breasts were really tender but I still didn't say anything to Shane. Then I bought a pregnancy test on the Monday and came home from work and took the test and passed!*

Missing a period is the first sign of pregnancy for most women. Nausea and sickness in the morning or at other times of the day, tender breasts, tiredness, needing to urinate more often, increased vaginal discharge, going off certain foods like coffee and fatty food, and a strange metallic taste, may all be signs that you are pregnant. Some women just know they are pregnant while others are unaware of any changes in their body.

Martha: *The only thing I went off was olives. Olives tasted like aluminium foil. It was strange, that awful sensation ... Olives are fine now.*

Anna, 27: *You become really protective about everything. You just sort of know you're carrying a baby. Everything you eat you want to make sure it's the best for her or for him. You're really conscious of what you put into it and being in a room which is smoky you're just conscious. Medicines, I just thought – cut it out – on everything. If I had a headache I wouldn't take anything. I was really conscious, maybe too much.*

It is often a mixture of emotions that flood in on discovering you are pregnant: pleasure, anxiety, fear and excitement. Even if the baby is planned you may have swings of mood and wonder if you are doing the right thing.

Your Due Date

January	1 2 3 4 5 6 7 8 9 10 11 12 13 14 15 16 17 18 19 20 21 22 23 24 25 26 27 28 29 30 31	January
October	**8 9 10 11 12 13 14 15 16 17 18 19 20 21 22 23 24 25 26 27 28 29 30 31 1 2 3 4 5 6 7**	**November**
February	1 2 3 4 5 6 7 8 9 10 11 12 13 14 15 16 17 18 19 20 21 22 23 24 25 26 27 28	February
November	**8 9 10 11 12 13 14 15 16 17 18 19 20 21 22 23 24 25 26 27 28 29 30 1 2 3 4 5**	**December**
March	1 2 3 4 5 6 7 8 9 10 11 12 13 14 15 16 17 18 19 20 21 22 23 24 25 26 27 28 29 30 31	March
December	**6 7 8 9 10 11 12 13 14 15 16 17 18 19 20 21 22 23 24 25 26 27 28 29 30 31 1 2 3 4 5**	**January**
April	1 2 3 4 5 6 7 8 9 10 11 12 13 14 15 16 17 18 19 20 21 22 23 24 25 26 27 28 29 30	April
January	**6 7 8 9 10 11 12 13 14 15 16 17 18 19 20 21 22 23 24 25 26 27 28 29 30 31 1 2 3 4**	**February**
May	1 2 3 4 5 6 7 8 9 10 11 12 13 14 15 16 17 18 19 20 21 22 23 24 25 26 27 28 29 30 31	May
February	**5 6 7 8 9 10 11 12 13 14 15 16 17 18 19 20 21 22 23 24 25 26 27 28 1 2 3 4 5 6 7**	**March**
June	1 2 3 4 5 6 7 8 9 10 11 12 13 14 15 16 17 18 19 20 21 22 23 24 25 26 27 28 29 30	June
March	**8 9 10 11 12 13 14 15 16 17 18 19 20 21 22 23 24 25 26 27 28 29 30 31 1 2 3 4 5 6**	**April**
July	1 2 3 4 5 6 7 8 9 10 11 12 13 14 15 16 17 18 19 20 21 22 23 24 25 26 27 28 29 30 31	July
April	**7 8 9 10 11 12 13 14 15 16 17 18 19 20 21 22 23 24 25 26 27 28 29 30 1 2 3 4 5 6 7**	**May**
August	1 2 3 4 5 6 7 8 9 10 11 12 13 14 15 16 17 18 19 20 21 22 23 24 25 26 27 28 29 30 31	August
May	**8 9 10 11 12 13 14 15 16 17 18 19 20 21 22 23 24 25 26 27 28 29 30 31 1 2 3 4 5 6 7**	**June**
September	1 2 3 4 5 6 7 8 9 10 11 12 13 14 15 16 17 18 19 20 21 22 23 24 25 26 27 28 29 30	September
June	**8 9 10 11 12 13 14 15 16 17 18 19 20 21 22 23 24 25 26 27 28 29 30 1 2 3 4 5 6 7**	**July**
October	1 2 3 4 5 6 7 8 9 10 11 12 13 14 15 16 17 18 19 20 21 22 23 24 25 26 27 28 29 30 31	October
July	**8 9 10 11 12 13 14 15 16 17 18 19 20 21 22 23 24 25 26 27 28 29 30 31 1 2 3 4 5 6 7**	**August**
November	1 2 3 4 5 6 7 8 9 10 11 12 13 14 15 16 17 18 19 20 21 22 23 24 25 26 27 28 29 30	November
August	**8 9 10 11 12 13 14 15 16 17 18 19 20 21 22 23 24 25 26 27 28 29 30 31 1 2 3 4 5 6**	**September**
December	1 2 3 4 5 6 7 8 9 10 11 12 13 14 15 16 17 18 19 20 21 22 23 24 25 26 27 28 29 30 31	December
September	**7 8 9 10 11 12 13 14 15 16 17 18 19 20 21 22 23 24 25 26 27 28 29 30 1 2 3 4 5 6 7**	**October**

This chart will help you work out your expected date of delivery. Pick out the date of the first day of your last period from the non-bold lines. The date your baby is due is immediately underneath in bold.

Pregnancy Tests

Pregnancy tests measure the level of the hormone, beta human chorionic gonadotrophin (B–hCG), in your urine which rises during pregnancy. They are usually reliable and you can test from the first day of a missed period, that is about two weeks after conception. If you think you are pregnant but test negative, try repeating it one week later as the test can occasionally give a false negative result. You can buy a kit at the chemist or have a free test at the doctor's surgery or a family-planning clinic. Do-it-yourself kits are the same as those used by GPs and just as accurate.

What to Do When You Are Pregnant

Once you know you are pregnant, see your doctor who will arrange various checks for you and refer you to a midwife. The Health Education Authority produces a comprehensive book about pregnancy which is available free for every mother in her first pregnancy. It also includes information on the grants and benefits to which you may be entitled. The book is available from your GP, midwife or health visitor.

Sarah, 28, seven months pregnant: *Take it easy. Don't try and be the first lady who just sails through it with no help from anybody. I thought I'd be one of these very independent ladies who would do everything exactly the same and I wouldn't let it affect me. Take the help. Anything: doing the shopping, doing a bit of ironing.*

Food

Marina: *It's incredibly confusing, all this modern dietary information ... you're supposed to ... give up eating anything remotely pleasurable before you even get pregnant. You have to stop drinking, give up smoking, take masses of vitamin supplements, drink three litres of water a day, run a mile before your All Bran, and try to remain emotionally stable, while looking like Pavarotti in a frock.*

It is not quite that bad. There is no 'correct' diet for pregnancy but there are certain foods to avoid. Soft cheeses such as brie or goat's cheese – especially those made with unpasteurized milk – may cause an infection with the bacteria listeria which sometimes causes miscarriage. Foods containing a lot of vitamin A such as carrots and liver can also harm foetal organs. There is some evidence that caffeine may lower your baby's birth weight.

It is good to eat plenty of fresh fruit and vegetables, starchy foods like rice, bread, pasta and cereals, lean meat, fish, beans and eggs (which should be thoroughly cooked to avoid the risk of salmonella infection), some dairy products such as milk and yoghurt. Cut down on sugar and fatty foods.

Eating for two is nonsense. Most of us get enough vitamins and minerals in our normal diet to sustain a healthy pregnancy, but if you are worried take a supplement designed for pregnant women. Whatever you do, this is not the time to start a weight-reduction regime. Also take extra care when preparing some foods. Cook meat thoroughly and wash fruit, vegetables and salads. This helps reduce the small risk of infection from toxoplasmosis (see page 266).

Everyone will give you advice about what to do and especially what not to do. Keep things in perspective. Most women do not have problems during pregnancy and most women have healthy babies. Some advice will be helpful while some will worry you unnecessarily. Remember it is your pregnancy, so listen to people whose opinions you trust.

Exercise

Lise, 38, and due any day now: *I went to the gym the first six months, and the last two months I did swimming, which is the best thing. If I was to give advice, swim. You feel great in the pool because you don't feel the weight. I have a feeling that the movements of swimming which stretch your whole body are good for the muscles that eventually give birth.*

Exercise is good for you all the way through pregnancy. The fitter you can keep during pregnancy, the more stamina you are likely to have during labour. Do whatever you feel comfortable doing. If you are a runner, run. If you never exercise normally this is not the time to become a marathon runner. Even skiing, aerobics and cycling should be OK if you are used to doing them. Gentle exercises such as swimming or walking are good if you are not a regular exerciser. If you enjoy it, it will decrease stress. There is no evidence that exercise is associated with problems in pregnancy or an increased risk of miscarriage.

Antenatal Classes

Antenatal classes provide an opportunity to meet other expectant women and couples as well as to learn about pregnancy and birth. NHS classes are usually run by midwives or health visitors. Private classes, for which you pay, are organized by tutors specially trained by the National Childbirth Trust. In some areas there are also yoga and other exercise classes for pregnant women. Check out what is available in your neighbourhood.

Antenatal Check-ups

Routine tests and regular check-ups are available to you during your pregnancy. They can help spot trouble, but it is also reassuring just to hear everything is fine. Most of the check-ups will be at your GP's surgery but you may need to be seen at the hospital at some point. Most pregnant women, provided the pregnancy progresses smoothly, have contact with a midwife every four weeks, then every fortnight once they reach twenty-eight weeks of pregnancy, and finally every week for the last month. Antenatal checks are designed to follow the baby's development. They also provide an opportunity to ask questions, discuss worries and make plans for the birth. The National Audit Office recently claimed that ten million pounds is being wasted on unnecessary checks in pregnancy. But many women disagree, relying on them for reassurance. Some doctors are also concerned that fewer checks will mean warning signs of eclampsia will be missed (see page 271).

Weight

Most women gain between 10 to 12.5 kilos or 22 to 28 pounds during pregnancy. Some women have their weight checked regularly during antenatal checks whilst others will only be weighed at the beginning of pregnancy. Some doctors do not think there is any need for regular checks. Weight gain in pregnancy varies tremendously.

Andrew, 39: *We have a small house with three floors. It's a skinny house and it's 120 years old. Vicki put on 70 pounds. She weighed 200 pounds by the end of the pregnancy. She used to do aerobics on the top floor and I used to sit downstairs and shudder when she did them. I thought she would come through the ceiling and the bedroom floor would give way underneath when she walked. You couldn't tell her ankles from her thighs. It was really something.*

Vicki gave birth to healthy twins and regained her figure, but if you do gain too much weight it can be difficult to lose.

Blood Pressure

This needs to be checked every four to six weeks in the early stages of pregnancy and more frequently as the pregnancy advances. During pregnancy blood pressure is usually between 90/50 and 125/80 (see page 385). A rise in blood pressure to 140/90 in the last three months, for example, can be the first sign of pre-eclampsia, a condition which can lead to problems for the baby and the mother if it is not treated. Eclampsia is a dangerous type of raised blood pressure which infrequently occurs in pregnancy. Pre-eclampsia is the first early sign of this and can be treated to prevent eclampsia developing.

Urine

This is routinely checked for sugar, protein and infection. The presence of sugar may indicate the development of diabetes in pregnancy. This can be treated by a change in your diet or taking insulin. Protein or albumin in the urine may indicate pre-eclampsia if it is associated with a rise in blood pressure. It can also mean you have an infection which can be treated with antibiotics. Check with your doctor that those prescribed are safe to take if you are pregnant. Tetracycline, for instance, stains the baby's teeth.

nine months: pregnancy & childbirth

Routine Antenatal Blood Tests

There are several routine blood tests usually done in early pregnancy. They check for anaemia, syphilis (see page 193) and hepatitis B. At present some clinics screen pregnant women for the HIV infection, but tests are anonymous and the results are not linked to your name. This is to try to find out how common the virus is in the general population. If you want to be tested for HIV ask for it to be done. Your blood is also screened for the blood diseases sickle cell anaemia and thalassaemia and for rhesus antibodies and rubella immunity (see pages 264–5). Sickle cell anaemia is an inherited disease of the red cells which mainly occurs in people of African origin. Thalassaemia is also inherited, and is mainly found in the blood of people of Mediterranean origin. There are other tests which are not routine but may be offered in your area.

Optional Tests

There is no test to guarantee a perfectly healthy baby but most babies are born perfectly healthy: 97 per cent of UK newborns are normal. Only 2 per cent arrive with a serious problem and 1 per cent have a problem that can be at least partially fixed. As good as the odds are though it is very common to worry that something is not right, or will go wrong.

> **Janet:** *I was really nervous I was going to miscarry the whole time because of the previous miscarriage but once I got to thirty weeks I started to really enjoy it. I felt brilliant and had lots of energy.*

There is an array of tests for abnormalities. But rarely is any test 100 per cent accurate. And there are enough tests available to make it difficult to decide which ones, if any, to have. Furthermore, what the NHS provides depends on where you live. Each test answers only a limited number of questions and some of them only give you an idea of the risk of your baby having an abnormality rather than a yes or no answer. There are tests for structural abnormalities (e.g. spina bifida – see page 275), heart problems, chromosomal abnormalities (e.g. Down's syndrome), and tests for some genetically transmitted diseases such as haemophilia, muscular dystrophy and cystic fibrosis.

Anna, 27: *I arrived at the hospital for my first appointment, my booking-in appointment. The first thing they hand you is the Down's syndrome leaflet about the tests and about Down's syndrome in general and what it involves. Me and my husband decided we didn't want to have it. If the baby did have Down's or was mentally handicapped ... I knew I wouldn't have an abortion anyway so I couldn't see why we should worry for the next nine months so I had a trouble-free, really relaxing pregnancy. I was very relaxed throughout. I have this sort of feeling the more you worry about things, it's worse for you. I think you get more problems when you're under stress.*

Martha, 31: *The only test I had was the one they take to find out your odds for Down's. My odds were one in 350. That's the only test I agreed to. It was a tough decision because I'm Catholic and my husband's Catholic. I would not have terminated the pregnancy. I guess it was to prepare myself mentally for every possibility. If they said it's one in a 100 chance at least I could have prepared for that and maybe taken some counselling before.*

Before making a decision to have any test make sure you understand the implications.

Ultrasound Scans

Most pregnant women will have at least one ultrasound scan. Some doctors think they should be done routinely, whilst others believe they are not needed unless there is a specific concern. Many women want a scan for reassurance that everything is alright, and also for the thrill and pleasure of seeing a picture of the baby.

Lynn, 37: *I felt anxious in case they found the baby was dead or abnormal. Although I tried hard to see the baby and follow what they were pointing out, I found it hard to visualize and interpret. It wasn't that obvious. But it was very reassuring once they said it was normal, and lovely to have the photo afterwards.*

An ultrasound scan performed at about eight weeks tells whether there is a live foetus which is especially reassuring if you have had bleeding early in pregnancy (see page 291) and are worried you may have miscarried. Once a heartbeat is heard at about six weeks there is a 96 per cent chance that the pregnancy will continue unless you have a history of miscarriage. A dating scan done between eight to twelve weeks can accurately assess how far the pregnancy has gone. It also reveals whether you have twins.

nine months: pregnancy & childbirth

Andrew, 39: *She went for her three-month check and I was sitting at work and she telephoned and said, 'I'm at the doctor's, are you sitting down?' and I said, 'Yes, but I know you're pregnant'. Then she told me it was twins and I said, 'I can't believe it, oh my God ...'. I guess I turned a different colour and I got off the phone and everyone said, 'What's wrong?' and I said, 'Vicki's pregnant with twins' and everyone just mobbed me ... I decided I should go home and I felt like I was going to faint or something like that ... But it was great, just great. Telling everybody was so much fun. I told my parents and they just sat there stunned.*

A dating scan is also useful if you are uncertain about the date of your last period or your periods are infrequent. However, it is still too early at this point to detect most foetal abnormalities. Later ultrasound scans for foetal anomalies are done at eighteen to twenty weeks of pregnancy when the heart, kidneys and other organs can be seen in greater detail. But sometimes needless anxiety is caused by the suspicion of a problem in what may well turn out to be a healthy baby. These scans can also tell the sex of the baby since a boy's penis can usually be seen, although sometimes mistakes are made in interpretation.

Lise, 38: *I just can't imagine why you wouldn't want to know. People say I want the surprise at the end but there's enough of a surprise at the end. My God, it's a huge moment! And you're able to prepare yourself. I'm really glad I've known it was a boy because I grew up in a family of girls and I think if I had found out on birth day I would have been shocked. I don't know any little boys. I've never babysat a little boy so I've had to sort of think about little boys. You really do want to meet the little guy, that's the overall feeling right now.*

Pam: *I would never want to know the sex beforehand. It would take the excitement away, like choosing your own Christmas present.*

Some clinics now use ultrasound to detect some chromosomal abnormalities. Studies are in progress to assess the accuracy of scans at twelve to thirteen weeks to detect Down's syndrome by measuring the nuchal fold, the neck of the foetus. More training and equipment are needed to make this available throughout the UK. Ultrasound appears to be safe for women and their babies, but we do not know the long-term risks – if there are any. Research shows that more left-handed babies are born to women who have had multiple scans. Some countries, like France, scan more routinely than others. Many doctors in the UK want to limit the number of scans. For some women there may be very good medical reasons to have a scan or even a series of scans to check that the baby is growing normally, but try to avoid unnecessary ones.

Beverley Beech, Honorary Chair of AIMS, the Association for Improvements in Maternity Services, and co-author of the report *Ultrasound, Unsound*: *Ultrasound is the biggest unevaluated medical experiment of all time, and it has been used in an uncontrolled manner on the whole population, and it should be restricted to those who really need it.*

Peter Sanders, Obstetrician and Author of *Your Pregnancy Month by Month*: *We live in the era of the unborn child. We can diagnose all sorts of things, we're making a lot of problems for ourselves. Wonderful ultrasound, wonderful testing ... but so often you do a routine test, someone sees something, and the operator doesn't even know whether it's significant or not because we're not that far advanced ... and then there's anxiety for the next month or six weeks.*

But there is no doubt that for some mothers and babies detecting problems early using ultrasound makes all the difference. It can mean that if necessary, a baby can be delivered early and treatment started. Sometimes operations can even be carried out to correct an abnormality while the baby is still in the womb.

Alison: *I had ultrasound like a lot of people just to really see my baby ... It revealed that my baby had a post-urethral valve – this is an eighteen-week scan – and that valve could eventually have caused some kidney damage but ... I was induced, he was born five weeks early, and avoided any long-term damage to the kidneys.*

AFP Blood Test (Alpha Fetoprotein Test)

This is offered free at sixteen weeks to all pregnant women. Most mothers who have a high AFP count will have a normal baby but a high count may indicate that the baby has spina bifida, and a scan or amniocentesis (see page 277) will be offered to exclude this possibility. A low AFP level in a woman over twenty-eight years may mean an increased risk of Down's syndrome.

Fiona, 29, and nine weeks pregnant with her second child: *I was in two minds whether to have the tests mainly because I'm Catholic and the attitude seems to be amongst the medical profession that it's only worth having the test if you're going to consider terminating if there's any abnormalities. My attitude was that though it's difficult to say until you're in that position I didn't think I'd want a termination in that event but I'd like to be forewarned and prepared ... if there's any possibility of say Down's syndrome then I'd like to be aware of that before the baby was born ...*

There should not be any pressure on you to have a termination if you are found to be carrying a Down's baby.

Triple Test

This is called a triple test because it measures three chemicals – AFP (see page 275), oestriol, and HCG (human chorionic gonadotrophin) – in the blood. It is a test taken as close to fifteen weeks of pregnancy as possible and this is most accurately estimated if an early ultrasound scan has also been done. The risk of having a Down's baby is calculated from the levels of the three chemicals but, again, this is only a calculation of lower or higher risk. With a higher-risk reading, a subsequent amniocentesis test (see page 277) can confirm virtually 100 per cent whether the baby has Down's or not. A low risk means it is unlikely the baby will have Down's, but it is not a guarantee. A higher risk is considered as greater than a one in 250 chance of the baby having Down's. If the risk is lower than one in 250 no further investigations are recommended. Scientists hope to develop a definite Down's test soon. Whether you are offered the triple test on the NHS depends on where you live. It costs about £18 to have one privately. The problem with the test is that it is not a yes or no test and the results can cause unnecessary anxiety. Jane had one, but she would never have another.

> **Jane, 34:** *We went off on holiday and when we got back there were about four really frantic messages from my midwife on my answer phone ... obviously something had gone wrong ... she told me our test had indicated I had a one in eight chance of Joseph having Down's syndrome. We didn't know he was Joseph then, all we knew is that our unborn baby had this very very high chance of having Down's syndrome ... I just cried and cried and cried. We were devastated both of us ... we saw the registrar ... and it was a youngish guy we saw and ... he said the situation was very serious, I had to have an amniocentesis to discover for certain whether or not the baby had Down's. He said something really callous ... I was at the 'earlier end of having to have an amnio' ... and he said that was a good thing. He said if a termination is necessary it can be that much sooner. We hadn't got our heads round this at all and he was talking termination ... I went down for the amnio I think a couple of days later ... we both distanced ourselves from the baby. We stopped using the pet name and started calling it 'it', and referring to it as something that might end ... it was an emotional shift away from the pregnancy.*

Before having a triple test consider whether you want to know the risk, and what you would do if you find your baby is at risk. Then think through whether you would want to proceed with an amniocentesis test (see page 277) and what you would do if your baby has Down's. Jane opted for amniocentesis.

Jane, 34: *We decided for sure at one point that if the baby had Down's we would keep it, and then a couple of days later we agreed that we wouldn't necessarily keep it ... our family life completely turned on its head. The awful thing about an amnio is you have to wait for the results and this was all happening in the run up to Christmas ... so we were in this awful limbo. Then on the 23rd December I had a telephone call from the hospital and it was this blessed woman ringing to say the results were through and your baby's fine. I said, 'You're sure you're talking to the right person?' and she said not to worry ... I said, 'Brian, the baby's fine,' and he sat down on the bottom step and he just cried and cried ... It was really moving. The relief was just phenomenal.*

Amniocentesis

Amniocentesis is usually performed at about sixteen weeks with a local anaesthetic. It involves putting a needle through the wall of the abdomen to extract a sample of amniotic fluid which surrounds the baby. An ultrasound scan is done at the same time so that the needle does not go into the wrong place, harming the baby. The fluid is sent to a laboratory to be tested for spina bifida. Some cells are also grown so the chromosomes can be tested for Down's syndrome, a process which can take up to three weeks. This test also confirms the sex of the baby, which is important to know if there is a problem with inherited diseases which only occur in one sex. You can ask for the baby's sex to be kept a secret if you prefer. Before you decide to have an amniocentesis test you need to be aware that there is a risk of miscarriage in the procedure with one in every 100 tests resulting in the loss of the baby, regardless of whether the baby is normal or not.

Chorionic Villus Sampling (CVS)

This test analyses a tiny sample of placental tissue to test for Down's syndrome and is particularly useful in spotting certain inherited diseases such as sickle cell anaemia or thalassaemia (see page 272). The test can be done very early, at ten to eleven weeks. The test usually involves passing a small tube through the vagina and cervix into the developing placenta known as chorionic tissue. The test result is almost immediate and if there is something wrong you can, if it is your choice, have an earlier termination (see Chapter 9). But CVS has a higher miscarriage rate of 2 to 3 per cent. CVS can also cause facial deformities in some babies. It does not test for spina bifida.

nine months: pregnancy & childbirth

Side Effects of Pregnancy

> **Anna, 27:** *As soon as I found out I was pregnant I went out and bought stretch mark prevention cream from Selfridges and I put that on every time after I had a bath and applied it to my belly area and I was very lucky, it worked for me anyway. I read a lot about it beforehand, I got my magazines, and books, and I read about what happens to your body and I tried creams and it worked. They say it works for some women and some women it doesn't.*

Some women really do bloom during pregnancy, but even the best of pregnancies come with side effects.

Stretch marks depend on the type of skin you have. Some women have none, others have lots of them. There is no evidence, apart from women's testimonials, that any of the creams marketed to prevent or stop them actually work, but nor are they likely to do you or your baby any harm.

Backache, haemorrhoids (piles), indigestion and urinary incontinence are all common problems in pregnancy. Varicose veins often develop too. The increased oestrogen levels during pregnancy dilate the walls of the veins. The extra weight we carry is also a factor in varicose veins.

Insomnia can also be a nuisance. Sometimes towards the end of pregnancy it is linked to the difficulty of finding a comfortable position in bed. If you are used to sleeping on your front, being nine months pregnant makes this difficult. Try lying on your side with an extra pillow under the bump.

Sickness

Most women experience some sort of nausea or sickness. It may arrive as soon as you get pregnant and it usually starts to decrease at about three months. For some women it is morning sickness, for others it carries on all day. There is no easy cure, though frequently eating small amounts of food sometimes helps. You can take anti-sickness tablets if the nausea and sickness are very bad. In a small minority of women the sickness is so bad they become dehydrated and need to go into hospital. Some people believe diet is a factor.

Nicky Wesson, Author of *Morning Sickness: A Comprehensive Guide to Causes and Treatments*: *In this country people suffer from it a lot, but there was a survey done of eighty-three different societies right round the world covering the entire globe, and interestingly in quite a few of those societies they didn't know what it was, they didn't have it at all. And it seemed that the reason was because of their diet ... the three things that people ate in the societies that didn't get it were: green vegetables – quite a high level of those – fats, and maize ... it was vitamin B6 which has been shown to help, but I think it's actually the zinc.*

Incontinence and Cystitis

Women often get symptoms like cystitis, meaning they need to urinate a lot during the first few months of pregnancy because the enlarging uterus puts pressure on the bladder, irritating it. We are also more susceptible to urinary infections during pregnancy. The pelvic muscles also stretch and slacken because of the hormonal changes in pregnancy.

Amy, 30: *I peed a lot. I had to get up a few times during the night to pee and not a great volume but my bladder was just so smushed that I had to keep emptying it. But no leakage ... I was very religious about doing my Kegel exercises [see below] when I was pregnant and even within twelve hours of when she was born I started trying to do those exercises again. And it was a very odd feeling for the first few days after she was born, going to the toilet and realizing I couldn't stop my flow of urine. I would try to contract those muscles and nothing would happen. The pee would just flow out. That was a real shock but very quickly those muscles came back. And I continue to do those Kegel exercises and it seems to have helped because I have never had a problem with leakage.*

Kegel exercises, also known as pelvic floor exercises, help to strengthen the muscles you need to control your bladder. You can do them anywhere without anyone knowing (see page 336 for how to do them). Do these exercises regularly and enjoy the benefits of better bladder control in pregnancy and throughout your life. Incontinence is now called the forgotten epidemic. Childbirth is a major cause but it also happens to many women who have never had a baby. Surveys show that up to one-third of women aged 35 to 44 suffer some incontinence and the exercises can help.

Memory Problems

Some women complain of memory problems during pregnancy whilst others feel their minds sharpen. Some research has shown that brain size in pregnant women decreases, but there is no evidence that brain size itself has anything to do with how well we function.

Where to Have Your Baby

The important thing is to have your baby the way you want to, unless there are medical problems which affect your choice. You can have your baby at home or in a hospital, lying down or squatting. You can ask to have your baby in a pool of water. Your partner can be with you if you want, or you can have a friend. In North America you can hire a labour coach. In the UK, most women have their babies in hospital under the nominal care of an obstetrician, while the midwife plays the main professional role, unless the delivery is complicated. Most of the antenatal care takes place in the community with a midwife and/or a GP.

There are other choices available, but the options open to you will depend on where you live and whether there are any complications in your pregnancy. In some areas obstetric care is organized by small teams of midwives so you get to know them. Obstetricians are then only involved if something goes wrong. Some areas have small maternity hospitals whilst others have GP/midwife units. It is also possible to have a birth at home attended by midwives. Home births have been painted as dangerous, but research shows that this is not the case. Fifty per cent of births in Holland take place at home. Only 2 per cent of UK babies are born at home and some of their mothers have difficulty arranging it. Other women who would like to have a home birth are put off by the difficulties in finding health professionals to help them. Also professionals differ in how they assess the risks involved. If you want to explore the possibilities of having a home birth, talk to the Independent Midwives Association (see Useful Addresses page 390).

Wherever you decide to have your baby, the most important thing is to feel complete trust in your carers.

Labour and the Birth

Fiona, 29: *I had this tremendous satisfaction, look at what we made, look at what we produced. This lovely little human being and she'd just been inside me a little while ago.*

> **Valma, 50:** *I remember when I had Helen I just couldn't wait to have a cup of tea afterwards. I can remember lying on that delivery table and thinking, 'I wish I could have a cup of tea now!'*

The figures for methods of delivery in England for 1994–5 show that 73 per cent of women had their babies vaginally without assistance, 12 per cent needed forceps or a ventouse (vacuum extractor) to help the delivery, and 15 per cent had a caesarean section. The proportions vary depending on whether it is a first or second baby. There is a great variation in the type of pain relief available, should you want it. These include:

- Relaxation and breathing control.
- Breathing nitrous oxide (gas and air).
- 'Tens' machine, a nerve stimulator to increase the body's natural painkillers called endorphins (see page 103).
- Pethidine which is a painkiller given by injection.
- An epidural anaesthetic which is injected into your spinal column and numbs you from the waist down.
- If you have a caesarean section you will need an epidural or general anaesthetic.

> **Lynn, 37:** *I was incredibly lucky to have such a straightforward birth. I'm a wimp when it comes to pain and had lined up an epidural in my mind as the only way to cope with childbirth. I even secretly fancied a caesarean. But when it came to it I found it was really quite manageable until near the end. The first few hours of labour felt like bad period pains but there were gaps between to recover and it was exciting to think the baby was on the way. I found a warm bath helped. I also used a Tens machine fairly early on which I think was beneficial.*

Whichever method you choose, discuss the various options with your carers beforehand. Keep an open mind as pregnancy and birth do not always go according to plan.

There are three stages of labour. They begin when your uterus starts contracting:
- During the first stage your cervix dilates and your baby's head is pushed down into your pelvis.
- The second stage starts when your cervix is fully dilated and your baby is pushed out through your vagina.
- The third stage is after the birth of your baby when your placenta is pushed out through your vagina.

How easily labour proceeds depends on a number of factors – how well your uterus contracts; how well your cervix dilates; whether your baby is being delivered head or bottom (breech) first; how tired you become; whether there are any other medical problems.

Josie: *Because of the earth mother era, I remember not daring to confess to my friends that my baby was delivered with the help of vacuum extraction, which I felt to be my failure and something to be ashamed of. It amazes me now that, even as a doctor, this peer pressure was so strong I didn't have anyone I could really talk to about it.*

Anna, 27: *We had to write up a birth plan and I tried to have it as natural as possible without any medication or pain relief. I managed without and it was about ten hours start to finish ... there was no complication whatever. I had a tape playing in the background throughout.*

Birth Facts You Should Know

A series of booklets have been published about pregnancy and birth based on the best available research evidence. (These booklets are available from Informed Choice – see Useful Addresses on page 390.) Recent research shows:

- If you have someone with you all the time during your labour you are less likely to need painkillers, or a delivery helped by forceps or ventouse, and are less likely to have a caesarean section. You may also be less likely to get postnatal depression.
- Being as upright as possible – walking, squatting, sitting – can make labour shorter and lessen the pain.
- Being upright during the second stage of labour lessens the chance of needing forceps, a ventouse or a caesarean. It also helps with the pain, decreases the chance of infection in the uterus, or of tearing the vagina, but you are likely to lose more blood if you use a birthing stool and it also increases your chance of a tear of the labia (the lips of the vagina).
- If your baby appears bottom first (breech position) instead of head first (cephalic position), at thirty-seven weeks of pregnancy, the baby is the wrong way round for an easy delivery. If nothing is done to correct this and your baby starts being delivered via your vagina, you have a 50 per cent chance of ending up with a caesarean section. No one actually knows whether having a caesarean is safer for the breech baby than having a vaginal birth.
- If your baby is breech, the doctor can usually turn your baby round by pushing with his or her hands on the outside of your tummy. This is successful in 70 per cent of cases,

although the success rate depends on the skill of the person doing it. It also decreases the chances of you needing a caesarean by over a half.

- One in four women has an epidural. This is the most effective form of pain relief available during labour and there appear to be no long-term effects on the baby. But labour can take longer, you are more likely to need drugs to speed up your labour and you are three times more likely to need forceps or a ventouse. You are also more likely to need a caesarean.
- Heavy bleeding and haemorrhaging after birth is less likely if you have an injection of syntometrine as the baby is born.

Lynn, 37: *I needed a wheelchair to get into the delivery suite because I couldn't walk. The midwife examined me and to my amazement and relief said the head was just visible ... The pain was very intense and all I really wanted was for the baby to come out as quickly as possible. I found the midwife's calm advice reassuring and helpful. She told me when to push, when to stop, when to pant. The baby was born very quickly ... I felt utterly exhausted. To my surprise I didn't particularly want to hold the baby at that moment. I just wanted to lie back and be told that he was all right.*

Elaine C. Smith, Comic Actress: *The second one was a lot easier I think because I knew what was about to hit me, and I wasn't as afraid ... I think with the first one there's incredible joy and excitement about being pregnant, but you're really going into no-woman's land, you know, you have no idea what's about to hit you ... My advice to everybody was always: have drugs ... epidurals are fabulous things as far as I'm concerned.*

Fiona, 29: *Emily was two weeks late, I was highly emotional and asked if I could be induced so I was induced at forty-two weeks and one day. They used pessaries and my labour took off straightaway and Emily was born within ten hours. She was a ventouse delivery ... it was a really positive experience, better than pregnancy any time. I'd give birth any day, I'd just rather not be pregnant.*

Episiotomy

This is when a cut is made to widen your vaginal opening to ease delivery. Almost every woman used to be given an episiotomy, but now they should only be done when the skin does not stretch sufficiently and would otherwise tear badly on its own. They may also be done when the baby needs to be extracted very quickly or when forceps are in use. The incision usually heals quickly, but some women do have problems with the stitches which can be very uncomfortable. Sometimes scarring can also become an irritant, during sex for instance, but this can be treated (see page 169).

Rosalie's firstborn was delivered with forceps, and the perineum, the space between her vagina and back passage, was badly torn:

> **Rosalie:** *I was so swollen and so bruised that for eleven weeks they couldn't tell exactly what damage had been done to me, and I realized that my vagina had been stitched up inside out. The inner linings of the vagina were facing outwards, which was uncomfortable, and we'd been told to try and have sex to see if things were normal, and you can imagine what that felt like. It wasn't normal at all.*

Even after that trauma Rosalie decided to have another child, but the caesarean way.

> **Rosalie:** *I know so many women who have been traumatized by childbirth. I find it curious that it's natural, because it's so unnatural to me to put someone through such pain and exhaustion with horrible consequences if things don't go right. It just doesn't seem natural to me. Now that modern medicine allows us to be awake, and feel as though we're part of a delivery process when you have a caesarean, I think it is great!*

Caesarean Delivery

> **Martha, 31:** *Someone in the next bed described it as feeling like someone's doing the washing up in your tummy. It only felt like ten minutes and she came out and she was gorgeous. It was kind of bizarre. There was a sheet up between me and her and one minute I was pregnant and next minute there was this baby and I started crying and Shane started crying and it was really lovely.*

Delivery by caesarean section involves making an incision through the walls of the abdomen through to the uterus to deliver the baby. Nowadays most caesareans are carried out with an epidural anaesthetic so the mother is conscious during the procedure. The number of caesarean births depends on the hospital, the obstetrician, and which country you live in. There is concern over the increase in caesareans in the UK. If you are told that you need a caesarean section, and you are in any doubt about the reasons, discuss them with your doctor and midwife. Some caesareans are performed if complications develop during labour and delivery needs to happen quickly to avoid damage to the baby, but obstetricians do not always agree over when this point has been reached. Some obstetricians think all breech births should be delivered by caesarean, others do not. Mothers who have caesarean deliveries have an increased chance of other complications and need to spend more time in hospital after the birth.

Janine: *I made this plan with my husband. We spent hours discussing it. I wanted a low-tech birth. No drugs, no episiotomy, no epidural. Low lights. The midwife was pretty supportive but kept telling me to keep an open mind ... I'd really wanted to have it at home but Jim felt a bit worried in case anything did go wrong. And it did. My waters broke and I didn't go into labour, I spent most of the day running around to try and make it happen. After thirty hours they put up a drip, then contractions started. Wham. The pain was so bad I just couldn't cope and I begged for an epidural which was a real relief. I thought, 'It won't be long now'. But then things just didn't go as they should, the baby was facing the wrong way. Well, I ended up with a caesarean as the baby's heart rate went down. It was all panic stations. I was glad I'd had the epidural as they could just do the caesarean. I was already all numb. Sometimes I feel a bit of a failure when I hear women going on about their perfect birth but in the end it didn't matter. Jack's pretty perfect even if it wasn't how I planned it.*

Going Home

Most women stay in hospital for one to two days after having a baby, but some go straight home. A midwife visits you regularly until the baby is ten days old, after which a health visitor will visit.

Valma, 50: *I can remember coming home and panicking and they give you all these classes about going into labour, breathing here and breathing there and you get sent home with this tiny little bundle that is totally dependent on you and I don't think it's changed these days either.*

Baby Blues

Some form of mild depression or baby blues is incredibly common after giving birth. Serious postnatal depression occurs in around one in ten women.

Amy, 30: *I knew it was coming but I wasn't prepared for the strength of it and how quickly it would happen. I found two days after she was born I was writing in my journal ... about her birth and how beautiful it was and I just burst into tears and I couldn't control myself ... it was very frightening to realize how powerful the hormones were that were rushing through my body and how they had really taken over in many respects and for a number of weeks after she was born I would just burst into tears for no reason ... Sometimes it was happy crying, especially when I thought about the moment of her birth because it was such an emotionally charged experience ... at other times I was just so totally overwhelmed. You know I couldn't feed her properly, she was crying and I didn't know how to console her. I was exhausted, my husband was exhausted. We really didn't know what we had gotten ourselves into. It was a very overwhelming feeling and I would just cry because I was in pain and I was tired and I didn't know how to calm her down. It all sort of blurs into one now. I didn't feel guilt about it. It lasted longer than I thought it was going to.*

A lucky 20 per cent or so of mums do not get the blues at all.

Maria: *I haven't had one single down patch. The midwives did warn me I might feel down when the milk comes in but I just feel ecstatic. Fantastic, absolutely fantastic. Totally in love ... it is extraordinary. I don't think anything has ever come anywhere close to it.*

Between 10 and 15 per cent of women get more than the baby blues and can become quite depressed after the birth. It often comes on so gradually that it is difficult to say when it begins. Half of the women who have it notice they are depressed by the time the baby is three months old, but it can start up to a year after the baby is born. Most women recover in a few weeks, but it can last several months.

When you have a baby everyone expects you to be happy so it is particularly difficult to admit to feeling tearful, despondent, tired, anxious, panicky, lacking in energy, disinterested in sex and irritable with everyone around. Postnatal depression is connected both to the changes in our hormones and to the altered lifestyle a new baby brings. Getting enough help, sharing the chores with your partner, not trying to be superwoman, talking to a close friend, not expecting everything to be perfect, will all lessen your risk of getting depressed. But giving up work, being isolated at home, marital problems, a baby who does not sleep, previous depression, problems with breast-feeding and the death of one of your parents recently or before you reached the age of eleven, can make you more vulnerable.

How Do You Know if You Have Got Postnatal Depression?

It can be difficult to know whether or not what you are feeling is actually postnatal depression. It may be hard to think objectively if you are overwhelmed by all the emotions you are experiencing at the birth of your new baby. Thinking about the following questions may help you recognize the signs of postnatal depression, and take the first steps to feeling better about yourself and your situation, or seeking outside help. If your answer is 'yes' to some or most of these questions, it is very likely that you are experiencing some degree of postnatal depression. Sometimes, simply being aware that you are going through something that is very common to women after the birth of a child can be a comfort. If, however, the feelings do not lift, or they get worse, it would be a good idea to discuss them with somebody.

These questions may help you recognize symptoms of postnatal depression:

- Have you felt unable to cope?
- Have you felt like crying all the time for no apparent reason?
- Have you felt unhappy a lot of the time?
- Have you had trouble sleeping?
- Have you been feeling guilty that you are not coping as well as you think you should be?
- Have you felt constantly anxious and worried about things that you normally take in your stride?
- Have you felt like you would prefer to be left alone most of the time?
- Have you felt unmotivated and unenthusiastic about things you would normally enjoy?
- Have you felt like it is all just not worth it?
- Have you experienced loss of appetite?
- Have you felt unusually irritable?
- Have you been feeling constantly tired?

All of these questions reflect the typical symptoms of milder forms of postnatal depression, which in most cases, and with reassurance and support from health workers, family and friends, disappear by themselves within a few weeks. In more extreme cases, women may experience feelings of dislike or disgust towards their baby and, very rarely, they may feel like hurting themselves, or even harming their baby. But you should not feel you have to battle through any of these feelings alone – there is help available.

It can be hard to admit you are feeling down and finding things difficult, but we know that talking to someone regularly – like a health visitor, your doctor or a counsellor – can help to get you back to feeling good about yourself and enjoying life again. Some women will need to take antidepressants to get over the depression. Rarely, you may need to see a psychiatrist or go into hospital because the depression is very bad. Fortunately this only happens in one in 1000 women.

Feeding

Jane: *I got such a surge of love for my baby whenever I breast-fed. I felt almost guilty that my husband could not really know what it is like.*

In England and Wales two-thirds of mothers breast-feed their babies, a figure which has hardly changed in the past twenty years. In Scotland about 50 per cent of mothers breast-feed their babies and in Northern Ireland 36 per cent of women breast-feed. The higher the mother's education the more likely it is she will breast-feed her baby (see page 232). Older women are also more likely to breast-feed than younger women.

We know that breast milk is best for babies. It contains the right mixture of nutrients, and your own antibodies which help the baby fight off infections. Breast-fed babies get fewer tummy upsets and are less likely to develop eczema and allergies. Women also gain from breast-feeding. It makes you feel close to your baby, there are no bottles to sterilize and prepare, and it helps your womb get back to normal as hormones which return your uterus to its usual size are released during breast-feeding.

Sue, 42: *As corny as it sounds there is this huge bonding between mother and child ... the physical sensation of the child sucking would bring a tingling feeling to me, deep within – just a real closeness with the baby and very sensuous as well ... They always say one of the good feelings about starting to breast-feed immediately is it starts to pull in your stomach muscles again and you do have that feeling ... as if your muscles are being pulled back into shape.*

Ann, 27: *It's not the sucking that's so nice. It's the little head you cradle in your hands and there's a huge feeling of bonding when you realize this child is dependent on you for survival.*

Some women have no trouble with breast-feeding, but many women do need some help especially at the beginning. It is quite normal to have a few problems, to wonder if you are doing it right, and to worry whether the baby is getting enough milk. Midwives and health visitors should be there to advise you. There are also self-help groups, the National Childbirth Trust, Breast Feeding Network and the La Leche League who can put you in touch with other women who can help (see Useful Addresses on page 390). Sometimes advice can be contradictory, so consider the information and try to do what feels best for you.

> **Amy, 30:** *Every doctor, mainly male doctors, I talked to about breast-feeding said, 'If you're doing it right it shouldn't hurt', and every mother I've talked to who's ever breast-fed has said 'Of course it's going to hurt'. I first developed blisters, very quickly, within a few days after she was born. She was just sort of sucking asymmetrically I guess and there was this ridge right down the centre of my nipple and by the end of the first week it had become scabs and they were bleeding and the horror of seeing this baby at my breast and seeing her turn her face away and seeing blood on her cheek! It was a very frightening experience and very painful and I can remember early morning feeds just dreading latching her on to my breast. But everybody I've talked to who has ever breast-fed has said that they all experienced pain. Not to the same degree that I did. Not everyone gets scabs. But the first week your boobs get really tender. It's much more enjoyable now, it's still painful, but not as painful and sometimes it's even pleasurable.*

If you decide not to breast-feed, only want to do it for a few weeks, or find it just does not work for you, feel positive about the decision. Women who do not or cannot breast-feed are often made to feel guilty or inadequate, which is wrong and unkind. Part of this has developed to counter pressure by baby-milk manufacturers, especially in developing countries, to encourage people to bottle-feed. There is also a positive side to not breast-feeding. You may feel less tired, and there is some evidence that women who bottle feed are less likely to be depressed. Bottle-feeding also allows your partner or other children to take part in feeding the baby. As with most areas of pregnancy and childbirth there are choices and you need to make the best choice for you based on the available information. Millions of babies have been bottle-fed successfully and the modern infant formula milks are specially treated to make them easier for the new baby to digest.

Sex after Childbirth

> **Trish:** *Just after I'd had the baby this family planning nurse came round wanting to talk about contraception. I told her, she must be mad. I was in such agony, I wasn't going to let him near me for months.*

Elizabeth, 30, a few months after giving birth: *It's getting there. It's still painful. It takes a while. Secondly it's very difficult to find the time.*

Susan, 41: *Sex is less pleasurable since childbirth. The general stretching of my vagina makes it less sensitive and less stimulating. An Italian friend of mine asked me about this after I had my first child because she wondered if it only happened to her and I told her the same had happened to me. I'm not devastated by it but I think I would have liked to be prepared. These are all the things that no one ever talks about.*

For some of us sex may be the last thing we want to think about. In 1994, the National Childbirth Trust asked 1000 of its members – 'Is there sex after childbirth?'. Forty-five per cent of women said they started having sexual intercourse again four to eight weeks after the baby was born, a few had started earlier and a small number were not ready even after a year. Most of them felt they had got it right, 17 per cent felt they would have liked to start sooner and about the same number felt they had started too soon. Pain and discomfort were the main reasons for any problems, though tiredness, loss of interest, lack of privacy and not feeling emotionally ready were other reasons given. Sixteen per cent felt their sex lives improved after the baby because they felt good about their body, they were less inhibited, their relationship was better and they felt more relaxed. We vary in all sorts of ways and our sexual preference after childbirth is no exception.

Miscarriage

Vivienne: *I've had two miscarriages myself ... There's this overwhelming sense of failure, of not being able to do what other women do very successfully, and I think the trouble is now that we invest so much of our hope and our aspirations into pregnancy and we sort of forget, that, even in the best of circumstances ... pregnancy would still go wrong, there would still be miscarriages. But we tend I think to think that miscarriages are our own fault in a way, and that we must have done something to make them happen.*

Spontaneous miscarriage is nature's filter, a way of making sure most babies are born normal. As sad as it is, it is a very efficient method since 97 per cent of babies are indeed born healthy. When pregnancy spontaneously ends in the first twenty-four weeks this is called a miscarriage. Any later and it is considered a stillbirth. In these later cases, when a baby dies, labour usually needs to be induced as it is the safest way for the mother and avoids a caesarean operation. This loss is discussed in our section on grief on pages 123–4.

About 70 per cent of conceptions probably end in miscarriage and half of these are lost before the first missed period so you never know you have miscarried. About one in five known pregnancies ends in miscarriage, mostly before twelve weeks of pregnancy. It is estimated that 95 per cent of miscarriages happen before sixteen weeks of pregnancy. They usually happen because the baby is not developing properly. Chromosomal abnormalities account for over 60 per cent of miscarriages before eight weeks. Other abnormalities account for most of the rest.

Carrying heavy shopping or falling over does not cause miscarriage. A woman's body is robustly built to protect a healthy foetus. There is no evidence that computer screens or microwaves cause miscarriage either. Some people say having an orgasm can cause miscarriage but this is not proven. There is an association of an increased risk of miscarriage in women who drink heavily or contract listeriosis from soft unpasteurized cheeses (see page 269) but for each individual woman it is very difficult to link cause and effect.

An early miscarriage can be like an extremely heavy period. There are often clots.

> **Ginnie, 50:** *I've had two miscarriages and three normal pregnancies. The first miscarriage was at six weeks. I was a bit disappointed but I'd hardly adjusted to being pregnant again as my first baby was only eighteen months old. I think I'd have been much more upset if it was my first pregnancy. I knew I could have a baby so at least there wasn't that worry. I had a few period pains and then suddenly started bleeding really heavily with great big clots. It all came away and the doctor said there was no need to go into hospital unless the bleeding didn't stop. The second one was at twelve weeks. We were just about to go on holiday. I'd just stopped feeling sick with the pregnancy when I felt that dragging period type pain. It wasn't long before the bleeding started. Once I'd started to miscarry I just wanted it to happen. If the pregnancy had carried on I'd have worried all the time that there was something wrong with the baby.*

Sometimes you get no bleeding or just a little bleeding. If the baby has died but has not come away and is still inside your uterus, this is called a missed abortion or missed miscarriage. A scan will show that there is no live baby and no heartbeat will be visible on a monitor. Sometimes very early on in pregnancy it can be difficult to be 100 per cent sure and you may need another scan a week later. If you do have a missed abortion you will probably need to have a D and C to empty your uterus (see pages 356–7). If not the contents usually come away naturally or are reabsorbed after about two weeks.

> **Lynn, 37:** *When I was ten weeks pregnant, I suddenly felt I wasn't pregnant any longer. My breasts lost their tenderness. I felt depressed and despite lots of reassurance, I had a horrible suspicion the baby had died though I had no bleeding. I wasn't surprised when one evening I did start to bleed and I noticed some dark blood on my pants. I had a scan the following day. It confirmed the worst. There was no heartbeat and the baby was only eight weeks in size so it must have died a few weeks before.*

Late miscarriage may occur because there is something wrong with the baby, or sometimes the placenta is not developing properly. It may also be due to a weakness in the cervix called cervical incompetence which is not very common. There are no easy tests to find out if this was the cause of a later miscarriage. If no other cause is found some obstetricians may suggest putting a special stitch into the cervix which is supposed to help stop the cervix opening before time. It is rather like a drawstring on a bag. But there is no guarantee that it will save the baby.

The later the miscarriage – and especially after sixteen weeks when you may have felt the baby move – the harder it is to get over. But whenever it happens many women feel depressed for months, especially if they have never had a baby. An expectant mother imagines the foetus as a real person very early on. One can feel a strong sense of failure and bereavement when it is lost. The trauma of miscarriage is often made worse when friends and family did not even know of the pregnancy. Chance remarks like, 'It was for the best' or 'You can easily get pregnant again', though often said with the best of intention, can be upsetting and hurtful at the time. And treatment in hospital is not always as supportive as it should be. Support groups such as the Miscarriage Association and the National Childbirth Trust (see the Useful Addresses on page 390) can help.

If you have had a miscarriage you will want to do everything possible to try to prevent it happening again. This is especially so when no cause is found. It can be very difficult to accept that there is often nothing to be done, but unfortunately there is no certain way to prevent miscarriage in the majority of cases. Making sure you are eating well, taking some exercise, not smoking and only having a little alcohol, will at least give your body its best chance of succeeding.

One of the worst things about having a miscarriage is all the conflicting advice that will come your way. There may be hints that you were working too hard, or doing too much generally, although these have never been shown to be a cause. Such suggestions will no doubt make you feel guilty and blame yourself. Advice is more likely to be conflicting when there are no good facts available and this is certainly the case when it comes to knowing how long to wait before trying to get pregnant again. You will be told to wait one month, three months, or even six months. No one knows what is the best time to wait from a medical point of view, so this is another area where you should trust your feelings and try when you and your partner both feel ready.

Recurrent Miscarriage

Most women who have one or more miscarriages eventually do get pregnant and deliver normal babies, but a small percentage have recurrent miscarriages. Surveys show that after one miscarriage the recurrence risk is 25 per cent, after two 30 per cent, after three 35 per cent and after four approximately 40 per cent. Recurrent miscarriage is defined as three or more miscarriages before twenty weeks of pregnancy. Most doctors will not investigate the reason for a miscarriage unless you have had three early miscarriages. However, if you are older, over thirty-five, it is important to start investigations earlier, say after two miscarriages.

In 60 per cent of cases no reason is found despite lots of tests. In 5 per cent of cases it may be due to a chromosomal problem in one of the parents. Anatomical problems, such as an abnormally shaped uterus, or fibroid growths in the uterus (see pages 36–7) may be responsible 10 per cent of the time; endocrine problems in the mother such as thyroid disease or progestogen deficiency, in 17 per cent; infections – possibly chlamydia (see pages 186–7) or mycoplasma – in 5 per cent; and immune problems such as a disease called SLE (systemic lupus erythematosis) in 3 per cent.

It is important to see a specialist unit if you have suffered recurrent miscarriage. There are treatments available depending on the cause. Immunotherapies and progestogen injections may be suitable for a small percentage but it has also been shown that, once you are pregnant, you are less likely to miscarry if you get a lot of support and monitoring of the pregnancy from the health professionals looking after you.

Lynn, 37, had two miscarriages before she had a healthy baby boy: *I was anxious anyway when I found I was pregnant the second time. I was looking out for any signs of miscarriage so it was with fear and dread I again ... started bleeding heavily. I didn't need a scan to tell me the baby was dead. The chromosomes [of the baby] were checked and found to be abnormal. I found this reassuring as it was nature's way and the baby would never have been normal anyway so that one I don't mind at all. Although I wasn't tested I suspect the first one was probably abnormal as well.*

nine months: pregnancy & childbirth

Even after several miscarriages, if you get pregnant and a heartbeat is seen on ultrasound at about six weeks, there is a 77 per cent chance of the pregnancy continuing without any problems.

Ectopic Pregnancy

An ectopic or tubal pregnancy is a type of miscarriage. Many of the same feelings of loss are experienced after an ectopic as after a miscarriage. Once the egg is fertilized it should travel down the fallopian tube into the womb, but sometimes it gets stuck in the tube, starts to grow there and cannot continue to develop properly. This is more likely to happen if there has been an infection or other damage to the fallopian tubes in the past (see page 303). Symptoms of ectopic pregnancy are pain on one side and a bit of bleeding, but if the tube and developing embryo actually rupture it can cause severe pain, internal bleeding and can be life-threatening. Treatment is surgery to remove part or all of the tube and surgeons make every effort to avoid removing the tube completely. You should still be able to get pregnant again, although once you have had one ectopic you may be at increased risk of having another one. If you are unlucky enough to have two ectopics and lose both fallopian tubes you will need to have IVF treatment to try to get pregnant (see pages 310–12).

Janine, 41: *I had a miscarriage, an ectopic, and the next time I got pregnant I had another ectopic. To start with I had no concerns that it was anything but a miscarriage. But after 6 weeks from the start of the miscarriage I was still bleeding and I was still in quite a lot of pain. I still felt hormonal, very tired and ill. I felt different from the last time I miscarried. The doctor put his hand on my stomach and it hurt when he took it off. I saw the gynaecologist and had a scan immediately from his clinic. The scan couldn't see anything except a bit of blood. I was taken down to theatre and had an operation straight away. There was a pint of blood in the abdomen and it was a nine week ectopic which I was told was quite advanced. The next time I got pregnant, I was told to have an early scan at 6 weeks. Before I had the scan I was in M & S and I did feel a pain, wondered whether there was something wrong, but I felt so nervous that I thought that was why I had the pain. I wanted to pretend everything was alright This time I collapsed, I couldn't get off the floor. It felt like something had just exploded. I was carried back to the car and taken to hospital.*

chapter 12

one in six: infertility

Gail: There is nothing I wouldn't go through to have a baby. They could tell me to do anything they wanted and I would do it … because I am desperate to have a baby.

A newborn baby girl begins her life with an enormous number of eggs – two million of them. Only 300 to 500 of these eggs will develop to maturity during our reproductive years. A healthy man produces around 40 million sperm each time he ejaculates. With all of these eggs and millions of sperm it seems amazing that we do not get pregnant every time we have intercourse. Conception ought to be guaranteed, yet *one in six* couples come forward for help because they are having trouble conceiving. And those are only the ones who ask.

We have, to a remarkable degree, mastered the art of having babies when we want them, and not having them when we do not. We often produce them even when it seems we are destined not to. With all the success stories emanating from the bedroom and the laboratory, it is perhaps all the more painful when nothing seems to work.

> **Catherine:** *It was my fault – I was letting him down. You can't tell people what it feels like to be infertile. You can't explain how inferior you feel, how unlike a woman you feel, how low you are inside you. There's nothing worse to me than being told, 'I'm sorry you can't have children'. There's a yearning deep down inside and everybody's pregnant around you and the feeling is awful.*
>
> **James:** *It's impossible to plan. You just don't know which way your future's going. You don't know whether you will have children in a year's time or whether you won't or never or maybe ... you just play each month, month by month, with the old time clock ticking away year by year, month by month, day by day. It's just awful.*
>
> **Rachel:** *When I was trying to have a baby I absolutely loathed pregnant women. I couldn't look at them.*

In this chapter we look at infertility and the test tube revolution. We discuss the need most of us feel to have children. We explore why infertility happens and what is involved in finding out why. We look at the range of treatments – their successes and failures – and the special difficulties lesbian couples face.

The Test Tube Revolution

> **Louise Brown, planning for her sixth birthday:** *I like to play pass the parcel which we might be playing this year, and musical chairs, and last time I played witches outside.*

Louise Brown, the world's first test-tube baby, was conceived in a laboratory dish in Cambridge and delivered in a hospital in Oldham in Lancashire on 25 July 1978. Louise was the creation of her mother's egg and father's sperm but they were brought together by two remarkable British scientists: Patrick Steptoe and Robert Edwards. Dr Steptoe handed Louise to her mother, Lesley, for the first time:

> **Lesley Brown:** *I don't think anyone else will ever be able to share that moment ... I thought she was lovely ... she was quite plump. She was a lovely little thing and I can remember after a while the only thing I could think to say to him was 'thank you'.*
>
> **John Brown, Louise's father:** *I suppose every father feels the same when they first see their daughter but to me it was totally different because we were told we would never have any children and it was oh, tremendous. Tremendous feeling, I can't really explain it. How do you feel when somebody says you win the pools or something? ... I had the same feeling ... we waited nearly fifteen years. And it's a long time to wait.*
>
> **Dr Robert Edwards:** *It was really fantastic to see the delivery. We'd seen scans and X-rays beforehand so we knew what was going on inside the uterus of course. But it was amazing to see the little girl, most startling when she started crying. I think that perhaps we hadn't thought about that. And when she started crying and shouting and screaming we knew then that somebody else had arrived on the scene with her own point of view.*

Louise's safe and healthy arrival was the result of ten years' work by a team headed by gynaecologist Patrick Steptoe and physiologist Robert Edwards whose efforts revolutionized the way women can have babies. After the success of Louise, Steptoe and Edwards went on to oversee more than 1000 baby deliveries by women who had previously had little hope of becoming mothers. Their work has inspired new generations of scientists to continue the search for solutions to fertility problems. It has also launched a new age in the reproduction industry.

Scientific advances since Louise's birth have made it possible to manipulate our bodies, our eggs and our hormones to ever greater powers of procreation. If our partner's sperm is not able to fertilize our eggs we can borrow or buy (in some countries) someone else's. We can use another woman's eggs when ours fail us. Fertility drugs give us twins, triplets, quintuplets or more – although sometimes at our own, and the babies', peril. The largest surviving bundle to date belongs to the American couple Bobbi and Kenny McCaughey. Bobbi delivered septulets – seven babies – in 1997.

Surrogate motherhood – rarely used in Britain but a brisk business in the United States – means someone else can even carry a child for us. In April 1997 an American grandmother gave birth to her own grandchild, acting as surrogate mother for her daughter. And the cloning of Dolly the sheep, in Scotland in 1997, made the possibility of cloning human beings seem even closer.

The Desire to Have Children

Having children can sometimes seem the very reason for our existence. Some women are more philosophical about motherhood and take the wait-and-see approach. Some of us actively choose not to have children.

The Biological Urge

Without this urge there would be no human race at all. Our existence and continued survival depends on it. This need is reinforced by the selfish gene concept which says the survival of our genes is all important. It is a straightforward matter for Professor Richard Dawkins who coined the phrase 'Selfish Gene': 'We are descended from an unbroken line of fertile women and we have inherited what it takes to procreate.'

So that is what we try to do. The idea is that our genes are programmed to drive us, as individual living organisms, to have sex, to become pregnant and, by reproducing ourselves, reproduce our genes.

Sarah Biggs, co-author of *The Subfertility Handbook*: *I had never had a child, I'd never been pregnant so I remember at the time I was going through many years of great pain, trying to define it, trying to understand why I felt so very unhappy and thinking, 'Well, there must be a reason. I must be able to understand this.' And I think the truth is it's so instinctive, it's so primeval it defies definition. I really didn't know what I was missing. I just knew I missed it very much and was out of kilter with everyone else.*

The Social Urge

The urge to have children comes from outside our bodies too – from parents, grandparents, friends and society itself. The majority of people in all societies tend to pair up and have children. If you happen to be one of the childless minority – either by choice or because of fertility problems – you may feel isolated, even discriminated against. Having children, and how many we choose to have, varies with trends and the times in which we live. In the sixties, 2.4 children per family was the norm. The average number of children now is 1.88. In the 1980s boom, childless couples were in. Couples without kids were called 'dinks' (double income no kids). In the supposedly more caring nineties children are, in some circles, considered proof that we are not so selfish and greedy after all.

Why So Much Talk About Infertility?

With one in six couples asking for help, and controversial new reproductive techniques, infertility is news. But this does not necessarily mean infertility is on the increase. We do not know if it is or not partly because we have nothing to measure today's rates against. One hundred years ago women were dying at the age of forty. Today many women at the same age are just getting around to considering having a baby. And we have no fertility rate records from fifty or 100 years ago. There has been plenty of publicity about men's falling sperm count, but the extent of this finding is now being questioned. We do, however, understand much more than we used to about fertility and what can go wrong with it.

The big change in our fertility pattern is *when* we are choosing to have children, and the fact that we can choose at all. Women are working, both for career satisfaction and for financial necessity, so they are putting off having their babies until much later than they used to. On average, we are now having our first child when we reach thirty. Fertility clinics see many, many prospective mothers in their late thirties and forties. This is because our fertility begins to decline at the age of thirty-five (see page 302).

Claire: *All those years bothering with contraception. I had a very successful career as a lawyer and babies would have got in the way. Now I'm thirty-six and all I can think about as the months go by and I still haven't got pregnant is the cruel T-shirt marketed in America which has a picture of a successful woman saying, 'Oh my God, I've forgotten to have a baby'.*

one in six: infertility

Another problem is marriage. With one in three marriages breaking down many women want children with their second or third partners – later in life – which can make conception and pregnancy more of a challenge.

Adoption of newborns, the solution for so many women in the past, is now only available to a tiny minority of childless couples after very rigorous screening procedures. Effective contraception and legal abortion have drastically reduced the number of available newborn babies for adoption.

Finally, massive media attention to new fertility treatments encourages many infertile couples to seek help including those who might have accepted their childlessness in the past. Even post-menopausal women have been able to have a child through the wonders of the laboratory.

When to Seek Fertility Advice

When everything is working properly and the woman is under the age of thirty-five, nine out of ten couples can expect a pregnancy within the first year of trying. Five per cent will conceive in the second year, and the remaining 5 per cent will take longer. The chances of getting pregnant in any one month are one in three at best. Most couples do not need to consider infertility tests until well into the second year of trying, although some couples may want to seek help before this.

If you know there are problems from the start, do not delay. If you do not have periods, if you have a history of pelvic infections, or if you are approaching the menopause, investigations should begin early. If the man has trouble getting an erection (see pages 173–5), difficulties ejaculating or he has had an operation on his testes for whatever reason in the past, he should see his doctor. Until fairly recently – and even now – men's fertility problems have been overlooked, to the detriment of a couple's chances.

The first port of call is the GP who should take a detailed medical history from both partners, carry out an examination and do some initial blood tests on the woman to check that the hormones involved in ovulation are all OK. Analysing a sample of semen will make it possible to check the sperm. Sometimes referral to a specialist is arranged immediately, but sometimes it is better to wait. If you are anxious, ask for an early referral since it often takes a long time to get an appointment.

The Causes of Infertility

As women age they become less fertile, with fertility in women taking a definite downturn after the age of thirty-five. Sometimes the most obvious problems are overlooked because people assume everyone knows how to make love, and that everyone understands what is going on in sexual intercourse. But this is not always the case and when couples do ask for help it is not uncommon to find something is going wrong with the sex itself. Sometimes a man and woman are not performing the act properly. His penis may not be fully penetrating her vagina. In rare cases he might not be entering her vagina at all.

> **Celia, 41:** *I was very young, about nineteen, and he was about twenty-one but he had a lot of inhibitions from his strict Catholic upbringing. I hadn't had much experience but I was not a virgin and he thought this was his chance to lose his virginity. He thought he had found where you put it but it was actually just sort of between my legs up almost between my buttocks! He had no idea of a woman's body. As it happens the last thing we wanted was to try and get pregnant but just imagine if he'd seriously thought this was it!*

So, assuming you are having intercourse, check that your partner is:

- Getting an erection.
- Putting his penis all the way into your vagina.
- Ejaculating inside your vagina.

And make sure you are having intercourse regularly, although there is no point in doing it more than once a day apart from for the pleasure of it. There is no evidence that restricting yourself to once every two or three days helps to conserve sperm in cases where the man has a low sperm count. Try to give conception the best chance by making love at the time of ovulation, which occurs approximately fourteen days *prior* to your next period. The best way to calculate this is to chart your periods (see page 33). You will soon know your next start date, if your periods are regular. Once you do, count fourteen days backwards from what you expect to become day one in your next cycle. The few days around this time will be your optimum conception time. Women often count forward from day one, but counting backwards is more accurate. There are also kits available from the chemist which help to identify when you ovulate. If your periods are not regular, obviously it will be more difficult to work out when you will ovulate. Ask your doctor for help in finding out why.

The causes of infertility are with the woman 41 per cent of the time and with the man 35 per cent of the time. Both partners have trouble 10 per cent of the time. And in 14 per cent of cases no cause is ever found. However, it soon becomes a couple problem.

> **Dr Tim Hargreave, specialist in male infertility, Edinburgh University:** *You can only really say that a couple has a fertility problem. It's extremely difficult to say that a man or a woman is infertile ... the problem is that if a man has a low sperm count, whether that couple are successful or not very much depends on who he's married to ... it's the way we interact. If his partner is very fertile then despite his low sperm count they have a better chance.*

Female Fertility Problems

The likelihood is that you are not ovulating (see page 30). This is the case for about 40 per cent of women seeking help. Blocked or damaged fallopian tubes are the second most common problem, troubling nearly one-third of women who are infertile. Other problems include uterine abnormalities and endometriosis (see pages 38–40).

Ovulation problems

Women who have regular periods are likely to ovulate most months. You know if you are not having periods or if they are very irregular or infrequent and this will help pinpoint the problem. The good thing is that absent or erratic periods can nearly always be treated with hormone drugs (see Chapter 2), which will regulate ovulation.

Blood tests will indicate whether your progesterone hormones (see pages 30–1) are at the right level at the right time in your cycle. You can even check this yourself with an ovulation kit available from chemists. The kits come with sticks which change colour when they are put in urine samples, indicating when you are ovulating. This is caused by changes in the levels of the luteinizing hormone or LH (see pages 30–1) in your blood and urine. If you have a problem it can be treated with a pill – usually clomiphene which your GP can prescribe. This works for eight out of ten women, but these drugs also give a sixfold increased chance of having twins. Another drug – bromocriptine – is used to stimulate ovulation when there is too much of the hormone prolactin, which is produced in the pituitary gland in the brain.

Gertie, 42: *I didn't get a proper period for five years before I had the children. So I was on bromocriptine to give me a period which you are meant to take orally [by mouth] but I couldn't take it orally because it made me nauseous so I had to stick it up vaginally every morning ... we were trying for about three or four years and then I finally went on clomiphene which is a drug that stimulates ovulation. I fell pregnant the first time.*

Anorexia or other eating disorders (see pages 141–7) can stop ovulation, as can excessive exercise or polycystic ovarian syndrome (see page 43). These conditions all need to be treated first. More rarely, some women have no eggs at all. This can happen for several reasons. Turner's syndrome, a chromosomal abnormality, prevents your ovaries from fully developing. Some chemotherapy treatment can also make your ovaries sterile. Premature menopause also leaves you sterile. Women who fall into any of these categories can try egg donation, which means using another woman's egg. The problem here is the severe shortage of available eggs. If you are interested in becoming a recipient, or want to donate your eggs, contact the Human Fertilisation and Embryology Authority (see Useful Addresses on page 390). Donors are anonymous and are usually between the ages of eighteen and thirty-five.

Fallopian Tube Problems
If your fallopian tubes are blocked or damaged, sperm cannot travel to their destination. This may be caused by infections, the most common being chlamydia which is a sexually transmitted infection (see Chapter 7). IUDs (see pages 208–9) may promote the passage of infections from the vagina into the fallopian tubes which may in turn block them.

Endometriosis (see pages 38–40) can sometimes cause so much scar tissue damage to our fallopian tubes that eggs cannot travel through them.

Clare, 40: *I had been using the coil for years ... I went to see what was wrong with my tubes and was told they were very blocked up. I could have had surgery but my husband was ill so coming to terms with that and deciding not to intervene was the moment I realized that I wasn't going to have children ... I was very sad about it for a time but there is life on the other side.*

Blocked or damaged tubes can be checked with a laparoscopy. This minor operation is done while you are under general anaesthetic. An optical instrument is inserted through a small slit in your stomach, usually just below your navel, enabling the doctor to see inside. Your tubes are checked by blowing dye up through the cervix. The laparoscope allows the doctor to see if your tubes are blocked or open. During the operation you are also likely to have your uterus examined with another optical instrument inserted up through your vagina. The fallopian tubes can be unblocked by blowing air through them or by surgical procedure. Success rates of operating on blocked tubes are very variable depending on where the tube is blocked, the extent of the damage and the skill of the surgeon. Surgery on the tubes should be carried out with the aid of a microscope and overall success rates using this technique vary from 30 to 65 per cent. You may not get pregnant immediately after tubal surgery. There is an increased risk of ectopic pregnancy if you do get pregnant. Some studies show that after fertility surgery there is a 10 per cent chance of conception each month.

Some procedures to examine the fallopian tubes can be done even while you are awake. Donna conceived after her treatment.

> **Donna:** *While it was being carried out I was linked to a TV monitor ... you could actually watch it on the TV as it was happening ... you actually saw the blockage in the tube ... and you could see it open and the dye suddenly flow through ... it's less hassle than going to the dentist.*

If it is not possible to repair the fallopian tubes then IVF should be considered (see pages 310–12).

Uterine Problems

Fibroids in the uterus may interfere with conception by preventing the implantation of a fertilized egg in the uterine wall. An odd-shaped or double uterus can have the same effect. Investigation into this takes the form of looking inside your uterus via the vagina using an optical instrument called a hysteroscope – sometimes under general anaesthetic but not always. Treatment is by surgical removal of any obvious abnormality such as a fibroid (see pages 36–7), or you may be given LHRH agonists to shrink the fibroids. An odd-shaped or double uterus can still carry a foetus. Only when it is severely malformed is there a real problem. If there is no uterus at all pregnancy is not possible.

Faulty Orgasms?

As scientists delve deeper into the mysteries of reproduction they have become interested in our orgasms. They have found that there is sometimes a connection between orgasms and fertility, with women with unexplained infertility having fewer orgasms. Although women do get pregnant without orgasm, it may be that the contractions of the vagina that take place during our orgasms play a role in helping the sperm on its way. See page 156.

Male Fertility Problems

Fertility problems in men are nearly as frequent as in women, yet men are often neglected when it comes to treatment. Mary-Claire Mason, the author of *Male Infertility – Men Talking*, found that when men *do* learn they have a problem they are taken aback:

> **Mary-Claire Mason:** *The news was unexpected. They weren't prepared for it. They'd assumed that because they were sexually potent they could get their partner pregnant ... that was part of their job ... and when they find that things aren't going their way, that they perhaps have failed in some sense, they feel vulnerable but they can't acknowledge this and they don't know what to do about it.*

> **Tom:** *I didn't deal with it very well at all ... when I did start to talk about it I realized that I had tremendous feelings of guilt, feelings of failure and I had no idea how to deal with those feelings. I had a great need to try and keep things on a normal footing ... obviously for my wife she wanted to try and sort it out but I always wanted life to go on as normal. I wanted our sex life to carry on as normal and of course it wouldn't ... our sex life stopped being so easy and so normal and for me that became even harder and the guilt and the feelings of frustration and failure became even more difficult.*

Poor Sperm or No Sperm

When a man ejaculates, the fluid which comes out of his penis, the ejaculate – or semen – is made up of two ingredients: seminal fluid and the sperm itself. The fluid is the transport medium for the sperm. Problems start when there are not enough sperm or, rarely (in fewer than 5 per cent of men) no sperm at all. Another problem is that the sperm are sometimes not well formed, or they have what is called low motility. Peter discovered that this was the case with his when he produced a sample at an NHS clinic:

> **Peter, 48:** *Let's face it. Men spend half their lives masturbating. So in principle it's no great hardship ... On that day it took closed eyes and gritted teeth to produce something ... Two problems were highlighted: not enough sperm and low motility – an ambivalence of ambition in those that could be counted. In other words, there weren't many to start with and those that there were showed very little inclination to go in search of an egg to fertilize.*

Most men will have trouble ejaculating or maintaining an erection at some time in their lives. It can happen for many reasons – anxiety, stress, relationship difficulties, lack of sexual arousal. This is quite normal unless it persists. For some men the anxiety associated with an episode of impotence can make the problem worse (see pages 173–5).

Sometimes impotence is caused by an illness such as diabetes, or because of problems with the nerve supply to the penis. Sometimes it is a side effect of drugs being taken, for example, with some drugs used to control high blood pressure. Whatever the cause, if it persists and is causing problems, see your doctor for help before it becomes a bigger problem. If it is the side effect of a drug, the drug can be changed. If it is psychological, sex therapy may help.

Sperm quality can also be affected by excessive smoking, alcohol abuse, and wearing tight underclothes which keep the testes (where the sperm are produced) too close to the body and therefore too warm. In the instance of a man getting the childhood disease, mumps, and if his testes become severely inflamed, a low sperm count might, albeit rarely, result. Every baby boy is checked by a doctor for undescended testes at birth and again as a child. If the testes are not in the scrotum and are therefore undescended an operation is carried out to put them in the right place. This helps but does not guarantee their production of sperm in the future. Undescended testes which are not corrected will leave a man without any sperm at all. And operations on the testes, for whatever reason, can also interfere with sperm production. Most men are born with two testes, but one is enough for procreation. Finally, some men have antibodies in their semen which destroy their own sperm.

When sperm is tested it is checked for the quantity and the quality, to see how the sperm look and how mobile they are. Very accurate computer analysis provides a good picture of sperm behaviour and its penetration of the egg. To do a sperm test, the man masturbates into a sterile container after leaving a gap of three or four days since last ejaculating. The container must be delivered to the laboratory within an hour of production. The tests are done more than once as there is so much normal variability in sperm counts and behaviours. One sperm count by itself does not spell disaster. If the sperm counts are low, blood tests for hormones will be carried out. Hormone tests include measurement of testosterone, FSH, LH, and prolactin (some of the same hormones that are measured in women), which might help to identify the cause as they are involved in the messages the brain sends to the testes to produce sperm. For example, a high FSH level in a man suggests the testes are not functioning properly. If there are no sperm at all, then a biopsy of the testes (when a small sample of the testes is removed) will be offered to try to find out why no sperm are being produced.

Normal Semen

- Volume   2 ml or more per ejaculation
- Count   40 million sperm per ejaculation
- Motility   50 per cent or more of sperm swimming in the right direction`
- Appearance   30 per cent or more sperm looking normal

A 'post-coital test' is also available. This takes the sperm and mucus mixture from around the woman's cervix the day after the couple has had sexual intercourse around the time of her expected ovulation. Post-coital tests are nearly always done at the hospital, although there may be the occasional GP with a special interest in infertility who checks them in the surgery. The post-coital test checks for whether sperm are present, whether they are moving, and helps check that ovulation has occurred and that the mucus around the cervix is the right type. There are many reasons for a post-coital test showing negative. Most commonly it is the wrong time in the woman's cycle. You need to have the test checked again if the first one comes back negative.

Some drug and hormone treatments have been tried on men to increase their sperm count, as yet with little success. When the problem is low sperm count, the sperm are concentrated and then injected into the woman's uterus directly through her cervix (sometimes using a local anaesthetic). The woman usually takes ovulation-stimulating drugs at the same time. When there are severe problems with the sperm a specialized IVF technique may be used. This involves injecting a single sperm into an egg. After fertilization the embryo is placed in the woman's uterus.

If there is no sperm at all, you can consider a sperm donation. As with egg donation, the donor's anonymity is protected. Clinics which offer an insemination service try to give you sperm from someone who has similar physical characteristics to your partner. Donors and sperm are screened for disease. For information about local clinics, contact ISSUE (see Useful Addresses on page 390).

James: *It's very difficult for me to know that it's Caroline that's going to have to go through the treatment. It's very difficult for both of us. For my wife she feels a little bit bitter because it's her that has to give up her job, give up some of her social life and go through a long period of what can be sometimes painful treatment. It would be great if I could change places with my wife and actually go through the treatment myself ... having brought this stress and this problem to our marriage I feel like I want to sort it out.*

Combined Fertility Problems

Sexual Dysfunction

This term refers to a range of psychological, medical or drug-induced problems that get in the way of sexual intercourse. It can be that you are not making love in the proper way (see page 302), or that one or both of you has lost your sexual drive. Anxiety, stress and medications can interfere with sex and therefore fertility.

When you go for help a detailed sexual history, done in all cases of infertility, will be taken. If you are having trouble actually having sex, some sort of sexual counselling or even more general therapy may be offered, individually or as a couple.

Mucus Hostility

This is a relatively rare problem where a particular man's sperm is incompatible with a particular woman's cervical mucus. His sperm is rejected or destroyed, unable to survive the swim through the plug of mucus surrounding the woman's cervix. Our hormones are supposed to make it easier for sperm to get through the mucus at the time of ovulation, but if there is 'hostility' it is impossible. Remarkably, this disorder is specific to the couple and the woman's mucus would probably be receptive to another man's sperm. If you are chemically incompatible in this way you can try IVF using your partner's sperm (see pages 310–12). This helps bypass the problem of the sperm having to swim through such hostile territory.

Psychological Problems

There may be psychological causes for infertility but this is difficult to evaluate. We all suffer stress in our lives. What kind of stress and how it affects our ability to conceive is impossible to measure. There are anecdotal stories about women leaving stressful jobs and suddenly becoming pregnant, but it is not possible to link cause and effect. It is possible that the stress you feel when it seems to be taking forever to conceive works against you. Yet women can conceive in the most stressful situations. Birthrates jump during war, as was recently the case in Bosnia. Common sense suggests that the more relaxed you are, the easier it may be to conceive, and sex will certainly be more enjoyable too. One thing many people say is that sex is less fun when you are having fertility problems.

> **Francesca, 42:** *It definitely affects your love-making because I treat my husband like a sex object. I'm very aggressive about wanting to make love with him and there's a certain underlying mission there and it's not just playful spontaneous sex. I want something from him and I think to some degree he feels that ... he knows I have an agenda.*

one in six: infertility

When No Cause Can Be Found

Sometimes no reason at all for infertility can be found. We need more research to understand why some couples cannot conceive. In these cases IVF may help. It can be very difficult to take the IVF step after the emotional trauma of trying and failing to conceive, and the battery of tests can put you off. But some couples opting for IVF feel relief that at last tangible treatment is being given.

In Vitro Fertilization: 'The Test Tube Baby'

This is the treatment pioneered in Britain in 1978 by Steptoe and Edwards. Since the birth of Louise Brown in that year more than 30,000 IVF-conceived babies have been born in the UK alone. IVF, and variations on it, are now on offer around the world.

IVF involves:

- A woman taking hormones by injection to stimulate the release of several eggs from her ovaries at one time.
- The release of these eggs being monitored by using an ultrasound technique.
- The eggs being collected using a laparoscope inserted into the top of the vagina through a tiny cut, while the doctor is guided by an ultrasound picture.
- The eggs being removed and put with the partner's sperm in a special solution, not in a test tube, but in a glass dish, for fertilization to take place.
- After fertilization, a maximum of three embryos is transferred back into the womb using a laparoscope.

IVF treatment is time-consuming and sometimes painful. It is expensive, costing from £750 to £2500, and the results can be disappointing. Every IVF clinic has a 'live birth rate', that is the number of births (multiple births count as one) resulting from every 100 treatments. Every woman who begins treatment must be counted in the clinic's statistics even if, for instance, she does not make it to the egg retrieval stage for whatever reason.

Maggie: *Everything I hated I had to go through. The injections every day, the blood test every week ... the worst part was the emotional trauma of IVF treatment, not knowing what the end result would be.*

Sarah: *I have twin boys who are a year old next week. I had two attempts at IVF. The first attempt I did become pregnant and I miscarried at three months. The second attempt resulted in my lovely boys.*

The Successes and Failures of IVF

Success depends in part on a woman's age as older women are less fertile. The average success rates for the UK as a whole are as follows:

- Under the age of thirty-five years, live birth rates are about 15 per cent for each treatment cycle, i.e. on average around fifteen women out of 100 will deliver a baby after treatment.
- For women aged thirty-six to forty, the live birth rate falls to about 11 per cent for each treatment cycle.
- For women over the age of forty, the live birth rate is 4 per cent for each treatment cycle. The chance of success from any single treatment appears to be the same for the first three or four tries. After that, it may be that too many problems stand in your way, and no amount of trying will help you succeed.

The Human Fertilisation and Embryology Authority or HFEA (see Useful Addresses page 390) will provide you with a guide so you can compare clinics' success rates.

Variations on IVF

Gamete Intra Fallopian Transfer (GIFT)
Here, the eggs taken from your stimulated ovaries are transferred to your fallopian tubes together with the sperm so that fertilization can take place in its natural environment.

Zygote Intra Fallopian Transfer (ZIFT)
This is a combination of IVF and GIFT where the retrieved eggs are fertilized by the sperm in the laboratory as in IVF but are then transferred to the fallopian tubes at the pre-embryo stage, instead of being placed in the womb as in IVF.

No laboratory fertilization is needed when GIFT is used, so it can be performed in less specialized units. GIFT is suitable for women with healthy fallopian tubes and where the sperm have already been shown to be able to fertilize an egg. The choice will depend to a certain extent on the availability of the services in the unit and the exact nature of the couple's problem.

one in six: infertility

The Problems of IVF

Drugs to stimulate ovulation are routinely used in IVF treatment in order to lead to the production of several embryos, because implanting more than one embryo increases the chance of success. However, this practice also increases the chance of multiple births.

> **Jack, 53:** *My wife really wanted a baby. So did I. But I couldn't cope with the idea of triplets and there didn't seem to be any way of controlling the outcome. I just thought really practically and I knew I couldn't handle three babies. We dropped out of the programme.*

Many clinics now advise implanting just two embryos because this does not greatly affect the success rate, yet it removes the risk of triplets – unless of course one of the embryos divides naturally. Multiple birth babies are more prone to disability, low birth weight, premature birth and have a lower survival rate at birth. Some women's bodies over-react to the drugs taken to stimulate their ovaries. When this happens their ovaries become large and cystic. This is painful and can cause acute nausea and cramping. Although surgery might be necessary the condition usually settles down on its own.

IVF is psychologically very stressful mostly because the failure rate is high, and even after a positive pregnancy test following IVF, a miscarriage or ectopic pregnancy is still possible. It is also, as mentioned, very expensive with a cost of up to £2500 per treatment cycle, depending on which clinic you attend. Sometimes the cost to you is reduced if it is shared with the NHS. And in a few places in the UK treatment is free under the NHS. Check with the HFEA for details on what is available in your area.

> **Jessica:** *We felt so desperate that I think we would have gone on until the money ran out basically ... when the first attempt failed we were determined to go again and if that attempt had failed I know we'd have gone again because we wanted a baby.*

> **Sian:** *I felt it was not fair on my husband to carry on and on and on having more and more attempts at IVF so I said, 'Right, as soon as I'm forty we'll call it a day if we haven't succeeded then.'*

Surrogacy

Surrogacy is legal in Britain, but it is illegal to profit from it. You may not advertise to be a surrogate mother or advertise that you need one. The surrogate mother may carry an embryo which has been developed in a licensed clinic, or she may be impregnated with the father's sperm. The latter is supposed to be performed in a place also licensed by the Human Fertilisation and Embryology Authority (see Useful Addresses on page 390). Surrogacy is sometimes a woman's only chance of having a baby but it is a risky business. The legal status of the participants can be confusing and uncertain, and the outcome is tragic when the surrogate mother herself changes her mind and wants to keep the baby. For more information, contact Childlessness Overcome Through Surrogacy (COTS – see Useful Addresses on page 390).

But it sometimes works. In March 1997 an obviously joyous north London couple took delivery of triplets from a surrogate mother of their choosing. The woman carried the couple's own eggs and sperm. Although the birth and 'handover' of the babies to parents went smoothly there was some public debate over whether the triplets can be considered Jewish, as their parents are, when the surrogate mother is a Christian.

Baby Cotton

In 1985 Kim Cotton became Britain's first known commercial surrogate mother. She was paid a fee of £6500 by a childless couple desperate to become parents. She worked through an American agency. The case of Baby Cotton, as the child was known, ended up in the high courts as social workers and lawyers wrangled over her well-being and the media scrutinized every angle of the story. It was a painful experience for Kim Cotton who had difficulty giving up the baby. She says her worry was that she did not know the couple who were taking the baby:

> **Kim Cotton:** *She wasn't handed over immediately so I went through one week of sheer hell that I don't think I'd wish on my worst enemy, but after that I had to put it behind me ... after I'd got everything into perspective I still came out saying, 'Well, I've helped a couple achieve parenthood and that's the main thing' ... I swore I'd never do it again.*

In 1991 Kim Cotton *did* do it again, this time to help a couple she knew. She was implanted with their egg and sperm which meant there would be no genetic link, unlike Baby Cotton who was created from her own egg.

> **Kim Cotton:** *The child is not genetically mine ... so I am not having to brainwash myself into saying, 'It's not your child, Kim'. I can quite honestly say this isn't my child. So that feels a lot cleaner emotionally to me. The main reason, Linda needed me. Her surrogate had dropped out at the last minute and I just found myself saying I'll help you, Linda.*

This time Kim had twins, a boy and a girl, born on 24 June 1991. This was her last surrogacy.

> **Kim Cotton, 1997:** *In 1983 I had never even heard of surrogacy, now my name is synonymous with it. I have been asked on many occasions would I still have done it knowing what I know now. The answer is yes but I would have done things just a little differently. Hindsight is a fine thing.*

Lesbian Parenthood

The ultimate reproductive challenge must be when two women – or two men – decide they want to become parents. The question here is not infertility, although it can be, but rather how do you surmount the challenge of turning a same-sex couple into a family of three?

There are very few clinics a gay couple can turn to in the UK. One of the most receptive to lesbian women is The Pregnancy Advisory Service in London (see Useful Addresses on page 390) which sees clients from across the UK and Europe. It takes inquiries from lesbians every day and of the 200 cases it takes on each year, half of them are lesbian couples who want to become parents. This private clinic offers donor insemination to women. It is licensed by the Human Fertilization and Embryology Authority (HFEA) and, under its regulations, the sperm donor must remain anonymous.

> **Janine, Fertility nurse and midwife:** *I don't believe any woman should be deprived ... you have to consider the welfare of any child first and foremost. People always have stereotypes ... the vast majority are just professional women with a decent lifestyle ... they have such a hard time getting accepted anywhere for donor insemination or any treatment because they've been to their GP and he's looked at them in horror and said, 'You can't!' Before women can get on our programme we need them to give us a letter from their doctor saying they are fit. But we have a lot of experience with doctors saying they won't get involved with any such thing. I believe that is really wrong. I'm pleased and honoured to help this group of people.*

But finding a donor, either through a clinic or through friends, is not the only problem. In the case of Susan and Louise the challenge of finding the right way to 'father' the child at times seems insurmountable. Susan does not like the idea of using anonymous sperm and a syringe.

> **Susan, 35:** *You have two incredibly broody women who can't figure out a way to have a baby. How do you do it? Louise doesn't want to know the father. She thinks it's too complicated in a relationship to have that third parent involved from the start … I don't see a problem in having a third parent … Louise has come as far as saying, 'I don't mind if it's someone you know but he's not going to be involved'. And I've come as far as saying, 'OK, I won't choose someone I have strong feelings for but I'll choose someone I like and you approve of but I still want him to acknowledge he's the father of the child.' I think it has a lot to do with your own experience and I didn't ever have a good relationship with my father and it's a real sadness in my life and I wouldn't like to deny my own child something that I think is really important for children just because I've chosen to live with a woman.*

Janet and Judy want a baby too:

> **Janet, 40:** *I called two sperm banks and they sent us a catalogue of specimens … with numbers, I think there were about seventy-five to 100 with one-liners about this specimen. Such as 'five foot eleven, big boned, blue eyes, dark hair, interest in music, studying psychology'. So we picked five of those off the original catalogue and sent away for some longer sheets on these guys … 3065, we really liked him a lot … we were trying to match up the guy that looked and sounded most like Judy and then for me she was going to match up the guy who sounded most like me.*

In the end Janet and Judy both went for donor 3065. They have no struggle with not knowing the father, but they are, however, struggling to conceive. The sperm came in a tiny vial packed inside a big case of liquid nitrogen.

> **Janet:** *We had to go pick it up at the doctor's office – I couldn't believe the size of it. We could hardly lift it together. And then we were driving home with it in the back of the car and Judy made this joke about we should have a sign that says baby on board! Plus liquid nitrogen can explode … So we got it home and we put it in our bedroom and then we just kind of looked at it for a long time, read the instructions … I forget who did it first.*

Janet and Judy have gone through the process of lugging the canister home, and using a syringe to try to inseminate themselves with donor 3065 four or five times, so far without success. There are no reliable statistics for the success of self-insemination but it certainly works for a lot of women. Donor insemination performed in hospital has a 3–17 per cent success rate depending on which hospital you visit.

Brave New Baby World

The fertility industry can now help to produce the longed-for baby – for the woman who no longer ovulates, for the man whose sperm swims backwards, for the gay couples and the single woman. It often succeeds. And it has also produced questions for heated debate. Critics are shocked that single women, and unmarried or gay couples should be allowed treatment. What about all the extra eggs and embryos generated by IVF treatment? And who is to say what is right and what is wrong? As Britain's Diane Blood pleaded for permission to be inseminated with her dead husband's sperm there was tremendous sympathy for her, and much criticism of the Human Fertilisation and Embryology Authority (HFEA) for denying her. There are questions about what to tell children about their genetic inheritance, and plenty of debate about selectively aborting some of the embryos in a multiple pregnancy (see page 226). There is outrage that a woman of sixty should want help in conceiving a child. Another view says, why not? Elderly men father children. And there is always the question, who should pay for it?

Hooked on Treatment?

Virginia Ironside of CHILD believes that sometimes people get hooked on treatment:

Couples can just go on and on and on and on and if they have the money or they can mortgage their house or whatever they cannot bear to stop. I think a lot of this is because some couples feel that there is actually ... a baby that is waiting in the clouds and it is waiting to come to them and by having more and more treatments they're keeping the door open for it coming and if they stop the treatment then they're almost murdering something that doesn't yet exist ... What makes it more difficult for couples now is that there is so much more treatment. There's always another step they could take.

D

growing old

Barbara Castle, Baroness Castle of Blackburn: I never look backwards. I always look forward. God knows where it's going to lead but it's ... interest in the curious evolutions of life that keeps me going ... now I have the glorious freedom of having other priorities.

Age cannot wither her
Antony and Cleopatra, Shakespeare

Maybe not Cleopatra, but the truth is age does wither. Our bodies droop, sag, flop and flag. Our breasts lose their firmness. Our hair turns grey. Skin wrinkles. We dry up inside, and out. We shrink. We have less energy. We hear less and see less. But we certainly have company. There are more old people – and older old people – than ever before. At the end of the twentieth century we can expect to live an average of twenty-eight years longer than women lived at the beginning of it. *Healthy* life expectancy, however, remained the same between 1976 and 1994, at sixty-two years for women, and fifty-nine for men. And women live longer lives than men. The challenge for us then is to find ways to make our extra years good ones. In spite of all the outward signs of ageing, women often find a new inner confidence.

> **Dame Thora Hird, 81, Actress:** *I never think I'm old. In fact it surprises me sometimes when I think, 'Thora, you're eighty-one'. It's very important not to let yourself go. I still look after my skin. I still manicure my nails. I'm still careful about my clothes.*

> **Julie Andrews, Actress, on her voice:** *Oh I think that as one gets older it shifts gears. It comes down a couple of tones. It seems my middle register and my lower register have really warmed up ... I am able to do a lot more with my voice than I used to ... I'm kind of glad that it's matured.*

But seventy-one-year-old May would gladly trade in her aching body for a younger model:

> **May, 71:** *I hate it. I hate it. My health's not good. I've got to rely on people. They're very good all around here, especially neighbours ... but I would love to be out, able to get out and go and do things and go here and go there. You feel you could be really enjoying yourself if you had your health.*

We begin to notice the ageing process when we are still young.

> **Susan, 41:** *You begin to notice subtle things. The beginnings of grey hair, crow lines around my eyes, sagging neck. And there are major differences in how you view yourself. Before you always thought of yourself as someone young. Now you begin to think of someone approaching middle age, when life is half over. I don't find it depressing, I find it inevitable.*

growing old

Marcy, 46: *You get used to the idea that men don't whistle at you or smile at you. I don't care as much about men now.*

Frankie: *We were coming up to sixty so we decided we'd go round the world on our 30-foot boat. We didn't think about old age. We just decided to go ... we were away for five years. We didn't think about being brave. We just wanted to have fun. We had a boat so why not use it. We didn't think about dying. The moment you start thinking about death you've lost the battle.*

Ageing is inevitable, but feeling bad about it is not. It is a time for adjustment: to retirement, to life after the children have gone, frequently to life alone after the death of your partner. Most of us have a say in how we are going to age. Assuming we have some control over our lives and therefore have a choice in the matter – although we cannot control when illness strikes – the quality of our older years can be affected by exercise, diet and friendship. In this chapter we look at what we can do to help keep ourselves healthy. We examine the illnesses and complaints which bother many of us as we age: osteoporosis, arthritis, high blood pressure, strokes and heart disease, cataracts, hearing loss, incontinence, insomnia, memory loss and Alzheimer's. We note the importance of friendships in staying happy, healthy and alive. Our silvery years ought to be a stage when there is, at last, time. Time to enjoy grandchildren, hobbies, and perhaps travel. Here, we emphasize how to make ageing positive, and how to get help when we need it, while keeping our independence and dignity right to the end.

Staying Healthy

Exercise

Doing nothing speeds up ageing. Women who are active have younger bodies than women who do nothing. The physiological age of an active woman can be ten to twenty years younger just because she exercises. The Health Education Authority (HEA) recommends thirty minutes of 'moderate intensity physical activity' five days a week. Any vigorous movement will do: brisk walking, house cleaning, gardening, dancing or any combination of activities we enjoy. Exercising regularly helps to keep our joints flexible, maintain muscle strength, improve circulation, and prevent constipation. It also helps to control weight. Our quality of life should improve, and we may live longer as a result. Physical activity also reduces the risk of heart disease, stroke and osteoporosis. See Chapter 6 for more on exercise. Remember, it is never too late to start exercising.

Diet

Eat lots of fresh vegetables and fruits as well as high-fibre breads and pastas. Try to stick to a low-fat diet but make sure you eat enough. Sometimes when we are on our own it can feel like it is not worth the bother but it is important.

Socialize

Stay in touch with your friends and make new ones. Being sociable can also mean exercise so there is a double benefit to walking, swimming, golf and tennis. They are all activities which keep us in touch with others. If you are in a relationship keep it fresh by spending some time apart each day to develop and maintain your own outside interests and friends.

Sadie is studying music, reading French and planning her next summer school residential course in gardening.

Fountain of Youth?

White mice have been found to live longer when given extra doses of melatonin, so what about us? Melatonin is a hormone naturally produced by the brain's pineal gland while we sleep and, in fact, it regulates sleep. The light of day shuts down production. You need a prescription to get it in Britain and Canada for use as a sleeping aid to fight jet lag for instance. But in the United States, where you can buy it off the shelf, it outsells vitamin C. This is because melatonin enthusiasts claim the drug holds the secret to eternal youth. They say it will make our old years healthier ones, and that melatonin can fight cancer, eye cataracts and heart disease. It is supposed to improve our sex drive and make bald men grow hair. Research is underway, but the claims remain unproven, except in helping jet lag.

growing old

Sex and Age

> **Adelaide:** *I think a lot of people when they get older feel they should give up sex. I think that's a terrible state ... you should not give anything up. I didn't find sex more difficult as I got older. I found that I had just as many orgasms as before and just as good and just as strong ... I had the same thrill, the same excitement. The same feeling of being in love which is one of the highest highs that you can have.*

Some of us lose interest in sex as we age. Some of us rev up, liberated from children, free of periods. Our sexual drives are remarkably variable. Whatever your appetite, there is no medical reason to stop having sex as you grow older. Some people swear by it.

> **Halina, 50:** *I'll tell you the big secret is being vegetarian and having lots of sex. You'll live forever.*

The 1994 *National Survey of Sexual Attitudes and Lifestyles* (see page 151) found that more than half of women between the ages of fifty-five and fifty-nine had not had sex in the previous month. The study found that fifty-something women are more often without partners than fifty-something men. This is because men often form relationships with younger women and because of widowhood. There are other reasons for the lack of sex in this age group. Around the time of menopause (see Chapter 3) some women do lose interest in sex, even if temporarily. See Chapter 7 for more details on sex – just about every sexual rule that applies to sex and the younger woman, applies in later life too.

> **Gwen, 81:** *When Billy died I did miss sex for a long time but it wasn't a thing I'd go look for because I didn't want it by anyone else. But I did miss sex. And it was a happy sex life that we had. I enjoyed sex and my husband enjoyed sex.*

> **Elizabeth, 68:** *Eighteen, twenty years ago I had my op. I had cancer of the womb. And my feelings changed then. Because I'd been messed around so much in hospital and all these old treatments ... now I feel I just don't want to be touched, bothered. It's a chore. Because you were properly messed about so much. ... Somebody touches me, I cringe, I can't help it.*

Your Limits

When you get older you do get tired more easily, so recognize your limits and give yourself a break. Take a cat nap in the afternoon so you can recharge for the evening.

It *is* frightening and things *do* go wrong more often as we age. But just about everything that might come our way has some solution even if there is no actual treatment or cure.

Osteoporosis

Low bone density itself is not a problem. Most of us will not even know we have it unless we have a fracture, which is what causes the pain and discomfort. Osteoporosis has only recently begun to get the attention it deserves, and it is good that our awareness has increased as a result, but the campaign has unduly worried some of us. One in three women develops osteoporosis.

Our skeletons are alive and growing all the time. In children new bone replaces old bone quickly but the process slows down in later life. When regrowth cannot keep up with the bone that is lost, osteoporosis develops. Post-menopausal women are at special risk because of the drop in the level of the all-important hormone, oestrogen (see page 55). Osteoporotic bone is fragile and pitted with large holes so it breaks more easily. If the osteoporosis is very severe a minor fall can lead to a bone fracture. One in four women who live to the age of ninety will suffer a fractured hip. In very extreme cases even a cough or a sneeze can break a bone. The symptoms include height loss, acute back pain or a curving spine.

Osteoporosis – Who is at Risk?

- Menopausal women because of the drop in oestrogen levels. Oestrogen helps to keep our bones strong.
- Young women or girls with low oestrogen levels caused by severe dieting and too much exercise. This can lead to a cessation of periods and an early menopause.
- Women who take corticosteroids over a long period, e.g. for asthma or rheumatic problems.
- Women with low bone mineral density due to a calcium-poor diet and lack of exercise.
- Heavy smokers.
- Women with a strong family history of osteoporosis.

Exercise

You can take active steps to help to prevent yourself getting osteoporosis. It is never too late to start exercising. According to Dr Joan Bassey of Nottingham University, in pre-menopausal women, jumping up and down fifty times a day increases bone mineral density in hips and therefore helps to prevent osteoporosis in later life. She does not recommend jumping for anyone with arthritis or joint problems of any kind or for anyone with back pain. This exercise is a prevention, not a cure. Beginner jumpers should start slowly. Try ten jumps the first day and build up slowly. When you reach your target of fifty jumps these need not be done all in one go. Jumping also improves balance and strengthens leg muscles.

Jogging improves bone mineral density in our spines, so it is excellent too, in combination with jumping, for the prevention of osteoporosis, but again this is only for women who are not suffering from arthritis or back pain. Other weight-bearing exercise, where our body takes the weight: walking, dancing, tennis, even shopping, is also beneficial. For older women, fast walking is the best exercise. The National Osteoporosis Society (NOS – see Useful Addresses on page 390) recommends taking a brisk twenty-minute walk three times a week to strengthen bones. Even better, walk daily. If you cannot do twenty minutes, do five or ten. It will all help to improve your mobility and balance and therefore reduce the risk of falling too. Exercise also helps bones absorb calcium better.

Calcium

Calcium is essential in our diet to maintain healthy bones. The NOS recommends 1000 milligrams a day for women aged twenty to forty, and women over forty should take 1500 milligrams. Nursing mothers are advised to take 1250 milligrams daily. Skimmed milk has slightly more calcium than higher-fat milks. Vitamin D is important too. Many women do not have a diet rich enough in calcium and vitamin D and it probably is a good idea to take supplements of both as a tablet as you get older.

Foods with High Calcium Content

Dairy Products	Quantity	mg of calcium
Cheese cheddar type	100g	750mg
Cheese camembert type	100g	382mg
Cheese cottage	100g	82mg
Milk – skimmed	(1 glass) 200 ml	240mg
Milk – semi-skimmed	(1 glass) 200 ml	240mg
Milk – full cream	(1 glass) 200 ml	232mg
Double cream	100g	75mg
Yoghurt – low fat	125g	225mg
Yoghurt – plain	100g	150mg
Egg – whole	x 1	26mg
Egg – yolk	x 1	23mg
Drinks		
Hard water	1 pint	114mg
Nuts, Seeds and Pulses		
Almonds	100g	234mg
Hazelnuts	100g	280mg
Sesame seeds	100g	670mg
Tahini	100g	680mg
Sunflower seeds	100g	120mg
Tofu	100g	510mg
Soya beans	100g	100g
Chick peas	100g	150mg
Fish		
Canned sardines in oil	100g	354mg
Canned pilchards	100g	300mg
Canned mackerel in oil	85g	221mg
Canned salmon in oil	85g	160mg
Cereal Foods		
Muesli	100g	220mg
Bread white	55g	100mg
Dried Fruit		
Figs (dried)	100g	126mg
Raisins	80g	62mg
Dried apricots	100g	67mg
Vegetables		
Broccoli (steamed)	100g	103mg
Baked beans	100g	45mg
Beans (green)	125g	45mg
Spinach	100g	106mg
Parsley	100g	203mg
Kale	100g	179mg

Information from the Geigy Scientific Tables Vol.1 and the John Radcliffe Hospital, Oxford.
The recommended daily amount of calcium is 800mg, or 1500mg after the menopause.

growing old

Smoking and Drinking

Avoid heavy smoking and drinking. Alcohol stops calcium from being absorbed and smoking lowers oestrogen levels. Caffeine interferes too, so drink coffee and other drinks containing it in moderation, or avoid it altogether.

Hormone Replacement Therapy

Hormone replacement therapy helps to prevent and treat osteoporosis as well as the other symptoms of the menopause (see Chapter 3). The National Osteoporosis Society advocates HRT, claiming it cuts the risk of fractures by at least a half if it is taken for five years after the menopause. HRT replaces the oestrogen we lose at the menopause, and it is this loss of oestrogen which adversely affects bone density. Vitamins and calcium supplements may be recommended for women who cannot take HRT, because they have had breast cancer or other medical conditions such as endometriosis or fibroids. Sometimes HRT can have adverse affects on fibroids and endometriosis.

There are nagging doubts about the extent of the effects of HRT on osteoporosis, partly because studies so far have failed to consider the type of woman who takes HRT in the first place. It may be that we would need to take HRT forever to enjoy the benefits of protection against osteoporosis. Much more research is needed.

Drug Treatment

There are also new drugs called biphosphonates which produce an increase in bone density of up to 4 per cent a year. We probably need to take these drugs for at least three years and possibly longer. These should be considered by women who have had fractures, have severe osteoporosis and do not want to use HRT. It is not known whether there is any advantage in taking HRT and biphosphonates at the same time.

Bone Density Tests

> **Susan, 50:** *I was a quarter of an inch shorter at my bone density test when my height was measured. I only recently started to pay attention.*

The thickness of our bones, the bone density, can be measured by a special type of X-ray. The density of the hip or lower backbone is usually assessed. The availability of scans varies across the country. The results help predict whether you are at risk of a future fracture, but many women with low bone density never have a fracture, while 60 per cent of women with good bone density do. It is probably more useful to have a repeat scan after a year to see how fast you are losing bone density. If you are losing it faster than the average it might help decide whether you should take HRT or another preparation to reduce the risk of osteoporosis.

Arthritis

Arthritis affects eight million people in the UK, but most of them live normal lives. It affects women much more than men partly because we live longer, but the incidence in women is also greater. There are two main types: osteoarthritis and rheumatoid. Whichever you have, it is good to keep mobile, stretch frequently and walk as much as possible to improve flexibility and mobility. Rest when you need to and make the most of the good days.

Osteoarthritis

This is the most common form of arthritis and it happens because of wear and tear on our joints. Almost everyone has some degree of osteoarthritis after the age of forty but only 10 per cent of us will notice it. It hits our hands and hips, feet and knees.

> **May, 71:** *Oh it's one long dead ache to go up the stairs. It's getting murder, I'm struggling. It's like all the muscles feel they're all tied up, tight.*

Physiotherapy can help treat osteoarthritis, as do cortisone injections into your joints. If you are overweight, losing excess pounds will help take the strain off your joints. Hip replacements to alleviate pain and regain mobility have become commonplace. Unfortunately many people have to wait in pain and for too long for a hip operation on the NHS.

> **Brenda, 77:** *I had to give up playing bowls, that was the worst thing. And the waiting to have the hip replaced, the pain was terrible, especially at night … I couldn't bend down to put my shoes on and as I live alone it was a problem. My doctor made a fuss about me not getting the operation and eventually I had it and a new hip put in. Oh the relief and being able to sleep.*

For most women with mild arthritis, painkillers such as paracetamol and anti-inflammatory drugs such as ibuprofen (Nurofen) do the trick. Remember to read labels carefully and check with your pharmacist to see if there is any reason you should not take a drug.

Rheumatoid Arthritis

This type of arthritis involves inflammation and swelling of the joints. It affects 5 per cent of women and 2 per cent of men and its severity varies. It can affect young people and old. White blood cells invade the lining of our joints causing the inflammation. No one knows why the cells do this – it seems they 'think' they are fighting an infection when in fact they are harming healthy body tissues. Rheumatoid arthritis can strike suddenly with intense pain and crippling stiffness, but this may be temporary and can be treated. Nearly one-third of sufferers will return to near normal within a few years. The rest will have flare-ups from time to time. One in ten will be severely damaged by the disease and could eventually become disabled. When it first strikes it can feel like the end of the world:

> **Bess, 74:** *I have a hard time even wanting to recall it. I woke up in the middle of the night and I was absolutely stiff like a board and terrified, wondering what had happened to me. As soon as I could I got on to my feet and started to move around and examine my muscles and try to figure out what had happened to me. I can't remember how long I was stiff but it was a shocking experience.*

Bess was treated by cortisone injection but she was also careful about her diet, eating plenty of fish and fresh vegetables. Fifteen months after her rheumatoid arthritis first struck she told us:

> *It's amazing because things seem to have settled down and I have movement back in my legs. I'm afraid to say it because the doctor keeps saying, 'It's always there, it'll come back.' I don't like to get negative statements from the doctor … The last time she saw me she said, 'Wow you're doing wonderful'.*

Drug Treatment

Various drugs are prescribed to help rheumatoid arthritis. Aspirin and ibuprofen relieve pain and inflammation if it is mild, although these drugs can cause indigestion and irritate the lining of the stomach. However, you may need more powerful drugs such as sulphasalazine, penicillamine or gold-based drugs. Unfortunately these have more side effects and you will need regular blood tests to check that everything is alright. There is some evidence that it is best to treat the symptoms with stronger drugs when the disease first develops to prevent damage to your joints.

Diet and Complementary Treatment

Some people prefer to try to control their arthritis by changing their diet or by using complementary medicines. Oil of evening primrose, mussels and ginseng oil are all used, but there has not been any good scientific research to assess their benefit. Some arthritis sufferers try eliminating certain foods from their diet, sticking to fish, fruit and vegetables for a week or so. Then they reintroduce foods, one at a time. Anything that seems to worsen the arthritis is eliminated. The process takes about six weeks. Scientifically tested or not, life improved dramatically for Angela.

> **Angela:** *I haven't taken any drugs for three and a half years. I haven't taken one single soluble aspirin or anything and that [diet] has enabled my arthritis to be controlled. I still have rheumatoid arthritis but I am controlling the activity in my joints by not eating foods that I am allergic to … I feel good.*

Alzheimer's Disease

> **Rosie, 44:** *Then she looked at me and said, 'Is your mother still alive?' I didn't want to frighten her by saying, 'Well you're confused, Mum, because you're my mother,' and yet at the same time I was upset for myself because you want your mother to know who you are and I said, 'Well, actually you're my mother'. And she said, 'I am?' And I said, 'You are'. And she patted my knee in that nice way my mother has and said, 'Well that's very nice dear but it's a little late to tell me.' Obviously I must have looked upset and she started comforting me and she said, 'No dear, really I'm very happy, it's just a little late to tell me.'*

About 650,000 people in the UK have some form of dementia. More than half of them are thought to have Alzheimer's disease. It affects more women than men, in part because women live longer. Alzheimer's usually strikes after the age of sixty-five but it can occur in people as young as forty. Its cause is not known, but it could be related to a breakdown in the brain's neuro-transmitters, the chemicals which allow the brain's nerve cells to interact with each other.

People with Alzheimer's disease find it progressively more difficult to learn, reason and remember. The first sign is usually memory loss. You may notice it yourself, when you find you cannot remember the names of people close to you or do not know where you have placed things. Forgetfulness is normal in people of all ages, but with Alzheimer's it becomes extreme. The sufferer has trouble concentrating and finds conversations difficult to follow. Eventually patients may become incoherent. Sometimes they can be very angry, even violent. There is no sure treatment for Alzheimer's disease and the patient may eventually need complete care. The disease can be hardest on the partner, children and close friends of the victim. There are support groups for families (see Useful Addresses on page 390).

> **Rosie, 44:** *You go through the same things you go through with a death. You go through anger, you go through deep depression, you go through denial ... The tragedy is that you're losing someone you love in a very prolonged way that is awful for them and awful for you ... there are times when the person is not the person that you knew. In other ways ... there's no masquerade, no mask – nothing – any more, so the person who she is, was, who I think was a very brave person and a very private person is still there.*

A drug called tacrine has been tested on Alzheimer's patients in the US, France and Sweden with some very modest results showing it helps to stop the breakdown of chemicals in the brain, in some patients. To date, the trial tests are inadequate with very short-term follow-up and we have no idea of any lasting benefits. The side effects of the drug include nausea and vomiting. Tacrine is not available in the UK. Here a drug called aricept is used and claims are made about its success with little scientific evidence to back them up.

Research teams around the world are looking for the cause and the cure for Alzheimer's. Several studies have linked aluminium in water and cooking utensils with Alzheimer's disease, but the current evidence seems to indicate this is not so. The hormone melatonin is also under examination to see if it can help people with Alzheimer's. An extract of Ginkgobiloba has recently been found to help people with dementia.

Heart Disease

'Britain's no.1 lady killer isn't a man'
Women are used to hearing about the risks for men when they hear about heart attacks so this British Heart Foundation slogan may surprise us. Coronary heart disease kills one in four women in Britain – five times as many women as die of breast cancer. And once we have reached the menopause heart disease is just as much a risk for women as for men.

A heart attack happens when one of the heart's main arteries is blocked and the oxygen supply to other organs is seriously reduced. The symptoms of a heart attack are severe and sustained chest pain which may spread to your arms, back, neck and face. You may also experience a very cold sweat and stomach pains.

> **Marlene, 57:** *Before the operation it was dreadful because I was short of breath. I was in so much pain ... I'd been ill on and off for years ... I kept having a numb feeling in my arms and the doctor said 'Oh it's alright, it must be the menopause.'*

Finally after a night of terrible pain, Marlene went to see her GP. He told her she was in the middle of having a heart attack.

> **Marlene:** *The pain was so bad you didn't know what to do. You couldn't concentrate on anything. All you wanted to do was crease up and get rid of the pain, to get some ease. I was all knotted up. You felt sick and you were perspiring. You didn't feel normal, you didn't feel natural. The oxygen wasn't getting to the brain.*

Pre-menopausal women have many fewer heart attacks than men at the same age, but women who do have heart attacks at this young age are more likely to die from them than young men are. Not enough research has been done on why this is so. It may be that women are less likely to think they are actually having a heart attack and therefore do not seek help immediately. When women do seek help, studies have shown they are less likely to be referred to the hospital for investigation and treatment of heart disease. Anyone who has had a heart attack should take a daily low dose (75mg) of aspirin (unless you suffer from indigestion or stomach ulcers) to help reduce the risk of a further heart attack.

Tips to Prevent Heart Disease

It Is Good to Eat:
- Fish (especially oily fish like tuna and mackerel).
- Fruits and vegetables – at least five pieces a day.
- Porridge, which lowers cholesterol.
- Potatoes, pasta (but leave out the rich sauces), rice, brown bread.
- Skinless chicken.

Avoid:
- Animal fats – use polyunsaturated oils (e.g. sunflower) or monounsaturated olive oils (but remember that even the much promoted no-cholesterol olive oil is 100 per cent fat and is therefore full of calories).
- Salty foods.
- Red meat – it is high in cholesterol. Ostrich meat is an exception.

growing old

Try to:

- Stop or reduce your smoking. If there is one thing you can do for your heart it is this. If you stop smoking it takes ten years to achieve the same lower risk status of someone who never smoked, but of course every year you do not smoke will reduce your risk.
- Watch your weight. Being very overweight is linked with heart disease, especially if you have put on three stone in four years.
- Walk as much as you can. Exercise helps control cholesterol levels, prevents heart attacks and helps in rehabilitation after one. But if you've been sedentary get fit slowly. If you experience chest pains, stop. If you have doubts about your fitness, see your doctor before you begin an exercise regime.
- Relax, have fun, make time for yourself.
- Enjoy sex. It doesn't cause heart attacks.
- Consider HRT – it may help reduce the risk of heart attack (see pages 60–71).
- Drink moderate amounts of red wine which helps to prevent heart disease. (Moderate means a small glass of wine per day.) Wine helps to break down cholesterol and reduce stress. More than moderate drinking can raise blood pressure.
- Consider taking vitamins E and C which may help to prevent heart disease (research is still continuing). They are called anti-oxidants and seem to stop free radicals oxidizing the good HDL cholesterol (see pages 386–7) which damages the heart.

High Blood Pressure

Madelaine, 41: *They often tell you that people don't feel high blood pressure but I do ... in the beginning it feels like a head cold to me in a way and you feel stuffed up and you can feel pressure on your eardrums from inside ... and that's when it's sort of moderately high but not out the window. But when it gets really bad then I have a headache up the back of my neck and up inside my head and over my eyes and ... then that eventually makes me sick to my stomach as well. It's more like a constant throbbing pain, it's not piercing.*

While Madelaine can feel her blood pressure rising, most people cannot. In a way she is lucky because high blood pressure – or hypertension – which goes untreated, can be dangerous. It can cause strokes and heart attacks (see pages 333–4 and 330–2) and damage the kidneys. Get your blood pressure checked every three years so that you can start treatment if it is getting too high. (For more on the causes of, and screening for high blood pressure, see pages 385–6.)

There are many different types of medicines available to lower blood pressure. Some women experience side effects. If you do, do not just stop taking the drugs but ask your doctor for another prescription. Make sure you get one that works and does not cause any problems because you will probably need to take them forever. Side effects may include cold hands and feet, a cough at night, swollen ankles and hot flushes. Some women lose their interest in sex. Some men become impotent and, so far, most of the medical concern about sex and side effects has focused on them.

There are other ways you can help yourself if you have high blood pressure. Make sure you eat lots of fresh vegetables. Cut down on red meat and fatty foods and do not add too much salt to your food. If you are overweight, see if you can shed a few pounds. If you are a smoker, stop or cut down. Make sure you exercise each day even if all you do is take a short walk.

Strokes

A stroke happens when the flow of blood to the brain is interrupted. High blood pressure and heart disease both contribute to strokes. Getting in shape can help to prevent a stroke and all the advice that pertains to the prevention of heart disease on pages 331–2, applies here too. Exercise and a low-fat diet should help to prevent or lower high blood pressure. However, some thin people with good diets have high blood pressure because genetic factors are also involved.

You may know you are having a stroke because you might feel numbness in your face, have trouble with speech and vision and you may feel dizzy. This is caused by a blood clot or bleed into the brain which kills brain tissue and, unlike many other body tissues, this does not regenerate.

Mary, 68: *I felt a bit peculiar, a bit dizzy ... I sat down sideways in the car but I didn't get right in because I felt dizzy again. Next thing I got out of the car and couldn't move. I lay down on the ground. I found I couldn't move because I was thinking I would crawl to the next house and tell them I was still conscious and it was very cold. One of the dogs got out and sat behind me and wagged his tail and I was lying there saying, 'Help, help'. It's a very quiet road and nobody could see me. After a quarter of an hour a neighbour came looking for me, she could hear me and couldn't see me ... I wet myself and I started being sick and they realized something was wrong and called an ambulance. And after that I don't remember ... it took a few days before I came round. I had funny hallucinations and all sort of things.*

The thought of having a stroke summons up absolute horror in most people. The idea that you could be trapped inside your body and have no control over it is very frightening. About half of the people who have a severe stroke will not be able to look after themselves afterwards without help. Ten per cent will have another stroke within a year. Thirty per cent will die within the first year.

Many specialists are negative about treatment after a stroke, but there has been some evidence to show that physiotherapy can help. Dorothy, eighty-seven, is in no doubt. Her husband had a stroke in 1990 and she nursed him until his death in 1996. During their last six years together Dorothy became his advocate, pushing for physiotherapy for him, since doctors were reluctant to offer treatment.

> **Dorothy:** *He just became unable to do the things that he normally did, quite helpless really. He couldn't lift his teacup and he was unable to walk properly ... In the end they sent around the local physiotherapist to see him at home, and she came once a fortnight for a couple of months but didn't stay very long ... she had far too much work to do for the amount of time they had given her ... I knew of a physiotherapist locally and she would come once a week and she gave him quite good physio. I had to pay for it privately of course. We went along like that for quite a long time ... I think he got quite a lot out of it ... He was able to walk a bit more and I am sure that helped ... The mere fact of giving him movement and doing some physiotherapy and managing to take him for a walk was just amazing.*

A tiny stroke called TIA (transient ischemic attack) may sometimes be a warning that a major stroke will follow, but not necessarily. Aspirin is used in the treatment of TIAs and may help after some strokes. It affects the stickiness of the blood, making it less likely to clot.

Eyes and Ears

Seeing

Practically all of us need glasses by the time we are fifty. This is a normal part of ageing and there is nothing we can do about it except to make sure we have our eyes tested and get the right spectacles. Laser surgery to remedy shortsightedness is being experimented with now and in the future it may limit the need for glasses. By the time you reach fifty you should have your eyes tested even if you have not needed glasses up until now, especially if there is glaucoma in your family. This is a condition caused by pressure inside the eyeball and it can lead to blindness if it is not detected and treated early. Macular degeneration is another major cause of blindness as we get older.

Cataracts are a common eye problem as we age. They are easy to treat and the operation is usually a great success (see Chapter 15 for details of the operation). Cataracts come on gradually and you notice that your vision starts to deteriorate. They are caused by changes in the cells of the lens in the eye which cause the lens to become opaque and make the world look blurred.

Hearing

Having a hard time hearing is frustrating. Wax build-up can be the problem and is easily fixed by having your ears syringed at your doctor's. As we age, hearing problems are usually due to nerve damage which is irreversible. This can be extremely distressing. Hearing aids are very helpful in this and new technology has improved their performance greatly. Many GPs can do a hearing test in the surgery. Hearing aids are available on the NHS, although in some areas there is waiting time. They are also available privately. Some are very expensive but not necessarily better than the cheaper ones.

Bladder Stresses

Moira, 50: *One of the down sides of having children is that ... sometimes when I sneeze I have to cross my legs, otherwise there'd be a little squirt.*

Weak muscles are the problem, not age. Incontinence affects many women, at all ages, although it is more prevalent in older women. Incontinence means a loss of control over urination. It can be as mild as a dribble after a sneeze or it can be a total loss of bladder control. It may occur after childbirth, or after gynaecological surgery. Serious weight gain can put stress on your bladder. It can also be related to an infection in the bladder or kidneys. Stress incontinence means you pass urine involuntarily when you sneeze, run or laugh. Urge incontinence is when you have to pass urine the minute you get the desire to and cannot hold it. But there is often a mixture of the two types. If treatment with exercises does not work, there are special urodynamic tests using a dye in the urine to find out what is really happening in your bladder and urethra.

Rosemary, 54: *Once I plucked up the courage to go to the doctor's you don't find it so hard to tell other people. It's erratic, it's not all the time ... Some days are fine and other days are dreadful. The worst is I'm going to the loo every hour and if you cough or suddenly laugh you lose water ... You don't control it at all, you can't. I'm not going to do anything about it. I've had the tests now and they've decided there's nothing wrong with my bladder. Apparently it can come from the bowel as well and there's nothing wrong with my bowel. I personally feel it's all tied up with the heavy periods and the fibroids. I've had it for a few years, it gets worse, it doesn't get any better. It's depressing until you can actually tell somebody about it. But once you tell somebody it becomes an inconvenience and not depressing.*

Many women – maybe most women – do not tell their doctors about an incontinence problem until they have suffered from it for a very long time. But there are many treatments for it, from simple exercises to surgery. Kegel exercises, named after Dr Arnold Kegel, a 1940s researcher into women's bladder stresses, can help to strengthen bladder muscles. These muscles are part of what's called the pelvic floor. You can do them anywhere without anyone even noticing. Just concentrate on the area around your vagina, tighten it, and pull up. Hold for a few seconds whilst continuing to breathe normally, and release. Do this repeatedly and regularly to help control leakage. If you cannot sense these muscles or quite imagine where or what they are, you can learn. Try stopping and starting whilst urinating and think about the muscles you are using to do this. Those are the ones you want to strengthen. For older women, or women who have trouble locating these muscles, try lying down to do the exercises until you get used to them.

There is an array of devices on the medical market: cones, sponges and aptly named plugs, all intended to help retrain and control the bladder so it is important to try to get over your embarrassment and ask for help if you need it. As far as surgical options for treating incontinence, which operation is suggested will depend on the cause of your incontinence. Some are done via the vagina and others involve cutting the abdomen. Success rates after surgery are very variable ranging from 35 to 85 per cent. In stress incontinence the aim of the surgery is to lift up the neck of the bladder and correct any prolapse of the front wall of the vagina.

Valma, 50: *I don't suffer from it any more. I used to get it when I laughed, when I sneezed, when I cried, when I swung the golf club. There would be a little dribble ... I went to the doctor. He sent me to the hospital and I've had a bladder repair and I'm quite perfect all over now.*

Sleep Patterns

Our sleep patterns often change as we get older. A baby can sleep up to seventeen hours out of twenty-four, older children usually need only nine or ten, and by the time we reach our seventies we may only need five or six. Many older women seem to need less sleep and manage on this amount. Others have trouble getting the sleep they need. If you are one of them:

- Try not to eat just before bed.
- Avoid caffeine and alcohol before going to bed.
- Try to have a ritual before going to bed – perhaps a hot drink, a bath and light read.
- Make sure you get exercise during the day.
- If you cannot fall asleep, read or get up and do something.

For more on sleep turn to pages 117–18.

The Elderly Intellectual

Old brains are almost as good as new brains but they do need exercise.

Professor Colin Blakemore, Physiologist, Oxford University: *Recent evidence indicates that 'Use it or lose it' does apply to brain function. Exercising your brain really does help to keep it functioning. No one knows what mechanism is involved. Anything that keeps the brain thinking – crosswords, reading, learning a new language, learning new computer skills, are all good in keeping one's mind alive. Cognitive defects, with confusion about time and space and memory loss, can indicate dementia or Alzheimer's. There is a gradual deterioration after the age of sixty-five to seventy. But there is no need to be concerned about minor lapses in memory, normal in everyone. It is not true that learning and cognitive function goes downhill after thirty. Verbal memory and IQ are preserved remarkably well throughout one's sixties.*

growing old

We have a capacity to learn throughout our lives. But our minds need exercising, particularly when we are older and we no longer have the stimulation of work or family routines. Our older years are a great time, then, for new activities – to take up the hobbies we always intended to, to travel and to read books.

> **Barbara Castle, Baroness Castle of Blackburn:** *I want to write a good book. I want to talk well to young people. I want to deliver good lectures when I'm asked to do it. And because I'm not looking over my shoulder, 'Ooh, is this going to advance my career? Or isn't it?' I'm speaking better than I ever did in my life.*

Looks

People have an idea of what old is supposed to look, like but frequently reality and stereotype do not match. We are living longer and feeling more comfortable with old age and we do seem to look younger. Fifty is not what fifty was. In fact at the turn of the century few women even saw fifty. As youthful as we are it can be a struggle to hold everything up, as writer and broadcaster Sue Margolis so perfectly captures:

> **Sue Margolis:** *Come on down – breasts, stomachs and faces! The only thing to look forward to is eyelid overhang and pelican neck as your nipples make a beeline for your knicker elastic and the corners of your mouth develop Nora Batty droop ... in bed you become aware that sex on your back rather than on top seems to look, well, just that bit more tidy really, that is of course, if you can bear to let a fellah see you in your full thread-veined glory.*

You can keep it up – to a degree – with exercise and a balanced diet. We do need help. Moisturizer to keep our skin pliable and extra calcium to keep our bones strong, for instance.

Looking After Others

> **Rosie, 44:** *It's not just my ill mother. It's also my father who's now really on his own. So it's trying to figure out and balance your role of being a good daughter and also taking care of yourself which I think women aren't taught to do very much. It's a real struggle. It's a real fight to know how much do I do for them. How much do I do for me.*

Vera, 66: *I've got a husband and I look after an old lady, ninety-two. And I've got four grandchildren I look after off and on. A woman never retires. Really. Not unless she's on her own.*

Francis Bacon (1561–1626) on marriage and single life: *Wives are young men's mistresses, companions for middle age, and old men's nurses.*

And old parents' nurses, he might have added. For there comes a time when the roles of parent and child reverse. You may be in need of care yourself but have to look after parents or in-laws. Resources for helping elderly people vary from area to area – from social services, doctors, nurses, psycho-geriatric services at the hospital to residential nursing homes. There are also more informal community services which most elderly people rely on as they become less independent: family, neighbours, voluntary organizations and the church, mosque or synagogue.

Social services should help by organizing a care package, although you may have to pay for the care depending on your own savings and resources. Make sure you are getting the right benefits such as attendance allowance, a non-means-tested benefit if you are being cared for or caring for someone at home. Financial constraints must be the single most common reason why we do not get sufficient care. Perfect solutions are not easy to find but there is a lot of support out there to tap into.

Most old people prefer to stay in their own home as long as possible, and good health increases our chances of continuing to look after ourselves until the end. Fifty-nine per cent of women over the age of seventy-five live alone.

The Statistics of Ageing

- Officially, women age faster than men. This is because women reach pensionable age at sixty, while men must wait until sixty-five. Over ten million men and women are eligible for pensions in the UK, nearly nine million of them are in England.
- Nearly two-thirds of over seventy-fives are women, and women make up more than three-quarters of the over eighty-fives.
- In 1994, 8000 people were over 100 in the UK – 7000 of them were women.
- Old men are more likely to be married than old women. In 1994, 60 per cent of men over seventy-five were married. But only 23 per cent of women over seventy-five had spouses.
- As the ageing population ages, older people are more often caring for even older people.
- Our life expectancy is increasing every year.

growing old

Thoughts on Ageing

Hannah, 41: *There is something good about ageing. The older you get the less you care about what others think of you. But the caveat is I do not imagine an age exists when I do not care what my mother thinks. I will be 105 and still worry what my mother thinks of me!*

Dusty Springfield, Singer: *I'm always a gypsy. There's always another motel down the road. I came from that kind of family who were restless. I'm actually quite glad I'm restless because it keeps me interested in life. There's always another challenge. There's always another place. There are always new people to meet and that keeps my head young, not necessarily my body but my head.*

Maeve Binchy, Novelist: *When I was twenty-four, I didn't know that at fifty-four you could still feel passion and love and regret and friendship and hope just as much.*

Barbara Castle, Baroness Blackburn: *I've never understood it when people talk about old age pensioners. I say, 'Yes those poor dears you know?' I don't think it belongs to me.*

Beth, 21: *I guess my main image of elderly people comes from my grandparents so in a lot of ways it's a very positive image because my grandmother's eighty-six and she's very fit and very active and does a lot and goes on courses and things. And I suppose my image of my grandfather is less positive because he was very ill for a long period before he died.*

Thinking About the End

Vera, 66: *I'd like to drop dead. I'd like to have my faculties right up to the end and literally drop dead. I'd hate to be a burden to anybody ... My mother went to bed. Never woke up. Lovely. The doctor said she'd literally died in her sleep. She had a bad heart. We were warned she could literally drop dead. But she went to bed this one night. I had to touch her next morning to convince myself that she had gone. She was so peaceful. Lovely.*

Gwen, 81: *I want to go out like a candle. I don't want to be a burden to anyone. And I'll have cremation. I am not going to be taken to the church where I was married and all the rest of it. I don't want my family to come and stand in front of a coffin of mine ... If you go down to the crematorium ... it's peaceful.*

Madelaine, 41: *I have discussions with my husband from time to time on pulling the plug if it gets to the point where it's not worth living but I think that's a little bit of a dangerous area because look at this guy in France recently that wrote the whole book by blinking, right? Now anybody looking at him would have thought, hey permanent vegetative state, pull the plug! Meanwhile he still had a book in him!*

Gwen, 81: *If you've got your health and all that it's quite alright. We've got to get old. We've got to go some time haven't we. Got to peg out some time! It comes to us all. We don't want it but we've got to accept it in the end. It worries me. I go to bed some nights and I perspire all down here thinking about it and I think I shan't see the children, I shan't whatever. And I think, 'Well once you're gone nobody's going to bring you back so that's it.'*

It is generally agreed by doctors and psychologists that the more we open up about death, talk about it, face it and our fears of it, the easier it will be for us to accept it. Half a century ago – in war – people did talk about death because it was right in front of them. Peace time and modern medicine have conspired to change the way – and when – we say goodbye. Euthanasia is defined as 'the bringing about of a gentle and easy death in the case of incurable and painful disease'. In this country it is illegal and yet allegedly widely practised. These contradictory positions have come about because there is a blurred line between helping someone with a terminal illness to die should they wish, and providing medical drugs to relieve their suffering – drugs which may also hasten death. In Holland the latter has been clearly decriminalized, but under strictly controlled circumstances. This reflects the fact that in our society there is an increasing acceptance that an individual has the right to decide on the time and mode of his or her death. However, others believe in the 'sanctity' of life and do not believe that an individual has any right over the time and mode of their death. There is, in the UK, no consensus about legalizing euthanasia. Many doctors do, off the record, admit to helping patients to die but there is a concern that, if legalized, this could be abused.

One of the problems is that death can also be delayed by heroic medical intervention in ways that can result in the patient surviving in a totally dependent, humiliating or undignified way. Because of this many people are now making living wills, asking that these heroic methods not be used on them. Although such living wills are not yet legally binding they help to let your family, doctors and lawyers know what you want. (See Useful Addresses on page 390.)

> **Vera, 66:** *Used properly I think it would be a godsend. My father ... had a massive stroke. He came out of it after about six or seven hours. The doctor said later it would have been kinder if he'd never come out of it. His brain had gone. He didn't even know me ... Now and again he'd have some lucid moments and he would say to me 'Vera I wish to God I was dead'. That last five years he had no dignity. It was cruel for him and for the rest of us.*

We all want dignity, not only in life but also whilst dying, and in death. The hospice movement has managed to bring this concept to the fore both in discussion and in practice but there are few hospices available. For those with cancer, Macmillan nurses can provide support and care. Many doctors find it difficult to accept they cannot do much more to help someone in a terminal illness. It can be easier to do another test or give another treatment than to talk openly to a patient about death, stop active treatment and give care and pain relief instead.

> **Anonymous Epitaph from Bushey Churchyard**
> *Here lies a poor woman who always was tired,*
> *For she lived in a place where help wasn't hired.*
> *Her last words on earth were, Dear friends I am going*
> *Where washing ain't done nor sweeping nor sewing,*
> *And everything there is exact to my wishes,*
> *For there they don't eat and there's no washing of dishes ...*
> *Don't mourn for me now, don't mourn for me never,*
> *For I'm going to do nothing for ever and ever.*

chapter 14

complementary medicine

Julia, 50: The argument for evening primrose oil was quite strong ... I boost that with vitamin C, vitamin B, and with a zinc complement as well. And then I have multi-minerals and I have cod liver oil.

Complementary medicine has been around forever. It goes in and out of fashion and, as we head for the turn of the century, it is most definitely in. Increasingly, GPs and specialists – traditionally sceptical about alternative therapies – are recognizing it has a place alongside mainstream medicine. The proof is in the patients who use it, often to manage a long-term condition, such as multiple sclerosis, or to seek relief for problems not cured or taken seriously enough by conventional medicine. It may not be so much a cure we seek, but a way of having some control over an illness ourselves.

Julia, 50, has MS: *When I was first diagnosed I read quite a lot of stuff about MS and my consultant told me that there wasn't really anything particular the usual medical practitioner could provide me with except maybe steroids if it got bad. I thought well I need to do something that gives me a feeling, whether it's illusory or not, that I am contributing towards keeping myself healthy.*

Sally, 43: *I've tried a number of different therapies: acupuncture, osteopathy, homoeopathy, healers, reflexology, a Chinese herbalist – and as far as MS is concerned nothing seems to get to the root of the problem. But on the other hand to be in the relationship with an alternative therapist … is almost always beneficial … on the level of maintaining my general health and well-being … what they do do is put me in a stronger position to deal with MS and its effects.*

Women visit conventional doctors more than men do, and they are also the main users of complementary medicine. The *Woman's Hour* survey found that 46 per cent of women see complementary medicine as something which can be a good addition to conventional medicine. Forty per cent said it was sometimes a good alternative. However, only 2 per cent regard it as better than the GP. Aromatherapy was found to be the most popular, with one in five women having tried it. Homoeopathy and osteopathy tied for second place.

Which Complementary Therapies Had Women Tried?

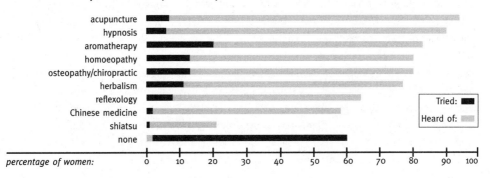

percentage of women:

There is no question that complementary medicine has great value for many. What is questionable is the evidence for why this is so. In many cases there is no scientific proof at all that a particular method is useful. Critics scoff at spiritual healers, but who can deny the pleasure of a relaxing aromatherapy massage for a weary body? The benefits of aromatherapy are now under study.

There are concerns too about a discipline which has few quality controls, where just about anyone can set up a business and call it complementary medicine. Opponents of complementary medicine argue that just because a medicine is natural rather than synthetic this does not mean it is safe. When you see a health professional, you count on their advice being good for you. You know that your own GP, the doctor in the hospital, or a nurse in a clinic, have had a certain standard of training. Their care and advice should be based on scientific knowledge and their experience. We tend to trust them and think of them as reliable and honest. But we also complain about them. We wish they had more time for us. Doctors' waiting-rooms are full of patient patients waiting their turn for a ten-minute consultation. Many of us want more than that and the complementary therapist often provides it.

> **Sally, 43:** *They've got more time than the doctor would have. That's true – you pay for an hour with these people, or half an hour and you don't get that with the doctor ... they tend to be very caring people though, I must say, so are a lot of doctors.*

Complementary therapists claim that conventional medicine pays too little attention to the whole person. They feel that doctors are often too ready to prescribe drugs which may have side effects, and may not be effective anyway. Conventional medicine has a remarkable track record with obvious successes in fertility treatment, kidney and heart transplants, immunization and the elimination of disease. But there are now concerns that our lives have become too medicalized, and with this has come some loss of faith in conventional medicine. Women with cancer often look to complementary therapy, both for the miracle cure conventional medicine has not yet found and for help in coping with the appalling side-effects of some conventional treatment.

Most people use alternative or complementary therapists in association with conventional medicine, often when the latter has failed to provide a cure for chronic or recurrent problems such as headaches, migraine, backache, arthritis, chronic fatigue syndrome, irritable bowel syndrome and premenstrual syndrome. Jeannette used a combination of complementary and conventional medicine in her fierce struggle against breast cancer and, as she wrote in her diary, it was not an easy road to take:

> **Jeannette, 36:** *There is a brick wall between practitioners of conventional and non-conventional therapy ... patients do massage, yoga, herbal stuff ... on the side – like children – because doctors frown on it ... wouldn't it be wonderful if the two worlds came together.*

Most, but not all, complementary medicine has to be paid for by the patient and is not available on the NHS. In 1995, 6 per cent of users did have their therapy paid for by the NHS. Most of this was for homoeopathy or acupuncture. Some GPs who have their own budgets purchase osteopathy for their patients. Complementary therapies are only likely to be available on the NHS where they have been shown to be effective through objective scientific criteria.

All new conventional medicines should be rigorously evaluated to see whether they work. The design of all trials for new drugs or treatments has to be approved by special ethics committees attached to hospitals, and patients are asked to take part. The best possible scientific test is a randomized controlled trial. This is done by comparing the new drug with the drug already commonly used, or the new drug and a placebo (a dummy pill that looks and tastes the same as the drug, but has no chemical effect). If it is a breast cancer drug, a group of breast cancer patients will be randomly split in two. One group will be given the drug currently in use. The other group will get the new one. Neither the patients nor their doctors will know who is taking what. The researchers, who do know which drug each patient is taking, observe which drug produces the best results. Scientists want subjects to remain unaware of who is taking what in order to eliminate bias. The mere knowledge that you are getting a certain drug may make you feel better. Critics of testing methods say depriving one group of a drug that may benefit them is unethical. But it can also be argued that it is even less ethical to prescribe drugs which are not yet proven to be effective.

Even though certain medicines and treatments have not been properly evaluated, and therefore there is no scientific evidence that something works, it does not mean that they are not effective. In the past most conventional treatments were not tested in this very rigorous way. Conventional medicine can therefore be accused of double standards.

Women's Opinions of Complementary Medicine

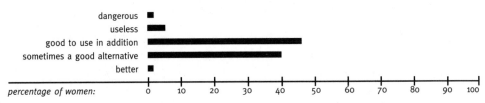

percentage of women:

In fact, much of conventional medicine has not come under close scrutiny, and complementary medicine even less so. Alternative therapists say it is too complicated to assess their treatments in this way and that it goes against the philosophy of complementary medicine – these therapies are supposed to have an effect on the whole body and mind rather than just on a particular disease. In order for patients to receive the best treatment possible, however, therapies (conventional or complementary) need, wherever possible, to be evaluated scientifically.

Much research into complementary medicine is, however, now being done, including one major study by the Cancer Research Campaign, looking into relaxation techniques versus aromatherapy massage. It wants to scientifically evaluate them and discover the difference between the two in reducing stress and anxiety for cancer patients. One obvious implication is financial. A single relaxation session can treat more than one person, while one aromatherapist can only do one massage at a time. A few studies are also being set up to examine the possible benefits of therapies such as acupuncture, homoeopathy, chiropractic and diets. The importance of allergies, the part that foods and food intolerance play in disease, the acceptance that osteopathy and chiropractic are good at dealing with many back problems, the emphasis on holistic medicine, and many other ideas that were once rejected or treated with scepticism by conventional medicine, are now accepted.

Choosing the right complementary therapy for you – and finding a qualified practitioner – can be a challenge. At least when you see NHS doctors you know they have had a basic minimum of training, although of course there are still bad doctors. We rarely understand what the letters after a doctor's name stand for and this is even more true of complementary practitioners. Talk to friends, read reputable journals, and ask your own GP to get the range of views on any one therapy and therapist. Find out what all the initials stand for and what training the practitioner has. And trust your own judgement.

A Short Guide to the Alternatives

The following is a guide to the main complementary therapies used by the women in our survey.

Aromatherapy

The *Woman's Hour* survey found 20 per cent of women have tried this.

> **Tracey Berry, Beauty Therapist:** *Aromatherapy can be used for all sorts of things. It's good for menopausal problems … you then choose the oils to suit that individual person. There are ones for mood enhancing, ones for migraine, and a whole host really.*

Aromatherapy involves massage with oils or bathing in oils derived from spices, woods, flowers or plants. Each oil may contain many different compounds and different oils are used for different problems. You can buy the oils yourself or you can go to a therapist who will choose the oils best suited for your needs.

There is a general acceptance that aromatherapy makes people feel better. Although there is no evidence that it is effective, aromatherapists claim it does much more than just provide a nice smell. It is being used in some cancer units for patients in chemotherapy to make them feel better.

> **Tracey:** *For home use the best possible oil you can ever have is lavender. It's so brilliant you can use it for insect bites, and stings. If you have sunburn you can use a few drops in your after sun cream and if you happen to catch yourself with the iron you can put it neat on to the skin. It really is the only oil that can be used neat. It actually heals the skin so there's less chance of any scar being left. You only need a drop or two and it lasts forever.*

It is recommended that all aromatherapy oils should be avoided during the first three months of pregnancy, after which you should always check with your doctor before use.

Homoeopathy

The survey found that 13 per cent of women have used homoeopathy. Homoeopathy uses very, very dilute solutions of substances derived from plants, animals and mineral sources. They usually come as pills. Homoeopathy is claimed to have a therapeutic effect, though this is highly individualized for each patient. Although it is not known how it works, some objective trials indicate good results for conditions such as hay fever, insomnia and asthma. There is a range of homoeopathic remedies available for premenstrual syndrome and the menopause. Some women find them helpful, although homoeopathy has not yet been scientifically evaluated. Some GPs are also trained homoeopaths, so they may be able to advise you. Larger chemists stock homoeopathic remedies and usually also have free leaflets which give more detailed information.

Homoeopathy and Irritable Bowel Syndrome
Irritable Bowel Syndrome (IBS) is a nuisance and nobody really knows why it happens. But because it is not dangerous and tends to be difficult to treat, conventional doctors are often accused of not taking it seriously. Wind, flatulence, diarrhoea and constipation, a feeling of distension and fullness in the tummy, are all problems associated with IBS. Often you will need to have a few tests to make sure there is no other cause, but once it is diagnosed as

complementary medicine

IBS, doctors try a range of antispasmodics, antidepressants and artificially produced fibre. None of these works very well and there is now much interest in diet and other therapies to try to control the symptoms. Changing your diet, by excluding certain foods from it and gradually re-introducing them, can help sort out what makes it worse for you. IBS is unlikely to be totally cured by any of the treatments but learning ways to manage it is a big help. Passing blood is not a symptom of IBS and you should always have this checked out by your doctor.

Celia has struggled with IBS for years. She is now experimenting with a variety of alternative therapies in the hope of getting rid of this condition:

> **Celia, 41:** *Its name is very very accurate. It's as if somebody's making your bowel or bladder pulsate and it's encouraging action when there really isn't any need for any ... I am sure it is stress related. It's as though some people carry their stress in their head and I carry mine right here in the middle of me ... I went to a homoeopathic doctor who identified it all in terms of the whole body and spoke in terms of having to divert your thinking to your head. He gave me a potion with phosphorus and other things in it and I had to put four drops in water before I ate. I can't tell whether it helped or not ... I went to an acupuncturist and he thinks I might have a wheat intolerance and so I've been off wheat, rye, barley and oats for a month and I have to say it's making quite a bit of difference.*

Celia suspects that her system may be intolerant of certain foods. And she is not the only one. There is growing interest in the notion that some of us have problem foods which cause upset tummies and painful joints. There is now evidence of a link between diet and conditions such as arthritis, migraine headaches and IBS. Linda is convinced that her new state of well-being has to do with eliminating certain problem foods from her diet:

> **Linda, 36:** *I was tired all the time – not ill – but just felt that something was not right and I had no real zest for life ... I had never been diagnosed by a doctor as having irritable bowel syndrome but thought that was it. At the gym I go to they had arranged for an allergy tester to come in ... I had the test and cut out wheat, sugar, tea and coffee ... I cut them out totally and after four weeks the improvement really started. I lost some weight, I feel so much better ... I know some people think food intolerance is rubbish and prefer to go to their GPs. They take any medication they are given, but what's the harm in eliminating something from your diet? If it doesn't work you haven't lost anything.*

Osteopathy and Chiropractic

In our survey 13 per cent of women said they had visited an osteopath or chiropractor.

Osteopathy

This involves manipulation of the muscles and joints. The balance between our muscles and bones, which make our musculoskeletal system, is important to their function. Osteopaths believe this balance is also important to the health of our body's organs. Some osteopaths only deal with musculoskeletal problems like back pain and joint problems. Others treat headaches and stress-related problems. The treatment of back pain by osteopathy has been found to be more effective than other treatments. Studies looking at the effectiveness of osteopathy for other conditions are rare, but anecdotal reports by patients indicate that it may be useful. Some physiotherapists also use manipulation to treat back problems.

Chiropractic

This concentrates on stresses, misalignments and problems of the joints in the spine which are thought to affect the nervous system, which in turn maintains the rest of the body's health. The therapist manipulates the spine and spinal joints to put things back in balance. It is especially useful for back problems. One study found it to be more effective than physiotherapy. Chiropractors also claim to treat more general health problems, including stress. There are various schools of chiropractor, some involving a four-year training.

> **Joan, 52:** *I had been gardening like a maniac ... My back got more and more painful and I ended up lying on the floor for three weeks, unable to do anything. Eventually I went to a chiropractitioner who manipulated my back several times and got me back to work.*
>
> **Jilly:** *I suffer terrible headaches. I thought it was something to do with my posture so I went to see a chiropractitioner ... It was all very impressive, particularly the couch which put me at every angle under the sun. He did a lot of manipulation of my neck and shoulders, so much that I thought it was bound to work, but I still have the headaches and I think they're more to do with stress.*

Herbalism and Chinese Medicine

Eleven per cent of women have been to see a herbalist according to our survey. The use of herbs and naturally occurring minerals to treat a variety of illnesses goes back thousands of years and is the oldest type of medicine known. Many modern medicines have been developed from herbs. There are different disciplines within herbal medicine with Chinese and Western herbal medicine following separate philosophies. Herbalists use whole plants rather than their individual chemical components. The herbs are supposed to relieve symptoms and hasten self-healing.

> **Halina St James, 50, Journalist specializing in alternative medicine:** *There are a lot of alternatives to hormone replacement therapy ... There are herbs like dong quai, a Chinese herb that women in China have been using for centuries to cure not only symptoms of menopause but PMS so it's a very good herb for women for their reproductive system. The other one that's really good is Mexican wild yams. Not yams you buy in the grocery store, but the medicinal root from Mexico ... and this will also help the symptoms of the menopause.*

There are many complementary therapies recommended for menopausal symptoms, including herbalism and diet. Some of the claims are based on scientific evidence but much more research is needed. Many women do not want to take synthetic hormones for premenstrual symptoms or the menopause, but neither do they want to suffer the symptoms. Chaste tree is another herb used to treat PMS and period problems. There is a scientific basis for this as it increases the hormone LH and stops the hormone FSH which changes the balance between oestrogen and progesterone (see pages 30–1).

Reflexology

Reflexology was tried by 8 per cent of women in the survey. This is a type of foot massage. Reflex points are mapped on the feet which are supposedly linked to specific parts of the body. By exerting pressure on the reflex points, by massage, the corresponding problem organ gets the benefit. Many people find reflexology helps with migraines and headaches.

> **Heather, Reflexologist:** *It's like taking a car to the garage, we take our cars to be tuned, so taking our body to the reflexologist is really like taking our body to be retuned and balanced.*

Acupuncture

Seven per cent of women in the survey have been to see an acupuncturist. Acupuncture is based on an ancient Chinese art. Fine needles are pricked into our skin, along supposed energy routes called Meridian lines. Our bodies apparently have positive and negative energy (Yin and Yang) and when we are ill the balance between the two is upset. Acupuncture aims to mend the balance by stimulating points along our energy lines. The needles may be inserted in our ears, arms and legs, abdomen or back, and may be left in place for up to half an hour. When acupuncture is used to treat tobacco addiction a tiny pin is stapled to the ear and left for days. When you feel like having a cigarette you are supposed to wiggle it to lose the craving. However, randomized studies have found no evidence to show acupuncture did help in the fight to give up smoking.

Acupuncture is used to treat a huge range of ailments including fertility, allergy, menstrual, abdominal and arthritic problems. It appears to be especially useful in the relief of chronic pain. Moxibustion is a treatment often done at the same time as acupuncture. Small amounts of moxa, the dried leaves of a herb, are burned in a little cup over the acupuncture points to treat and prevent disease by the application of heat. There are many variations of acupuncture. Acupuncture is part of a wider philosophy of healing which includes massage, herbal medicine and exercises.

> **Jo-Jo:** *I was offered a course of acupuncture. I wanted it for stress and anxiety because my job was over the top. It was terrific whilst I was having it. I went to sleep for the whole afternoon after it. Personally I think it was the therapist that relaxed me more than the needles. I'd really like to know as I'm thinking of having some more – but maybe it doesn't matter.*

Hypnotherapy

Six per cent of women in the survey had tried hypnotherapy. Hypnotherapy is based on the belief that both the conscious and unconscious mind can influence diseases. A trance-like state is induced by special relaxation techniques. During this state suggestions are made and implanted at a subconscious level. When you come out of the trance, the idea will be in your mind without you realizing it has been put there. Hypnotherapists claim they can help you to stop smoking, but a randomized trial on this did not show it was any more useful than other methods.

Shiatsu

Just 1 per cent of women have tried shiatsu. This massage technique involves the application of pressure using fingers, hands, elbows, knees, feet, and sometimes the whole body. The pressure is meant to unblock energy which is apparently stuck at certain points in your body, thus releasing energy and vitality. Any type of massage may be beneficial as it helps you to relax.

chapter 15

a guide to common operations

Sadie, 87: I had my eyes done. No trouble at all, just went in one day and came out the next. That was OK. I could see so much better. All I had to do was put drops in my eyes for a few weeks and it was wonderful. I could see immediately.

Over the years operations have become much safer. But even today, they carry some risk, both from the operation itself and from the anaesthetic. Some operations are riskier than others. Before embarking on any operation it is therefore helpful to be well informed about the procedure itself and the possible complications. Sometimes operations are essential and even life-saving. When they are not, the pros and cons must be carefully considered before making a final decision.

This is a quick reference guide to the most common operations. We include operations for women only as well as a few which are common to both sexes. You will also find the frequency statistics, information on why an operation needs to be done, what it involves and some of the problems that may occur. How often an operation is carried out depends not only on how prevalent the problem is, but also on the current medical and social trends and resources. The frequency of different types of operations varies across the UK and from country to country. The British government is cutting back on statistical services making it more difficult to track who is having which operations. The private sector does not provide overall statistics which leaves the picture incomplete. The statistics in this chapter are for England only.

The success of an operation depends on whether the problem or disease for which it is being carried out can be completely cured or not and whether there are any complications. Complications that occur during operations include wound problems such as infections, bleeding, and scarring. These are usually minor and are fairly common. Reaction to general anaesthetic varies from person to person. Some people become sick and nauseated immediately afterwards. Modern anaesthetics cause fewer problems, although they can make you feel rather tired or exhausted for a few days.

Chest infections can occur after an operation and may need treatment with antibiotics. More rarely you may get a blood clot in your leg. This is called deep-vein thrombosis and most people recover from such a blood clot. They are easily treated with anticoagulants which thin the blood. These drugs need to be taken for several months, during which time your blood will be regularly checked. Much more dangerous are blood clots in the lung which occur when a bit of the clot in the leg breaks off and goes into the lung. When the clot is in your lungs it is called a pulmonary embolus, and it can be fatal.

Unfortunately the information provided in hospitals and by GPs is often insufficient, and you may be left with many unanswered questions such as how long it will take to recover from an operation? Ask four doctors this question and you are likely to get four different answers. Recovery time depends both on the success of the operation and you, the individual.

It is best to wait to return to work until you are really *feeling* recovered. Colleagues will remember that you have had an operation for the first few days, but they soon forget and expect you to return to your normal duties. Similarly at home there is no need to prove yourself by coming out of hospital and taking on all the household chores instantaneously, then feeling a martyr and getting cross with everyone for not helping, or, worse still, finding that you get ill again because you were not fully ready to get back to normal.

Before any major operation you will be asked about your medical history and about what medication you are on. Women on the contraceptive pill will be advised to stop taking it because of the associated increased risk of blood clots. Women taking HRT can usually continue to take their medication, but this should be discussed with your doctor.

The Operations

D and C (Dilatation and Curettage)

Dilatation and curettage, or D and C, is an operation performed to try to find out the cause of heavy or irregular periods, bleeding between periods and to check the lining of the uterus for cancer. It is also used to remove the remains of a foetus after an incomplete miscarriage or ERPC (evacuation of retained products of conception). The operation involves the insertion of thin metal dilators of increasing size, up to 8–10 millimetres, which are passed through the cervix into the uterus. Once the cervix is dilated, an instrument with a tiny spoon attached to it is passed into the uterus and the superficial lining is scraped off. This is done under a general anaesthetic. It is now thought that this operation is too readily performed, especially on younger women. The number is decreasing as other investigations such as endometrial aspiration or hysteroscopy (see below and pages 358–9) appear to be more useful and can be done without any anaesthetic or under local anaesthetic.

D and C has also been used as a treatment. It was thought to be a cure for many menstrual problems, but has been shown to be ineffective – over the long term – in the treatment of period problems, especially heavy periods. It is only the first period immediately after a D and C which is likely to be lighter.

> **Margaret, 58:** *I had one after my fourth baby. I think it was because my periods were very heavy and irregular and I had a D and C to see if that would straighten it out. It felt fine afterwards. It didn't bother me.*

How Common? This is the most common operation women have. In England in 1994–5, 87,210 women had a D and C on the NHS. By the age of forty-three, 15 per cent of women have had a D and C. But the rate is decreasing.

Recovery Time? If the procedure is done as an outpatient you only need to take the day off work. If you need a general anaesthetic you may need a day or two to recover. You may bleed for a few days after the operation.

What Can Go Wrong? There are few problems associated with a D and C. However, the cervix can get damaged. Very rarely the instrument ruptures through the wall of the uterus, which can cause internal pain and bleeding, but it should heal itself.

Endometrial Aspiration Curettage

An endometrial aspiration curettage is similar to a D and C. It is usually done with no anaesthetic or sometimes under local anaesthetic. It does not involve stretching the cervix and is increasingly being performed instead of a D and C. A small tube is inserted into the uterus. A sample of the lining is sucked out and sent to the laboratory for testing of the cells. If you have never had a baby you may need to have a general anaesthetic because the neck of the womb will still be very tight making it difficult and very painful to insert the little tube. It sounds awful but most women report that, although it is uncomfortable, it is bearable and the sharp pain lasts only for a few seconds.

How Common? There are 10,000 of these performed annually on the NHS and this number is increasing.

Recovery Time? The procedure only takes a few minutes and most women recover almost immediately.

What Can Go Wrong? There are few problems, but occasionally the instrument punctures the wall of the uterus or there is excessive bleeding. If it is too painful and uncomfortable it has to be done with a local or general anaesthetic.

Abortion

See Chapter 9 for a full discussion of this.

Sterilization (Tubal Ligation)

Sterilization (see pages 211–12) gives over a 99 per cent 'permanent' method of contraception. The procedure, tubal ligation, stops the egg and sperm meeting. The fallopian tubes are sealed or blocked using clips or rings. It can be done under local or general anaesthetic, though most NHS procedures are carried out under a general anaesthetic because it is quicker. It involves making two small incisions in your abdomen near the fallopian tubes (see the diagram on page 211). Your womb, ovaries and cervix are left untouched and your sexual drive should be the same as ever. Some women find sex improves as they no longer worry about getting pregnant. Your ovaries continue to produce eggs, but they are absorbed into the bloodstream and destroyed by the white blood cells.

How Common? In 1994–5, 52,612 tubal ligations were performed on the NHS. Many others would have been done privately.

Recovery Time? It is done either as an outpatient or you may have to stay in hospital for one or two nights. If it is done under a general anaesthetic it may take a few days before you feel back to normal. The scar may feel uncomfortable for a few days.

What Can Go Wrong? This is a good method of contraception. It has a failure rate of less than 1 per cent. Reversal of tubal ligation is possible, with claims of up to a 58 per cent success rate, but this is not available on the NHS in all areas of the country. The results depend on the initial type of sterilization and the skill of the operator. Some women notice their periods are heavier after sterilization. This may be because they stopped taking the contraceptive pill after the operation and the pill had given them lighter periods. A small minority of women are sorry they had the procedure. About 4 per cent of women have regrets eighteen months after the operation.

Hysteroscopy

This is when a very thin telescope called a hysteroscope is inserted through the cervix into the uterus. The telescope is used to examine the lining of the uterus to try to identify a reason for heavy or painful periods or bleeding between periods. A fibroid or polyp (see pages 36–7) may be present and can sometimes be removed during the procedure. This is usually done as an outpatient under local anaesthetic or under general anaesthetic when you stay in for the day.

How Common? In 1994–5, 30,017 were performed on the NHS.

Recovery time? Recovery from the procedure itself is almost immediate, although you may need a day or two to get over a general anaesthetic.

What Can Go Wrong? It is unusual for anything to go wrong, though very rarely the hysteroscope is pushed through the wall of the uterus causing internal pain and bleeding.

Hysterectomy

Hysterectomy is the removal of the uterus or womb. There are two types of hysterectomy. Most UK hysterectomies are done by cutting through the lower wall of the abdomen. This is called an abdominal hysterectomy. It leaves a scar about four to six inches long, which usually runs horizontally along the bikini line. Alternatively, some surgeons will remove the uterus through a cut inside at the top of the vagina. This is usually undertaken if a prolapse (see below) is the problem.

Hysterectomies are now also being done using a laparoscope (see page 364). Which procedure you get mainly depends on your surgeon, but you should discuss your preference with him or her. There are many reasons for having a hysterectomy. Hysterectomies are performed to alleviate heavy periods when other treatments have failed. Forty-five per cent of hysterectomies are for heavy periods, and in many of these nothing abnormal is found in the uterus itself when it is examined after the operation. At least 50 per cent of women who have hysterectomies because of heavy periods lose less than 80 ml of blood during a period. Although this is not technically a heavy period some women feel it is heavy for them, since they are used to having lighter periods. Other reasons for having hysterectomies include fibroids (20 per cent), prolapsed uterus (9 per cent), cancer of the uterus (9 per cent), pelvic inflammatory disease (1 per cent). A few are done for endometriosis (see pages 38–40).

A prolapse is a dropping down of the uterus from the pelvis into the vagina. This can happen because the ligaments which support the uterus have got weaker, or because the walls of the vagina have become stretched and weakened. You can feel the protrusion into your vagina. The muscles in the pelvis are also sometimes repaired if they have got stretched. All the stitches used dissolve on their own.

> **Iris, 74:** *The alarming thing was that I had this bothersome piece of flesh that was protruding from me day by day – from my vagina – and I was nervous about even going to the doctor about that and what could be done about it. I went to a gynaecologist and ... I had a vaginal hysterectomy which was to have the uterus taken out and have this flesh cut off that was protruding.*

How Common? In the UK in 1994–5, 72,821 were performed – 57,293 were abdominal hysterectomies; 15,528 were vaginal hysterectomies. By the age of forty-three, one in ten English women will have had a hysterectomy. Rates of hysterectomy vary from country to country. Half as many Norwegian women have hysterectomies, but in the USA at least one in three women will have her womb removed by the age of seventy.

Recovery Time? Allow enough time. Most women need at least eight weeks before going back to work. Many women do not feel fully recovered until three months or more after the operation. Avoid heavy lifting and bending until you feel comfortable. Be guided by your body as to how much and how quickly you should start doing things after the operation. You may be told not to drive a car until you are out of pain. The rule is if it hurts do not do it. Recovery time appears to be shorter for women having a vaginal hysterectomy because there is no cut in the abdomen.

What Can Go Wrong? Although many thousands of women have hysterectomies the operation is not without complications. Forty-five per cent of women will get some complication immediately after the operation: pain, bleeding, a wound infection, urinary problems or vaginal discharge. Some women complain that sex, especially their sexual drive, becomes a problem. For some this is because the ovaries have been removed at the same time causing the immediate onset of the menopause; for others the blood supply to the ovaries might have been affected, which would also cause early menopause. HRT can help (see pages 60–71). There is also controversy as to whether it is better to remove the uterus only and leave the cervix since it has a role in orgasm. Discuss this with your surgeon.

> **Jan, 54:** *Being a theatre nurse I rehearsed the operation night after night after night so I knew exactly what was going to happen to me ... what I hadn't rehearsed was the grief over having lost something which had been such a nuisance ... for a while I didn't feel that I was a woman ... it was the end of an era ... it took me about six months to feel at ease and at peace with it ... I'm taking HRT and seem to feel fairly well ... I feel very feminine, although I do have bouts of tiredness.*

Although some women feel depressed after a hysterectomy, others report improvement in their well-being, especially if they no longer suffer from the problem for which the hysterectomy was done. Up to two women out of 1000 will die having a hysterectomy because of complications during or after the operation. The figure is lower for younger women because they are generally fitter.

Having Your Ovaries Removed

The ovaries are taken out at the same time as a hysterectomy in 50 per cent of cases, even though there is usually nothing wrong with them. They are taken out in case they should get cancerous in the future. It has been estimated that you would need to remove the ovaries from 200 women to prevent one case of ovarian cancer. If you are pre-menopausal and have your ovaries removed you will have a sudden menopause. You will need to consider taking HRT to stop the symptoms (see pages 60–71). Even women who do not have their ovaries removed at the same time as the hysterectomy are neverthless more likely to experience the menopause early. This may be within months of the hysterectomy or several years earlier than the menopause was expected. This may in part be due to the interference to the blood supply to the ovaries during the operation.

Gynaecologists have different views about hysterectomy, how often it is needed and whether ovaries should be removed at the same time. The decision to have a hysterectomy for a non-malignant condition should always be the woman's, but in cases where the woman is becoming extremely anaemic, she is likely to gain great benefit.

Possible Advantages of Hysterectomy

- Sorts out period problems.
- Stops the need for medication to cope with painful or heavy periods.
- Removes worries about contraception.
- Removes need for cervical smears.
- Eradicates risk of uterine or cervical cancer.
- Removal of ovaries at the same time avoids the risk of ovarian cancer and gets rid of premenstrual symptoms.

Possible Disadvantages of Hysterectomy

- Recovery time can take up to three months.
- There may be complications.
- You will never be able to have children.
- You may feel depressed.
- Removal of the ovaries produces an acute, immediate menopause.
- Earlier than expected menopause, even if the ovaries are left in.

a guide to common operations

Endometrial Ablation
(Transcervical Resection of the Endometrium – TCRE)

This is a relatively new operation for women with very heavy periods and it is still under examination to see how good it is in the long term. It involves removing the whole lining of the uterus, using different techniques such as electrosurgery, rollerball or laser. This is an alternative to hysterectomy and may stop periods altogether or make them much lighter. Under general anaesthetic an instrument is inserted through the cervix into the uterus, so no cut is made in the abdomen and there is no scar. It is not suitable for all causes of heavy periods such as those due to fibroids (see pages 36–7), or endometriosis (see pages 38–40). It cannot be done to treat uterine cancers.

How Common? In 1994–5, 9658 were performed.

Recovery Time? A big advantage of endometrial ablation over hysterectomy is that recovery time from the operation is shorter both in hospital and at home. The hospital stay is usually two to three days and you feel fit enough for work after two to three weeks.

What Can Go Wrong? The aim is to remove all the lining (endometrium) of the uterus but this is not always possible. Almost 50 per cent of women will have no periods at all during the first year after the operation, but after one year this figure is only 20 per cent. However, most women find their periods become light and manageable. A 1997 UK study found 80 per cent of women are happy with endometrial ablation, but 20 per cent need further surgery such as a repeat endometrial ablation or a hysterectomy for continued pain and/or bleeding. As the lining of the uterus is removed, pregnancy should not occur though there are concerns that if some lining is left a pregnancy could still theoretically occur. The uterus may be perforated during the procedure but this is rare.

Vaginal Repair

This involves cutting away some vaginal tissue and pulling what is left together to tighten the walls of the vagina. This is usually done for a prolapse which is caused by the uterus coming down into the vagina, or the vaginal walls getting baggy causing the bladder to flop forwards into the vagina. This often causes frequent urination and incontinence. Sometimes the ligaments which hold up the uterus are shortened to hold it in place. A prolapse is associated with being very overweight and having had several pregnancies. Sometimes the back wall of the vagina gets baggy and loose, with the rectum becoming displaced forward, making it feel uncomfortable and sometimes difficult to pass faeces. There are a variety of surgical repairs to treat this condition. Before you decide in favour of this operation, do try Kegel's pelvic floor exercises to strengthen your muscles (see page 336).

Elderly women particularly may not want to go through an operation. An alternative is to have a special pessary – a vinyl ring – put into the vagina which acts as a support. This can usually be inserted at a doctor's surgery and will need changing every year.

How Common? In 1994–5, 24,690 were done.

Recovery Time? It usually takes six weeks to recover (longer if a hysterectomy is done at the same time), but this will depend on the size of the repair required, the general health of the individual, and if and how the bowel and urinary systems are affected.

What Can Go Wrong? Infection of the wound, urinary infections and bleeding can occur. If you are still having sex, or want to in the future, make sure you talk about this with your surgeon so your vagina is not tightened too much to make sex difficult. Sometimes the operation is not successful and has to be done again.

Oophorectomy

One or both ovaries are removed under a general anaesthetic. It involves a cut in the abdomen, or more recently it is being done using a laparoscope (see page 364). Oophorectomy is carried out for ovarian cancer, non-cancerous cysts on the ovaries and endometriosis (see pages 38–40). It may also be done during a hysterectomy to protect against the development of ovarian cancer. Once the ovaries have been removed you are no longer able to have your own children. If you need to have an oophorectomy at a young age, it may be possible to have some of your eggs removed before the operation. These can be frozen and stored for use in the future using IVF (see pages 310–12) but this is still at the research stage and the procedure is not guaranteed.

How Common? In 1994–5, 11,433 operations were performed.

Recovery Time? This usually takes six to eight weeks but it may take longer.

What Can Go Wrong? There can be infection and bleeding of the wound. The menopause may happen overnight if both ovaries are removed. This can be remedied by taking HRT (see pages 60–71). An oestrogen implant, when a small oestrogen pellet is inserted into the skin at the time of the operation, is another option. This will need replacing approximately every six months under local anaesthetic. This method of giving oestrogen has become less popular as some women find they need to have implants inserted increasingly frequently. Our bodies appear to become resistant to the oestrogen when it is taken in this form, and women often experience a recurrence of hot flushes, night sweats and vaginal dryness, even though the actual oestrogen levels are high.

a guide to common operations

Laparoscopy

A laparoscope is a very thin telescopic camera and it is used to allow the examination of the uterus, fallopian tubes and ovaries, to help find the cause of heavy periods or pelvic pain without a major operation. It can be used to diagnose endometriosis, ovarian cysts or pelvic inflammatory disease. It involves making a little hole in the abdomen through which the laparoscope is inserted.

Laparoscopy-assisted surgery can sometimes also be done in place of a major operation, although one still needs a general anaesthetic. It can be used to treat endometriosis, infertility, and to perform a hysterectomy. It can also be used to perform sterilization (see pages 211–12). Laparoscopy leaves only tiny scars. During a laparoscopy-assisted hysterectomy, the womb is separated from surrounding tissue using tiny instruments. It is then removed through the vagina. This is a more complicated procedure than most laparoscopy operations, needing specialist equipment which is not available at all hospitals.

How Common? In 1994–5, 53,705 laparoscopies were carried out.

Recovery Time? Women are normally out of hospital in a day or two and back to work in a week. For minor laparoscopic surgery, you may need just a few days to recover from the anaesthetic. Some women recover quickly and return to their normal routines immediately.

What Can Go Wrong? There are the usual problems associated with any operation.

Mastectomy

Mastectomy involves removal of the breast tissue under a general anaesthetic. It is usually carried out because breast cancer has been diagnosed. Mastectomy can be partial when the tumour and some of the surrounding breast tissue are removed or total, when the whole breast is removed, including some of the lymph glands under the arm, but the muscle under the breast is left undisturbed. It is called radical when the breast, lymph nodes and muscle are all removed. The latter is done relatively rarely in the UK, since having this more mutilating operation does not add to a woman's life expectancy. (See also Chapter 10 for more discussion of mastectomy.)

How Common? In 1994–5, 12,561 mastectomies were performed. There were 40,297 lumpectomies done in the same year, reflecting the trend towards more conservative surgery.

Recovery Time? The hospital stay is four to five days after the operation, but most women need four to six weeks to recover. Recovery from the accompanying treatment of chemotherapy and/or radiotherapy after the mastectomy may take several months. You will need time off work and if you are at home with children you may need extra help.

What Can Go Wrong? There can be problems with the wound such as infection or bleeding. Some women get swelling of the arm after the operation (oedema) especially if the lymph nodes have been removed. Pain in the arm can also occur.

Cataract Extraction

The lens in the eye is what enables us to see. Cataracts occur in the lens and cause impairment of vision because the cells become opaque and light cannot get through. When to have a cataract removed depends on how much your vision is being affected. Your optician or ophthalmologist will advise you. You do not need to wait until the cataract is very severe before having this operation. It is a very safe procedure with good results.

Cataract extraction involves opening the lens capsule, removing all the lens contents and implanting a plastic lens inside the capsule. Different techniques are available. The most modern ones use phako surgery, where the lens is broken down and scooped out with ultrasound after a tiny incision is made in the eye. The new lens is popped in and there are no stitches. The operation is often carried out under local anaesthetic, when you will be awake. If you prefer to be unconscious during the operation it can be done under a general anaesthetic. You may not even need to stay overnight in hospital. You have your eyes done one at a time, perhaps a few weeks apart. It can make you feel a bit unbalanced until the other eye is corrected too, and then it can be a few weeks before your vision and any glasses you need are sorted out and adjusted.

How Common? There were 17,287 cataract extractions for men and women in 1994–5. By the age of eighty most people will have some degree of cataract in their eyes but in the early stages it will not affect vision. Some diseases, such as diabetes, make you more prone to developing a cataract.

Recovery Time? Many people get immediate improvement in vision after the cataract is removed but in others it can take several weeks. Once your sight is restored you will need to have a check to see if you need new spectacles. Some people return to work immediately though most will take one week off. You can behave quite normally after the operation. In the past, the advice was to keep still and not bend over after a cataract extraction but this is no longer necessary. Do try to avoid rubbing or hitting your eye. You will need to put in eye drops several times a day for one week to help reduce any inflammation.

What Can Go Wrong? The eye can get infected, red or sore, but this can be treated. In a few cases the back of the eye can get waterlogged and then vision does not improve. There is no way to predict who will have this complication nor is there any effective treatment for it.

Cholecystectomy (Gall Bladder Removal)

Cholecystectomy is an operation to remove the gall bladder, which is a small sac inside the abdomen attached to the intestines and which stores bile made in the liver. The most common reason for the operation is because gallstones have developed in the gall bladder causing pain, infection or jaundice. Ten per cent of all women will be found to have gallstones on ultrasound screening, but unless they cause problems, there is no need for an operation. We do not know why gallstones develop but they are more likely to occur in middle-aged women and women on the pill or HRT, though men also get them. Gallstones can be removed by keyhole surgery (removal using a laparoscope) with a tiny incision in the abdomen, or with a more major cut. In keyhole surgery, an instrument with a microscope is inserted through the small cut. The operation is then performed looking through the microscope, with small instruments. Rather like the appendix we seem to be able to live without the gallbladder quite happily. It is safer to have the operation after any acute attack or infection has settled. Gallstones can sometimes be treated without surgery. Certain medicines may help dissolve them or ultrasound can be used to break them up.

How Common? In 1994–5, 35,772 men and women had gall bladder operations.

Recovery Time? It varies from woman to woman. Most women find they need several weeks before returning to work. It takes less time to get over keyhole surgery.

What Can Go Wrong? The wound can get infected, or bleed. Only very rarely does something go wrong with the operation itself.

Haemorrhoidectomy

This procedure is to remove haemorrhoids – varicose veins which develop around the anus. At least 50 per cent of women will have them at some time, especially during pregnancy and/or after the delivery of the baby. They are also associated with constipation because of straining to pass a movement. Usually they can be helped or cured by eating more roughage, or applying creams which can be bought without prescription. If these measures do not work, the haemorrhoids can be injected (in hospital) with a fluid which shrinks them, or they can have bands put on them until they shrivel in size. If you continue to get a lot of pain and bleeding from haemorrhoids you may need a haemorrhoidectomy. The haemorrhoids are cut out under general anaesthetic.

How Common? In 1994–5, 12,086 haemorrhoidectomies were performed.

Recovery Time? It may be done as an outpatient but you have to stay overnight. It will feel sore and uncomfortable for some weeks, especially when you have a bowel movement. You may need to take painkillers and laxatives. It takes longer to recover than most doctors tell you.

What Can Go Wrong? Bleeding after the operation. Recurrence of the haemorrhoids, scarring around your anus and, as with all operations, the scar may get infected.

Varicose Veins

Varicose veins are very common, especially in women after pregnancy. They occur because of damage to the valves in the veins which cause a back flow of blood and increased pressure in the veins. There are several ways of managing varicose veins. If they are small and do not cause problems most women do nothing. Support tights or stockings can relieve discomfort. Some varicose veins are suitable for injections under local anaesthetic with a chemical which makes them shrivel. This is particularly successful if the veins are below the knee and if there are not too many of them. The procedure is still effective seven years later for 50 per cent of women. Varicose vein operations involve tying off the damaged veins to stop blood going through them. Instead it flows through other deeper veins. The procedure is called a ligation. Sometimes varicose veins are left in or they can be stripped out. Tiny thread veins are not the same as varicose veins. They are also common, but very difficult to treat. Laser treatment shows promise.

How Common? In 1994–5, 41,379 ligations were performed on men and women (mostly women) – 16,107 other operations were performed for varicose veins.

Recovery Time? Injections: You can go back to work the following day but your leg(s) will need to be bandaged for three weeks. Walking helps speed recovery.

Vein stripping or vein tying: You need at least one week off work, bandages stay on for three weeks and once again you should walk each day.

What Can Go Wrong? Injections: Brown stain marks at the site of the injections look unsightly and, although they fade, they often do not disappear completely.

Tying and stripping: Most women are happy with these operations but sometimes the varicose veins recur – or rather other veins become varicosed. Deep vein thrombosis can occur in the deeper veins after these operations. The scars can look unsightly.

chapter 16

well-woman check

Jan, 54: It was my first mammogram and it was a routine one ... I gave the letter to Ian to open – it was a routine thing but when [they say] you've got to come back for a repeat I felt panic stricken and I felt I'd already been given a diagnosis of breast cancer.

There is something very reassuring about being told you are healthy by a doctor. Your friend or partner tells you and you may not believe it, but when you hear it from a health professional you do. As a result, regular annual check-ups for women have been part of the North American scene for many years.

> **Madelaine, 41:** *In Canada I used to go once a year ... and I'd have a pap smear, an internal, she'd weigh me, she'd check my breasts and you'd come away from it thinking if there was anything seriously wrong with me she would have spotted it, right? But here I'm always confused about how things work and also the doctors always give me the impression that they don't have enough time so they'll see you if you've got something seriously wrong but you don't feel you should go in when you don't have anything seriously wrong.*

In the UK, doctors are sceptical about the value of the annual check-up. And there is no agreement about what one should involve if we did have them on the National Health Service. There is probably too much checking in North America, but not enough here. And some British women would like to see more.

> **Marina, 49:** *I would like to feel that the practice would offer an annual check-up ... I would certainly take advantage of it ... what I tend to do is bowl along every so often and just report symptoms and say this is what's happening to me, is this acceptable?*

One reason annual checks are popular in the US is because most health services are funded privately. A check-up is a service provided by a business and doctors get paid for each one. This may influence how often they think women should see them. In Canada many women go for annual check-ups which the state pays for, but in most parts of the country they are not invited. Most health care there is publicly funded, as it is here. British GPs are not paid for doing annual general check-ups, except in patients over the age of seventy-five. Doctors in the UK do get paid for carrying out certain screening checks such as cervical smears. In fact in the new era of cost-effective medicine, if doctors screen 80 per cent of their women patients between the ages of twenty-five and sixty-five, they get a financial bonus from the NHS.

Some women feel they do not want to bother their doctor for check-ups because the doctor seems too busy: in the *Woman's Hour* health survey carried out for this book we learned that, although women are generally happy with their doctors, they do feel their doctors are short of time. Some women do ask for check-ups and get rebuffed. But doctors' surgery practices vary across the country. Some GPs run well-woman clinics – see if yours does and

well-woman check

find out what is available to you. If yours does not, find out where there is one in your area – you may be able to visit a well-woman clinic even if it is at another surgery. Most family-planning clinics also give well-woman checks. Some GPs check your blood pressure and give advice on breast examinations when they call you in for a cervical smear, and some women take this opportunity to turn the appointment into a more general check-up and discussion about health, including diet and exercise.

The Usual NHS Checks

You should be able to get the following on the NHS:

- Weight check measured through body mass index (BMI) which links height and weight.
- Blood pressure test.
- Cervical smear every three to five years from the age of 20.
- Breast check when you are concerned (see Chapter 10).
- Mammogram every three years from the age of fifty (see pages 379–81).
- Family history consultation, paying particular attention to a history of heart disease, cancer and diabetes.
- Consultation on your eating, drinking and smoking habits.
- Cholesterol test (see pages 386–7).
- Consultation about hormone replacement therapy (HRT) and whether it is right for you when you reach the menopause (see Chapter 3).
- A urine test for diabetes or kidney infection.
- Consultation about any worries you may have, e.g. anxiety over the break-up of your marriage, depression, bereavement or problems with children.

Going Private

A routine minimum private health check costs around £200, takes about an hour and is much more comprehensive than the NHS could ever dream of. This will not necessarily be any better for you, but you will certainly feel it is. Private health checks include some or all of the following:

- A full physical examination, including listening to your heart and lungs, checking your pulse rate, feeling your tummy, examining your skin, and looking down your throat.
- An internal vaginal examination.
- Cervical smear.
- A bone density scan (see page 326).

- Blood tests for anaemia, any problems with liver or kidney function, calcium levels, gout, cholesterol.
- Electrocardiogram (ECG) to check the heart.
- Lung function tests (breathing into a tube and seeing how much air you can blow out).
- Hearing and eye tests.
- Chest X-ray.
- Bowel test.
- Mammogram.
- A leisurely conversation where the doctor asks you about your work and home life and your general outlook on life.

After the examination you will receive a letter detailing all the findings. The letter will certainly make you feel good, unless something untoward is found in which case you will be advised to see your GP. It will review the topics discussed, emphasizing the good things, highlighting anything abnormal, and making recommendations for action for your future good health. The doctor will tell you he or she looks forward to seeing you next year. A copy of the letter will be sent to your NHS GP if you agree.

Of course there is overlap between what you get on the NHS versus going private. If you need an electrocardiogram on the NHS you will get one. But private screening includes a battery of tests you would never normally receive on the NHS, unless your doctor had a special reason for ordering them for you. There is no evidence to show that giving *all* people *all* of these tests saves lives. Some tests are helpful in some circumstances. For instance, if you have high blood pressure it is a good idea to have an electrocardiogram (ECG). If you have a family history of ovarian cancer (see pages 382–4) you should be screened for this early. There is a big debate about who should get which tests when. Giving everyone the tests would cost billions, with little evidence to show that most people's health would benefit. Most but not all screening tests shown to be effective to date are now available on the NHS, although sometimes you do have to ask for them.

There is a downside to too much testing. Screening can cause unnecessary worry when slightly 'abnormal' results are found. With fast-paced developments in the world of testing (genetic testing for instance) it is essential that every new screening test be properly evaluated before it is introduced, to prevent further unnecessary investigations and anxiety.

Many women are reassured by thorough check-ups. If you want a private one either because you are worried about something or because you feel your own GP does not have the time, go for it. But make sure you visit a reputable clinic or see a doctor you know from others to be reliable. Private clinics are profit-making businesses which will love having your business and will encourage follow-ups.

Regular Screening Tests

'Screening' in health care is a medical test. This can be as simple as a doctor examining some part of your anatomy. It can also be a blood test, cervical smear, or mammogram. You, the subject, may either be apparently well and healthy, or someone who is considered to be at higher risk of something because of your own personal medical history. Part of the point of 'screening' is to try to get as many people in the population as possible to have a test, because the more people you test the better the chance of catching the few who have a problem needing attention.

The first step in screening is to identify a group of people who might be at high risk of getting a disease. Screening a population to find out who smokes and persuading the smokers to give up in order to prevent lung cancer is an example of primary prevention.

The next step in screening is secondary prevention. Here the aim is to find the disease itself and treat it early before it causes any harm. This stage often begins with a question from your family doctor who might ask: 'Do you have a family history of breast cancer?' Women who answer 'yes' are members of a particular group in the population who could be at a higher risk of breast cancer, so they become the target group for possible earlier testing in the mammography screening programme.

Screening is fraught with problems. The tests involved are rarely 100 per cent accurate. So some women may be told there is something wrong, only to find later they are fine. Such results are called 'false positives'. Other women are told things are all right, when the test actually fails to detect an abnormality. This is called a 'false negative'. In an ideal world screening tests would be reliable, with false positives and false negatives kept to an absolute minimum. They would be inexpensive and able to identify a problem early on so it could be treated effectively.

Screening tests available specifically for women include those for cervical cancer, breast cancer, and ovarian cancer. Screening is also available, to both sexes, for high blood pressure (hypertension), high cholesterol and bowel cancer. Pregnant women face an array of screening tests (see page 270–7) but the usual ones are for immunity to German measles, anaemia, diabetes, pre-eclampsia and syphilis. They are also offered screening to show whether they are at risk of carrying a baby with Down's syndrome. Newborn baby girls and boys are screened for thyroid disease, dislocated hips and other conditions.

Cervical Screening

> **Brenda:** *I felt really worried about having a smear and kept putting it off. My daughter kept nagging me. She'd had one and couldn't understand why I was making such a fuss. One day when I was at the doctor's for a pain in my elbow she said why didn't she do it there and then. I couldn't think of a good excuse and it seemed stupid to say I was embarrassed. I can't say I enjoyed it but it was very quick and apart from being uncomfortable wasn't as bad as having a blood test.*

In the UK, there is good news about cervical cancer. Over 80 per cent of women now have regular cervical smears and deaths from cervical cancer are going down. Since the national system was set up in 1988 to call all women aged twenty to sixty-five for regular smears, the rate of cervical cancer deaths in England and Wales has fallen from over 1800 in 1989 to fewer than 1400 in 1994.

There are two types of cervical cancer – squamous cell cancers, which account for 85 per cent of cases, and adeno cancers which account for the rest. The present cervical screening programme checks for the pre-cancerous squamous cell type. The screening test rarely picks up the adeno type, which develops from cells further up in the cervix. The best way to prevent squamous cervical cancer is by detecting and treating pre-cancerous changes in cells, which can occur in the cervix (the 'neck' or opening of the uterus) many years before they actually become cancer. Screening involves having a cervical smear, so called because a sample of cells is taken from the cervix and smeared on to a glass slide which is then examined under a microscope. The smear is taken by a nurse or doctor who inserts a speculum into your vagina to hold it open so your cervix can be seen. A considerate nurse or doctor will warm a metal speculum first. The best time to have a smear is midway between periods. A wooden stick is gently scraped on the cervix to get a sample of the cells which is sent to the laboratory to be examined. The procedure should not hurt but may feel a little uncomfortable. The more relaxed you are the less of an ordeal it is.

Cervical smears are available free of charge on the NHS and all women between the ages of twenty and sixty-five should have one at least every five years. Older women can have them free of charge too, although at present they are not routinely invited.

How often smears should be done is controversial. Most experts agree that once every three years is enough to spot a developing cancer in time. But in many parts of the UK, women are screened every five years, because of lack of money and because the professionals in those areas have given higher priority to other services. However, when an abnormality is discovered, smears should be done much more frequently – perhaps every three or six months depending on the abnormality – and certainly yearly until the problem is sorted out, wherever you live. An abnormal cervical smear does *not* mean there is a serious problem. This is one test which causes frequent but unnecessary alarm.

There is no scientific evidence to show that yearly smears significantly reduce the incidence of cervical cancer. Even so, there is fierce debate around the world over whether they should be done more frequently. For years, Canada, the country where people have the longest life expectancy on the planet, has struggled with this question. In the province of Ontario the cervical cancer rate remains steady (where ours is falling) even though many young women have annual smears. In fact it is common for young women there to have smears twice a year – every time they see their doctor to have their birth control prescription renewed. There is no recall programme in the province (unlike here) so the women who are most at risk – the over fifties – often go without, while those least at risk are having smears at a ridiculous pace. Any talk of ending the annual provision is met with opposition because women do not want to give up something they perceive as good for them. There is a strong movement of doctors who believe the annual smear should stay, but for reasons that go beyond cervical cancer screening. Dr Janice Willet is an obstetrician and gynaecologist in Sault Ste Marie in Northern Ontario. She has been studying screening procedures in the province. She favours the annual smear, simply because it gets women in to see their doctors.

> **Dr Janice Willett:** *Women have always used cervical screening as a reason to see the doctor ... but when they're going in they're also getting screening for breast and ovarian cancer. Cervical screening is just a small part of that exam. So my main concern about that [going to three-year intervals] is that women will not ... seek the services of their physician for other screening often because they perceive it as secondary to the pap smear. If they're only seen every two to three years that's a large window for screening especially for breast exams and also for ovarian malignancy which has little or no symptoms.*

So why are women in the UK only being asked to have smears every three to five years? Money plays a part but so does science. The NHS – these days – has to be cost effective and the advantage of yearly screening over three-year intervals is very small. A few more abnormalities will be found, but since cervical cancer takes years to develop the overall benefit will be negligible. Some doctors feel that having smears every five years is not frequent enough whilst others argue it is. However, if you have a problem like irregular bleeding or an unusual vaginal discharge, do not wait to be called, make an appointment to discuss it with your doctor.

If everything seems normal and you still want yearly smears, see your doctor about it. If necessary have them taken privately. This costs around £27. But beware of private firms targeting women in an alarmist way to have private smears, implying that the NHS does not provide a proper screening programme.

The Causes of Cervical Cancer

We are not absolutely sure what causes cervical cancer, but there is good evidence that it is the result of a sexually transmitted infection (STI), probably the human papilloma virus (HPV), commonly known as the wart virus. There are over fifty different types, but strains HPV 16 and 18 are the ones most implicated. The virus can be transmitted during sexual intercourse (see Chapter 7 for more on this). If you have never had sexual intercourse with a man the risk of cervical cancer is negligible, though it is still recommended to have smears. Every woman who has ever had sex should have regular cervical smears. Other factors are also involved. Starting to have sex when very young, not using condoms, long-term use (more than five years) of the contraceptive pill, and having many sexual partners or a partner who has had many partners, appear to increase the risk. Heavy smoking also increases the risk factor, if you are sexually active of course. It is possible that smoking affects our immune system.

Cervical Smear Results

The quality guidelines laid down by the NHS say it should take no longer than one month to get your results. Too many women have to wait longer. When you have your smear taken, check out how and when you will hear. Do not assume that no news is good news because sometimes results get mislaid. It is best if the doctor lets you know the result either way. A 'negative' smear means it is normal and nothing is wrong. A 'positive' smear *may* mean there is something wrong or abnormal.

There is plenty of confusion about the terms used to describe abnormal smears. The term 'dyskaryosis' is not cancer, but if left untreated a proportion of cells could develop into cancer over time, taking about ten years to do so. 'Carcinoma in situ' (CIS) is not actually cancer either, although it is more likely to develop into a cancer if not treated.

For every 100 cervical smears taken:

- Eighty to ninety will be normal.
- Five to ten need to be repeated for technical reasons – perhaps not enough cells were taken from the cervix or there was a problem with the preparation of the smear at the laboratory.
- About seven will show some abnormal cells of which: four to five will show a mild abnormality known as borderline or mild dyskaryosis; one a moderate abnormality called moderate dyskaryosis; and one more a severe abnormality called severe dyskaryosis.

- Only one in every 100 will show cancer in situ (pre-cancerous).
- Only one in every 500 will show the possibility of a cancer.

Sometimes a smear is reported as showing evidence of wart virus infection. Once again there is no need to panic. It means you have been in contact with a wart virus at some time which was probably transmitted sexually, but not necessarily (see page 185 in the STI guide). No specific treatment is available for the wart virus, but it usually goes away within a few years. If a wart virus is present you may need to have more frequent smears. It has been estimated that 20 per cent of women in their twenties may test positive to wart virus, but 90 per cent of these clear via the immune system within a few years and cause no trouble. We do not know which women with wart virus may go on to have problems, so for now more frequent smears are offered to women with the infection. But tests which can check for wart virus are now on the market and are being evaluated to see how reliable they are in predicting who might be more at risk of developing cervical cancer, therefore requiring more frequent smears.

If the Smear is Abnormal

One problem with having a smear is hearing that the smear is abnormal. This obviously makes us feel anxious. If you get a letter saying something is wrong with your smear this does *not* mean there is something seriously wrong. However, we tend to think of all the scare stories we have heard and read about cervical cancer.

> **Pam, 39:** *Whatever the letter actually said, my mind said 'cancer'. My husband had gone into the hospital for a minor operation and I said nothing to anyone for a couple of days. By the time he came home I'd chosen the hymns and the flowers for my funeral ... I know that women's lives have been saved by cervical screening but I don't think most professionals have any idea of the grief that can be caused by having a positive result.*

If a smear is mildly abnormal you should have another in six months. If it is still abnormal (or the first smear showed a more severe abnormality) you should have a colposcopy. This is done in hospital, at a family-planning clinic or other outpatient facility. The cervix is checked through a low-powered microscope called a colposcope. You are awake and the procedure does not involve an anaesthetic. It is similar to having a cervical smear. During a colposcopy a special solution is put on the cervix to identify any abnormal areas. This may sting a bit. A biopsy is taken so that the cells can be checked and any abnormal looking areas are treated immediately. This usually involves applying carbon dioxide laser, 'cold' coagulation, cryosurgery or electrocoagulation to destroy the abnormal cells, but large loop diathermy or excision is often used too. You will need a follow-up appointment for a check-up or more treatment.

> **Pam:** *The actual colposcopy was much less traumatic than I'd thought it would be. None of the procedures was painful, it was no more embarrassing or painful than any other vaginal exam and everyone was extremely kind.*

One year after the colposcopy Pam was clear of all abnormal cells.

Each of these treatments has an almost 100 per cent success rate. But if they are unsuccessful or the abnormal cells spread, a second treatment may be needed. Large loop excision is the preferred treatment as it is carried out under local anaesthetic, has far fewer side effects and has no effect on future fertility or ability to have a normal pregnancy and delivery. More rarely, a cone biopsy, which involves cutting out a conical ring of the cervix, is carried out under general anaesthetic. Only rarely is it necessary to have a hysterectomy.

Women who are told they have an abnormal smear sometimes worry because of the association with a sexually transmitted infection. This can have a strong negative effect on a woman's feelings about sex, especially if she needs treatment.

Scare Stories

Four million smears are taken in the UK every year. In recent years there have been many scares caused by errors in the laboratory or the smears being taken inaccurately with thousands of women having to be retested because of this. Poor training and human error are usually, but not always, to blame. Interpretation of the results does depend on human judgement and sometimes abnormally appearing cells are very hard to find. Also, the test is not 100 per cent accurate. Having regular cervical smears, however frequently, will not completely get rid of your risk of developing cervical cancer, but it does mean that four out of five cases that would have occurred will be prevented.

A national co-ordinating network monitors quality control in the laboratory to make sure that all the laboratories use a standard procedure. New and better tests are also being developed to highlight genetic abnormalities in the DNA of cervical cells which can then be measured by computer, reducing human error.

Breast Screening

Breast screening tries to spot breast cancers at a very early stage so that women can have treatment to stop the cancer spreading. It is the spread of the cancer – the secondary cancers – which causes problems. Screening for breast cancer involves a low dose X-ray of the breast called a mammogram. Like cervical screening it does not detect all breast cancers, but women who are screened are 30 per cent less likely to die of breast cancer than those who are not.

Joanna: *Each breast was squashed into this thing and I had to lean to the side. It is uncomfortable, it's just the pressure really and being stretched in a different way. Fortunately it didn't take long. But it's tolerable.*

All women between the ages of fifty and sixty-five should be invited to have a mammogram every three years on the NHS. If you are in this age group and have not been called, you should contact your GP. The statistics show that if all women in this category had mammograms, breast cancer deaths should fall by at least 1250 each year.

Jan, 54: *There's a note on the wall which says 'We squeeze because we care' and it was not a very pleasant procedure. It's quite painful, it's quite sterile and it's quite impersonal. I think they do the best they can.*

The aim of mammography is to find the tiny breast lumps you could never feel, lumps as small as half a centimetre. If 100 women have a routine screening mammogram (excluding women who come forward because they have found a lump):

- Over ninety will have normal results.
- Five or six will need a second mammogram to clarify whether something is wrong or not.
- One will be found to have something wrong enough to require having a biopsy.

A biopsy is done by putting a thin needle (sometimes using ultrasound as a guide) into the breast to remove some of the cells. This is called a fine needle aspiration and you do not usually need an anaesthetic for this. The cells are then examined under a microscope to check for cancer cells, often while you wait if this is done in the outpatient department of an NHS hospital. One out of two biopsies taken as a result of screening may show an abnormality. About one-fifth of the abnormalities found are pre-cancerous lesions and are known as 'in situ lesions'. Sometimes instead of doing a needle aspiration, or in addition to it, the lump that has shown up on a mammogram is actually removed under anaesthetic and some of its cells are examined in the laboratory. This is the most reliable way of knowing exactly what it is.

Mammograms not only show up changes that might be cancer, they can also show an abnormality which could be a fibroadenoma (see page 240) or a cyst, though the mammogram cannot distinguish between the two. Flecks of calcium may be visible which can sometimes, but by no means always, indicate a cancer or pre-cancer in the breast, but there is no need to panic as in 80 per cent of women with flecks of calcium there is no cancer. If anything is found to be wrong you should be called back very quickly to have another mammogram or a biopsy. The waiting and uncertainty can be the most difficult time. But even if something abnormal is found, it is not usually cancer. Where a cancer is found you should be able to see a breast specialist quickly to discuss what needs to be done and what your options are. For a full discussion of breast cancer see Chapter 10.

> **Jan, 54:** *What they'd seen were these little … T cells, little teacup-shaped things. And they explained to me that they were probably little calcium things that would disappear and even now to this day I am waiting to go for yet another regular check and I'm still quite nervous about it. It's a little shadow that … follows you about and every so often you remember that you were once a sort of possible … you want to go and you want to be told you're all right.*

Controversies and Breast Cancer Screening

There is discussion about who should be screened for breast cancer, how often and which sort of screening it should be. Some experts think younger women, under the age of fifty, should be screened. The mammograms of women in this age group are more difficult to interpret because breast tissue is more dense before the menopause. One mammogram in a younger woman may not be that helpful, but there may be a benefit from subsequent ones because they offer a comparison. However, this may carry a risk. The Canadian National Breast Cancer Study followed the progress of women under fifty who were screened, and discovered that women in this group had a higher breast cancer death rate possibly related to the X-rays.

A large study in the UK is now underway. Britain recommends women have a mammogram every three years after the age of fifty, but North Americans are often encouraged to have them yearly. Women over sixty-five are not routinely called for mammograms even though they are most at risk. The trouble has been that, traditionally, older women do not come forward when called for screening generally. Women over sixty-five are entitled to have mammograms. We hope they will soon be regularly invited. The best scientific evidence indicates that the safest option is probably once every two years after the age of fifty. This will catch most cancers without exposing women to too many X-rays. Women with a family history of breast cancer (at a young age) should start screening early. For example, if your mother had breast cancer under the age of fifty many experts recommend you should start ten years before this. So if your mother had breast cancer at fifty you should be screened at forty. If you do have a family history of breast cancer you should discuss it with your doctor.

Hormone Replacement Therapy and Breast Cancer Screening

Oxford scientists have found that it is more difficult to pick up cancers on mammograms in women on HRT. This is probably because HRT makes the breast tissue more dense and therefore cancers may be missed when the mammogram is read by the radiologist.

Ovarian Cancer Screening

> **Lucy, 51:** *What was interesting looking back was that my older sister and I both started to have severe tummy pains after we knew about the diagnosis of ovarian cancer in our younger sister. We were both convinced we had cancer but we felt foolish, did not tell each other about the pains until after the operation when we found we were clear. I knew I couldn't not have my ovaries out, I would never feel secure. As for my daughter, we will have her tested when she's older whereas that option wasn't available years ago. Our sons should also be tested as it was my father who was the carrier. There was nothing on my mother's side.*

Ovarian cancer is the fifth most common cancer in women in the UK. One in every 5000 women will get it and it accounts for 6 per cent of cancer deaths in women. It is rare in young women. Ninety per cent of women developing ovarian cancer are over the age of forty-five. The horror of ovarian cancer is that it tends to develop and spread before causing any noticeable symptoms. Seventy per cent of women who get it only know when it is far advanced and it is then difficult to treat and cure.

Benign Ovarian Cysts

We are born with two ovaries, situated in our pelvis on either side of the uterus, but attached to it by our fallopian tubes. Up to one in five women has small cysts on her ovaries. Most of these are harmless and are sometimes found incidentally on ultrasound examination for other investigations and may even disappear on their own. If they grow and cause pain, surgery may be required.

Cancerous Ovarian Cysts

When an ovarian cyst is cancerous it needs to be detected early and removed to ensure a healthy recovery. But screening tests available at present for ovarian cancer all have problems, in that they may be falsely negative or falsely positive. Ovarian cancer *may* be detected during an internal examination, an ultrasound scan using a probe inserted into the vagina, a blood test and various other more sophisticated checks. A combination of these tests improves the accuracy. But none of these tests is 100 per cent accurate (as Lucy's story shows below), and screening for ovarian cancer is not on offer to all women yet. But women with a family history of ovarian cancer (e.g. a mother or sister) and women who carry the breast cancer gene, BRCA1 (see page 253), should ask to be screened because they are at greater risk. Having the BRCA1 gene increases your risk of breast cancer and gives you a 40 per cent risk of developing ovarian cancer. These women should be offered annual screening with an ultrasound scan. They should also have the blood test CA125, from the age of twenty-five or from five years before the earliest age of ovarian cancer in the family. CA125 is a blood test which identifies a chemical protein which can be increased if an ovarian cancer is present. What you decide will depend on how old you are and whether you have had children yet. The oral contraceptive pill decreases the risk of ovarian cancer so if you have a strong family history it is worth considering going on the pill. Unfortunately the CA125 reading does not always show increased levels of the problem chemical protein in the early stage of the disease and may only show this in 80 per cent of women who have more advanced ovarian cancer.

When early ovarian cancer is detected, it is necessary to remove the cancerous ovary. Women with a strong family history of the problem, or women who are found to have the BRCA1 gene, sometimes opt to have their ovaries taken out, like Lucy did, which removes the risk of a cancer developing. You need to take into account that this will bring on your menopause immediately (see Chapter 3). After surgery, treatment for ovarian cancer nearly always involves chemotherapy. With modern treatment, early detection of ovarian cancer has a good prognosis.

> **Lucy, 51:** *My older sister is a doctor and she had kept records of all the women in our family who had had ovarian cancer: my grandmother, my aunt and many more distant ones on my father's side. She happened to read about a Dr Ponder at Cambridge who was studying this. She sent him the details and he wrote back saying that after looking at the family history it seemed we had a 25 per cent chance of inheriting the gene and that we all should have regular scans ... My younger sister had a scan in November and was pronounced clear. By the end of December she had been taken into hospital with ovarian cancer and secondaries ... Dr Ponder said we two sisters now had a 50 per cent chance of having the same problem. So we both immediately booked in to have our ovaries out. We staggered the operations, to have them at different times so we could help look after our younger sister who subsequently died.*

Sandra is fifty-six. She has recently been diagnosed with ovarian cancer and is in the middle of treatment.

Sandra: *It was two years ago. I hadn't felt well for a long time. I was diagnosed with IBS [Irritable Bowel Syndrome]. It didn't seem to be getting better so I went back to my doctor and he changed the treatment. I felt more and more bloated after food. Eventually I had a scan and I was told I had advanced cancer and it was all over my abdomen. Two days later they operated and took away as much as they could. I feel very bitter now, I felt I should have had a scan months ago. I ought to have insisted and thinking he [the doctor] knew best was a real mistake. I don't ask how long I've got because I don't want to know. I'm having chemotherapy with Carboplatin with Taxol. I don't mind about losing my hair, it's my life I'm worried about. I've never recovered from the oncologist asking me if I knew anyone with cancer. I said, yes a friend had breast cancer and she replied 'Oh yours is much worse than that'. It made me feel I was done for.*

Suzy, 49: *I'm potentially at high risk as my mother died of ovarian cancer when she was fifty. I'm not sure that I want to be screened. I have big doubts about the obsession of screening, with all the false negatives and false positives. If someone said to me, 'We've got this really great screening test, it doesn't miss any, it doesn't say you might have it when you haven't', and then the treatment was really easy, I might have done it. But I don't want anyone to ask me. I'd rather take the gamble. It's different with cervical cancer screening. Then it's pre-cancer they're looking for and the treatment is good and not worrying. It's not like you have to have a whole big operation. I don't want to be made into an invalid. We've just extended our mortgage and if they'd found ovarian cancer, I wouldn't have been able to do that.*

We all look at risk in different ways. How risk is explained will also affect how you make decisions. Being told you have a 95 per cent chance of being fine feels different from being told you have a 5 per cent chance of a serious problem.

Other Screening Tests

Other commonly available screening tests for women (and men) check blood pressure and cholesterol levels. In the future bowel cancer screening should also be available routinely (see page 386).

Blood Pressure

We should have our blood pressure checked at least every three to five years, although most of us will have it done more frequently. There are many opportunities for this to happen: during a check-up if you are taking the pill, during pregnancy, when having a cervical smear and during check-ups while on HRT.

There is a normal gradual increase in blood pressure with age, and sometimes your blood pressure goes up because of anxiety associated with seeing the doctor. Most women are unaware that their blood pressure is raised unless it is extremely high. The problem is that over many years high blood pressure can eventually cause problems. It affects your arteries and may increase your risk of a stroke and heart attack (see pages 330–4). Although women appear to tolerate high blood pressure better than men do, it does make us more vulnerable to stroke, heart disease, kidney disease and circulation problems in the legs. When you have your blood pressure taken you get two readings. One is for systolic pressure – that is the measurement taken when your arteries are working to push blood through your heart. The other is diastolic, the measurement taken when your arteries relax between spurts. In the UK you are considered to have high blood pressure (hypertension) when the higher reading is 150 or greater, and the lower reading is greater than ninety. An average reading is 120/80, but it varies from woman to woman especially when we get older.

A 1992 survey for the Department of Health showed that 37 per cent of women aged fifty-five to sixty-four had high blood pressure or were being treated for it. The figure rose to 52 per cent in women aged sixty-five to seventy-four and to over two-thirds in women over seventy-five. There is uncertainty just at what level of high blood pressure treatment should begin.

High blood pressure can be inherited. It is also linked to stress and being overweight. When routine tests are carried out on older women with high blood pressure, no other problem is

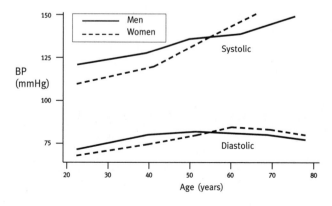

usually found. High blood pressure is also associated with pregnancy and sometimes occurs when you are on the birth control pill.

If your blood pressure is found to be raised, unless it is very high, it will need to be rechecked at least twice more before a diagnosis is made and treatment suggested. There are many things to do to help yourself. If you are overweight, the blood pressure may go down without any other treatment if you lose weight. Try to change your eating habits and do even just a little more exercise (see Chapter 6). Decreasing your salt intake will also help.

If these measures do not work, your doctor may suggest pills. There are various groups of drugs designed to lower your blood pressure. Unfortunately with hypertension you will probably need to take the tablets for the rest of your life. For most people this is an inconvenience in that we have to remember to take the pills and to go for regular check-ups with our doctor or nurse. For some of us the tablets cause side effects, like depression, cough, nausea, skin problems and in men, impotence. Drug-related trouble can usually be solved by changing to different pills.

Madelaine found an unexpected side benefit of her treatment for hypertension.

> **Madelaine, 41:** *Before I started taking pills for high blood pressure I used to get migraines, the kind that you would like someone to chop your head off. I don't get those migraines any more and I think they were in some way related.*

Cholesterol Screening

Cholesterol is a fatty substance in our blood and it comes in two varieties. The 'good' cholesterols are the HDLs – high density lipoproteins – which help to prevent heart attacks. The 'bad' cholesterols are the LDLs – low density lipoproteins – which are associated with an increase in our risk of heart attacks. Eating high fat foods increases our LDL level. However, some people inherit high 'bad' cholesterol levels and have too much of it even though they avoid fatty foods. In Britain, mostly because of diet, about two-thirds of our cholesterol is made up of the LDLs, the bad ones, which is why a high cholesterol reading usually means bad news. They clog the walls of our arteries promoting heart disease. Blood cholesterol levels are much higher in Western countries – where people eat high fat diets – than in countries such as Japan and China where low fat diets are the norm. Cholesterol levels also increase with age.

There is a blood test available that can easily measure your cholesterol level, checking for both LDLs and HDLs. In the UK at present there is no screening programme to offer everyone a regular blood cholesterol check, although some experts think there should be. However, it is a good idea to have your cholesterol checked if you have high blood pressure, have had a heart attack or angina, have a family history of high cholesterol or heart disease, for example, if there is someone in your family under the age of sixty who has, or has had, heart disease.

Although there is no ideal level for cholesterol, it is thought that one should aim for a level below 5 mmol/litre. Sixty per cent of women in the UK have a level higher than this. If you have a high cholesterol level, take a look at your diet. See if you can move away from foods high in saturated fats such as hard cheese, fatty meat (red meat in particular), butter and creams (see page 138).

Hormones also affect cholesterol levels. Oestrogen is beneficial but some progestogens adversely affect HDL ('good') cholesterol. This in part explains why women have lower cholesterol levels before the menopause while our oestrogen levels are still high. It may also help to explain the benefit of taking HRT (see pages 60–71) for some women.

If your cholesterol continues to be raised after modifying your diet for three to six months, you may need to take one of the cholesterol-lowering drugs. This is especially so if you have another risk factor for heart disease such as high blood pressure or angina.

> **Marjorie, 56:** *I have always been against taking pills. They're just a nuisance to remember all the time. It just reminds you that you're not as well as you should be. But when I got all the information about the dangers of my cholesterol being so high despite a mostly healthy diet and with the hypertension, the arguments were overwhelming. So I had to go for it.*

Bowel Cancer Screening

Bowel cancer is another common cancer which, if caught early, can be treated easily, but as with ovarian cancer we often do not know there is a problem until the cancer is advanced. Tests are being refined before a national screening programme is set up. One study asked men and women to collect their faeces to check for blood. If blood was found then a further test was carried out called a colonoscopy which involves passing a tube into the bowel with a tiny camera lens to look for any abnormal cells that might be early cancers which have caused the bleeding. They could then be treated at an early stage before developing into cancer. Those screened had fewer bowel cancer deaths. However, there are also lots of other causes for blood in the faeces, so many people had colonoscopies who did not really need them.

well-woman check

There is another study underway using a special tube called a flexible sigmoidoscope which is again passed into the bowel and has a special microscope attached to it. It is being offered to one group of sixty-year-old patients who are being compared with another group of sixty-year-olds who are not offered the test. Some doctors feel we know enough to start screening now without waiting for the results of this trial. The results will not be available until 2007. Bowel cancer can run in families so if you do have close relatives who have had bowel cancer it is a good idea to ask for this test.

If you bleed from your rectum this does not mean you have cancer. Haemorrhoids may cause this (see pages 366–7). But if you do bleed, get it checked out by your doctor, especially if you are over fifty.

Genetic Testing

There is an ever-increasing number of genetic tests available which will forecast some of your health risks as you get older. In the future, you will be able to know, if you want to, your chances of developing not just breast and ovarian cancer, but high blood pressure, depression and heart disease plus an array of other more unusual diseases. There are already tests for other specific complaints such as Huntington's chorea, a rare inherited brain disease.

The new genetic tests present us, as individuals, with a range of tormenting questions:

• Do I want to know about some future predisposition to a disease like breast cancer?
• Do I want to take action now on something that *might* happen in the future – like having a mastectomy before there are any signs of cancer?
• Do I want to know that I may carry a gene, which, if mixed with a similar gene from a much-loved partner, may mean that my child will die early – from cystic fibrosis or Tay Sachs?
• Do I even want to know that I carry familial hyperlipidaemia which makes me more prone to heart attacks, and which will make my children more prone to them?
• When do I tell my children about this – will it just worry them unnecessarily, and make them have to think about what they can and cannot eat all their lives?

There are, of course, benefits from the new genetics which are less troubling. Parents can be tested to find out if they carry the gene for the blood disease thalassaemia, common in some Mediterranean countries, or the gene for Tay Sachs disease which affects certain Jewish groups and causes early death due to disease of the nervous system. Knowledge about the risk of heart disease might put us off smoking, encourage us to eat a low-fat diet or take fat-lowering drugs. If you know you are at high risk of breast cancer you might decide not to take the contraceptive pill or perhaps start your family earlier rather than later (see Chapter 10).

But whether we really want to know what life – and ill health – have in store for us is an unanswered question and one with far-reaching consequences. The results of these tests will not only affect how we feel about ourselves but also whether we will qualify for life insurance or a new job.

How to Choose Your Doctor

The health service in the UK is set up so that everyone can be registered with a family doctor called a general practitioner (GP). In the survey conducted for our book 38 per cent of women had been to see their doctor in the previous month. At least 70 per cent said they see their GP every year. So obviously it is important to find a doctor you like and trust.

Many factors influence the choice of doctor, but often we end up with the one closest to home. The sex of the doctor is sometimes important, but our survey showed 43 per cent of women did not mind either way with 28 per cent saying it depended on what the visit was for. Whether you can find a woman GP or not depends on where you live. If your local GP's surgery does not have a woman doctor in the practice and you want one, ask whether there is a female nurse who specializes in women's health.

Lists of GPs in your area are available from the local library, post office, local health authority and the community health council. All practices should have a leaflet describing the services they offer. Once you know who is available (and in rural areas, this may be quite limited) ask your friends or neighbours – whoever you trust – and then make your choice. Arrange an appointment with the doctor to discuss registration before you make your final decision. It often helps to list the things you want to know about before that meeting. For instance, you could ask about screening services, annual checks, and so on.

Tips to Help You When You See Your Doctor
- Make a list of what you are worried about and what you want to discuss – to avoid missing the opportunity to talk about what really concerns you.
- Be ready to tell your doctor what you hope to get out of the consultation.
- Ask what might have caused the problem.
- Ask about the options for treatment.
- Discuss the advantages and disadvantages of different treatments.
- Make sure you know how to take any medicines prescribed and ask about the possible side effects.
- Find out if there is anything you can do to help yourself.
- If you have any tests, ask when and how you will get the results.
- Ask for a leaflet about your condition so you can read more about it.

Changing to Another GP

Many practices have a choice of doctors, others insist you see your own named doctor. If you want to change practices you may do so. We often feel awkward about this and worry that we will be labelled as a difficult patient. But it is your right. It is very easy to change doctors, if you live in a town or city, but for those in rural areas choice may be limited. If you find you constantly feel dissatisfied with each new GP and want to move to another surgery, you need to consider whether it might be you who is making unreasonable demands or being difficult. To change, you need to find another doctor whose practice has space on its list and then fill in a form to register.

Doctors also have choice in who they wish to take on their list of patients. If there is a dispute they can ask you to leave their practice. In spite of this you are always entitled to a doctor and if you have problems finding a GP contact the local Health Authority who will assign another one to you, but he or she will probably not be the one of your choice.

The Patients' Charter

The Patients' Charter aims to set standards of care within the NHS, but it also now puts greater emphasis on patients' responsibilities which range from remembering to tell your doctor your new address when you move, to only calling the doctor for a home visit when absolutely necessary. Doctors are obliged to make an assessment as to whether a home visit is necessary – they do not always have to visit when requested. The Patients' Charter includes target times for how long you should wait before seeing a consultant, how long you should wait to be admitted to hospital for an operation, and how long you should expect to wait in the outpatients' department. Of course if you need treatment as an emergency you should not have to wait at all, although even in emergency rooms cases must be ranked.

Seeing Another GP for a Special Reason

GPs get paid separately for contraceptive and obstetric services so if you feel shy about seeing your own doctor for contraception or feel he or she is not interested in helping you with contraception, for example, you may go to another practice. You can also visit a family-planning clinic. You may also see another doctor for care during pregnancy.

If you are dissatisfied with your GP's advice concerning a medical problem, unhappy with a hospital doctor you have seen, or you if simply want another opinion, your GP should be able to arrange this under the NHS. We often feel embarrassed to ask as we are afraid of upsetting the doctor concerned and worry whether future treatment and the relationship might be affected. It should not be and it is far more important to get another opinion if you are worried.

If You Have a Complaint about Your GP

From a patient's point of view there is nothing worse than professionals being defensive and secretive about a badly handled incident. Every practice should have a written complaints procedure. Ask the receptionist or, if you feel embarrassed asking, write a letter to the practice manager. Most complaints should be able to be sorted out with an explanation and an apology. If you are unhappy with the practice's written response, ask to meet the person concerned so that you can talk the matter through. The trouble very often turns out to be one of lack of communication between the doctor and the patient.

Jane Hanna, Lawyer specializing in medical complaints: *At the top of the list of complaints is misunderstanding between the doctor and the patient so complaints really only happen when there hasn't been good communication. It nearly always comes down to that, a situation, for example, where the patient may perceive the doctor as being in a rush and where the opportunity doesn't really present itself for the patient to ask all the questions they really want to. That's certainly true if you're dealing with a diagnosis of a new condition, especially if the patient is quite fearful, and often you don't know what to ask either.*

If you have a complaint you want to take beyond the doctor's practice, you can discuss it with your local community health council or the local health authority which should have someone in charge of complaints. There is also the Health Service Ombudsman who investigates some complaints about the NHS if you remain dissatisfied with the reply from the practice and/or the health authority.

Useful Addresses

Chapter 1:
Women's Health Concerns
Quit
Victory House
170 Tottenham Court Road
London W1P 0HA
Quitline 0800 002200
Tel. 0171 388 5775
Fax 0171 388 5995

Chapter 2: Periods
The Endometriosis Society
50 Westmintster Palace Gardens
Artillery Row
London SW1P 1RL
Send large SAE for information.

Margaret Pyke Family Planning
Centre
73 Charlotte Street
London W1P 1LB
Advice line 0171 530 3636
Appointments 0171 530 3650 /
0171 530 3600
For contraception and general
advice on women's health.

National Association for PMS
PO Box 72
Sevenoaks
Kent TN13 3PS
Tel. 01732 741709

National Endometriosis Helpline
Tel. 0171 222 2776

See also Women's Nutritional
Advisory Service in **The
Menopause** section below.

Chapter 3: The Menopause
Amarant Centre
80 Lambeth Road
London SE1 7PW
Tel. 0171 401 3855 (for
appointments only)
Helpline 01293 413000, 12–7pm,
Monday–Friday (staffed by trained
nurses).
The centre offers a consultation
about the menopause which will
include an examination. There are
also menopause clinics at some
hospitals but you will need to be
referred by your GP.

Wells Spring Trading Ltd
PO Box 322
St Peter Port
Guernsey GY1 3TP
Write for details on ordering
natural progesterone cream.

Women's Nutritional Advisory
Service
PO Box 268
Lewes
East Sussex BN7 2QN
Tel. 01273 487366 (general
enquiries)
They have a number of helplines
on a variety of subjects,
including:
Overcoming PMS Naturally
0839 556 600
Overcoming the Menopause
Naturally 0839 556 602.
For a full list of helpline numbers
call 0839 556615.

Chapter 4: On the Surface
The British Association of
Aesthetic Surgeons
The Royal College of Surgeons
35 Lincoln's Inn Fields
London WC2A 3PA
Tel. 0171 831 5161
Phone for a list of plastic
surgeons.

Cosmetic Surgery Network
Cindy Jackson
PO Box 3410
Highgate
London N6 4EE
Tel. 0181 209 0862
Send a large SAE for information.

National Eczema Society
163 Eversholt Street
London NW1 1BU
Tel. 0171 388 4097

Chapter 5: The State You're In
Al-Anon
61 Great Dover Street
Lonon SE1 4YF
Tel. 0171 403 0888
Support group for friends and
families of alcoholics.

Alcohol Concern
Waterbridge House
32-36 Loman Street
London SE1 0EE
Tel. 0171 928 7377
Publishes a directory of services
and provides information on where
to get help in your area.

Alcoholics Anonymous
PO Box 1
Stonebow House
Stonebow
York YO1 2NJ
Tel. 01904 644026

British Association for Counselling
1 Regents Place
Rugby CV21 2PJ
Send an SAE for a list of
registered counsellors in your area.

Cruse Bereavement Care
126 Sheen Road
Richmond
Surrey TW9 1UR
Tel. 0181 940 4818
Helpline: 0181 332 7227, 9.30am–
5pm, Monday–Friday

Drinkline 0345 320 202
Helpline for information on alcohol
misuse, whether you are the
drinker or not.

Marie Curie Cancer Care
28 Belgrave Square
London SW1X 8QG
This organisation runs eleven local
Marie Curie Centres (hospices),
provides nursing care in patients'
homes and offers bereavement
counselling. To access these
services you will need to be
referred by your GP or consultant.

Mind
The Mental Health Charity
15-19 Broadway
London E15 4BQ
Tel. 0181 519 2122
Fax 0181 522 1725
Mind Info Lines: London 0181 522
1728 / Outside London 0345 660
163, 9.15am–4.45am,
Monday–Friday *(continued over)*

The Mind Info Line gives information on counselling services, local support groups, drug information, hospital rights, sexual abuse and suicide. The information line also offers Language Line, an interpreting service over the phone covering more than 100 languages for people whose first language is not English.

The Promis Recovery Centre
Old Court House
Pinners Hill
Nonington
Kent CT15 4LL
Tel. 01304 841700
Promis deals with a range of compulsive behaviours.

Samaritans
National helpline number 0345 909090, or check your telephone directory for local numbers.

SANDS (Stillbirth and Neonatal Death Society)
28 Portland Place
London W1N 4DE
Tel. 0171 436 5881

Seasonal Affective Disorder Syndrome Association (SAD)
PO Box 989
London SW7 2PZ
Tel. 01903 814942
For information and advice on obtaining lamps.

UK Council for Psychotherapists
167-169 Great Portland Street
London W1N 5FB
Send an SAE for a list of registered psychotherapists in your area.

Winston's Wish
(Weekend camps for bereaved children and families)
Gloucestershire Hospital
Great Western Road
Gloucester GL1 3NN
Winston's Wish are happy to respond to professionals and families around the country by letter. The service they provide working directly with families is only free in Gloucestershire. They

can help a small number of families from outside the area but these will need to have financial help from their own health authority.

Chapter 6: The Shape You're in
The British Heart Foundation
14 Fitzhardinge Street
London W1H 4DH
Tel. 0171 935 0185
The foundation produces excellent leaflets and books on diets, dieting and healthy eating.

Eating Disorders Association
1st floor, Wensum House
103 Prince of Wales Road
Norwich, Norfolk NR1 1DW
Helpline 01603 621414
Youth Helpline (for those aged 18 and under), tel. 01603 765050, 4–6 pm, Monday–Friday.
Recorded message for general information about eating disorders, anorexia and bulimia (lasts about 9 minutes – 50p per minute): Tel. 0891 615466
The Association also has a booklist and books can be ordered through them.

The National Sports Medicine Institute of the UK
Charterhouse Square
c/o Medical College of St Bartholomew's Hospital
London EC1M 6BQ
Tel. 0171 251 0583
Funded by the Sports Council, it provides a wide range of fitness tests ranging in price from around £10 to £50.

Chapter 7: Sex and the STI Guide
Body Positive
51b Philbeach Gardens
London SW5 9EB
0171 835 1045 (reception)
Positive line 0800 616212
7–10pm, Monday–Friday; 4–10pm, Saturday and Sunday .
Also runs self-help groups for people with HIV.

The British Association of Sexual and Marital Therapists (BASMT)
PO Box 62
Sheffield S10 3TL
continued above

Send SAE for a list of sex therapists in your area.

HVA (Herpes Viruses Association)
41 North Road
London N7 9DP
Tel. 0171 609 9061
Recorded message giving information of when and who to call for advice.

Jewish Marriage Council
23 Ravenshurst Avenue
London NW4 4EE
Tel. 0181 203 6311

Lesbian Helpline
Tel. 0171 837 2782

London Rape Crisis Centre
PO Box 69
London WC1X 9NJ
Tel. 0171 916 5466
Counselling line: 0171 837 1600

Marriage Care (Previously Catholic Marriage Advisory Council)
Clitherow House
1 Blythe Mews
Blythe Road
London W14 0NW
0171 371 1341
Helpline 0345 573921, 3–9pm, Mondays and Thursdays

Marriage Counselling Scotland
105 Hanover Street
Edinburgh EH2 1DJ
Tel. 0131 225 5006

National Aids Helpline
24 hours a day, freephone 0800 567123

Positively Women
(for women with HIV)
347–9 City Road
London EC1V 1LR
Helpline 0171 713 0222
10am–4pm, Monday–Friday, and 5–9pm on Mondays and Thursdays only. The helpline is run by women who are HIV positive.

Relate (Marriage Guidance)
Herbert Gray College
Little Church Street
Rugby, Warwickshire CV21 3AP
Tel. 01788 573241 for referral to local centres.

Relate (Northern Ireland)
74-6 Dublin Road
Belfast
BT2 7HP
Tel. 01232 323454 for referral to
local centres.

Scottish Women's Aid
(for women suffering domestic
violence)
12 Torpichen Street
Edinburgh EH3 8JQ
Tel. 0131 221 0401

SPOD (Association to aid the
sexual and personal relationships
of people with a disability)
286 Campden Road
London N7 0BJ
Tel. 0171 607 8851

Terrence Higgins Trust
52-54 Grays Inn Road
London WC1X 8JU
Tel. 0171 242 1010
Every day from 12–10pm
website: http//www.tht.org.uk
Helps on a wide range of HIV and
Aids related problems and is for
men and women.

Women's Aid Federation of
England (for women suffering
domestic violence)
PO Box 391
Bristol BS99 7WS
Tel. 0117 944 4411
Helpline 0117 963 3542

Chapter 8: Contraception
The Brook Advisory Centres
(central office)
165 Gray's Inn Road
London WC1X 8UD
Tel. 0171 713 9000
Only for young people up to the
age of 25. Phone for details of
local centres throughout the
country.

The Family Planning Association
(central office)
2-12 Pentonville Road
London N1 9FP
Tel. 0171 837 5432
Helplines, 9am–7pm, Monday–Friday:
UK 0171 837 4044
Wales 01222 342766
Scotland 0141 576 5088
Northern Ireland 01232 325488

Marie Stopes House
(and Daycare Centre)
108 Whitfield Street
London W1P 6BE
Tel. 0171 388 0662
(clinic number only)

Natural Family Planning Service
Catholic Marriage Advisory Council
Clitherow House
1 Blythe Mews
Blythe Road
London W14 0NW
Tel. 0171 371 1341
It is not necessary to be Catholic
or married to use this service.

See also Margaret Pyke Family
Planning Centre in the **Periods**
section, above.

Chapter 9: Abortion
British Agencies for Adoption and
Fostering
Skyline House
200 Union Street
London SE1 0LX
Tel. 0171 593 2000
Fax 0171 593 2001
website:
http://www.vois.org.uk/baaf

British Pregnancy Advisory Service
Austy Manor
Wootton Wawen
Solihull
West Midlands B95 6BX
Tel. 01564 793225
e-mail:
marketing@bpas.demon.co.uk

Support around Termination for
Abnormality (SAFTA)
73-5 Charlotte Street
London W1P 1LB
Tel: 0171 631 0280
Helpline: 0171 631 0285, 10am–
6pm, Monday–Thursday,
10am–4pm, Friday. Outside these
hours, a message will be left on
the helpline giving emergency
numbers for parents to phone.

Chapter 10: Breasts
Breast Cancer Care
Kiln House
210 New Kings Road
London SW6 4NZ
Tel. 0171 384 2344
continued above

Nationwide free helpline:
0500 245345
e-mail:
breastcancercare@bccare.demon.
co.uk

Breast Care Campaign
Blythe Hall
100 Blythe Road
London W14 0HB
Tel. 0171 371 1510
Fax 0171 371 4598
Also gives information about non-
cancer breast disease.

Bristol Cancer Help Centre
Grove House
Cornwallis Grove
Clifton
Bristol BS8 4PG
Tel. 0117 9809505

CancerBACUP (British Associations
of Cancer United Patients)
3 Bath Place
Rivington Street
London EC2A 3JR
Administration 0171 696 9003.
Ring for information leaflets.
Helpline: 0171 613 2121 or
0800 181199, 9am–7pm, Monday–
Friday.
The helpline is staffed by
specialist cancer nurses and offers
advice to people with cancer, and
to families and friends of people
with cancer.

Cancer Care Society (CARE)
21 Zetland Road
Redland
Bristol BS6 7AH
Tel. 0117 942 7419
Telephone and personal
counselling by trained counsellors.

Cancer Link
11–21 Northdown Street
London N1 9BN
Tel. 0800 132905
e-mail:
cancerlink@canlink.demon.co.uk
Gives information on all forms of
cancer.

Cancer Relief Macmillan Fund
15–19 Britten Street
London SW3 3TZ
Tel. 0171 351 7811
continued over

Provides nurses and financial grants for people with cancer and their families. It funds the Macmillan nurses whose services are available free of charge for home care and hospital support.

RAGE (Radiotherapy Action Group Exposure)
c/o Joyce Pritchard
24 Edgeborough way
Bromley
Kent BR1 2UA
Tel. 0181 460 7476

UK Breast Cancer Coalition
PO Box 8554
London SW8 2ZB
Tel. 0171 720 0945
Fax 0171 720 8877

Women's Nationwide Cancer Control Campaign
Suna House
128–30 Curtain Road
London EC2A 3AR
Tel. 0171 729 2229
email: wnccc@dial.pipex.com
website:
http://dspaca.dial.pipex.com/town/square/gm40/

See also Marie Curie Cancer Care in **The State You're In** section, above.

Chapter 11: Nine Months: Pregnancy & Childbirth

The Active Birth Centre
25 Bickerton Road
London N19 5JT
Tel. 0171 561 9006
e-mail:
mail@activebirthcentr.demon.co.uk

AIMS (Association for Improvement in the Maternity Services)
40 Kingswood Avenue
London NW6 6LS
Tel. 0181 960 5585
Voluntary group which aims to improve maternity services but also gives advice on choices in maternity care and complaints.

Association for Postnatal Illness (APNI)
25 Jerden Place
London SW6 1BE
Tel. 0171 386 0868
Network of volunteers who have suffered from postnatal depression and can offer advice and support.

Breast Feeding Network
PO Box 11126
Paisley PA2 8YB
Advice and network of counsellors who can give practical help with breast-feeding. Send SAE for details.
e-mail: bfn@btinternet.com

Independent Midwives Assocation
94 Auckland Road
Upper Norwood
London SE19 2DB
Send SAE for list of registered independent midwives.

Informed Choice
PO Box 669
Bristol BS99 5FG
Tel. 0891 210400
Provide a series of leaflets based on scientific evidence about the choices available to pregnant women.

La Leche League
BM 3424
London WC1N 3XX
Tel. 0171 242 1278
(24 hour answer phone)

MAMA (Meet-A-Mum-Association)
26 Avenue Road
London SE25 4DX
Tel. 0181 771 5595
Support for mothers who have postnatal depression or who are feeling lonely and isolated.

Miscarriage Association
c/o Clayton Hospital
Northgate
Wakefield
West Yorkshire WF1 3JS
Tel. 01924 200799

National Association for Maternal and Child Welfare
40-42 Osnaburgh Street
London NW1 3ND
Tel. 0171 383 4117

National Childbirth Trust
Alexandra House
Oldham Terrace
Acton
London W3 6NH
Tel. 0181 992 8637, 9.30am–4pm, Monday–Friday.

Toxoplasmosis Trust
61-71 Collier Street
London N1 9BE
Tel. 0171 713 0663
e-mail: info@toxo.org.uk

Chapter 12: One in Six: Infertility

CHILD (National Infertility Support Network)
Charter House
43 St Leonards Road
Bexhill-on-Sea
East Sussex TN40 1JA
Tel. 01424 732361
e-mail: office@email2.child.org.uk

Childlessness Overcome Through Surrogacy (COTS)
Loandhu Cottage
Gruids, Lairg
Sutherland IV27 4EF
Tel. 01549 402401 (general information)

Human Fertilisation and Embryology Authority (HFEA)
Paxton House
30 Artillery Lane
London E1 7LS
Tel. 0171 377 5077
website: http://www.hfea.gov.uk

ISSUE
National Fertility Association
114 Lichfield Street
Walsall
West Midlands WS1 1SZ
Tel. 01922 722888

The London Women's Clinic
113-115 Harley Street
London W1N 1DG
Tel. 0171 487 5050
e-mail: lwc@lwclinic.co.uk
Donor insemination and assisted conception services.

See also British Agencies for Adoption and Fostering in **Abortion** section, above.

Chapter 13: Growing Old

Age Concern
Astral House
1268 London Road
London SW16 4ER
Tel. 0181 679 8000

Alzheimer's Disease Society
Gordon House
10 Greencoat Place
London SW1P 1PH
Tel. 0171 306 0606
website:
http://www.vois.org.uk/alzheimers
e-mail:
101762.422@compuserve.com

British Diabetic Association
10 Queen Anne Street
London W1M 0BD
Tel. 0171 323 1531
website:
http://www.diabetes.org.uk

British Heart Foundation
14 Fitzhardinge Street
London W1H 4DH
Tel. 0171 935 0185

The Continence Foundation
307 Hatton Square
16 Baldwins Gardens
London EC1N 7RG
Helpline 0171 831 9831
website: http://www.vois.org.uk\cf

Hospice Information Service
St Christopher's Hospice
51-59 Laurie Park Road
Sydenham
London SE26 6DZ
Send an SAE for details for hospice and palliative care services.

National Osteoporosis Society
PO Box 10
Radstock
Bath BA3 3YB
Tel. 01761 471771
website: http://www.nos.org.uk

Royal Association for Disability and Rehabilitation (RADAR)
12 City Forum
250 City Road
London EC1V 8AF
Tel. 0171 250 3222

Voluntary Euthanasia Society
13 Prince of Wales Terrace
London W8 5TG
Tel. 0171 937 7770
e-mail:ves.london@dial.pipex.com
Charge £3 for copy of a living will.

Chapter 14: Complementary Medicine

Association of Chartered Physiotherapists in Women's Health
Dunston House
Dunston
Lincoln LN4 2ES
Send SAE for details of services.

British Acupuncture Council
Park House
206–8 Latimer Road
London W10 6RE
Tel. 0181 964 0222

British Chiropractic Association
29 Whitley Street
Reading
Berkshire RG2 0EG
Tel. 0118 975 7557

British Society for Allergy and Environmental Medicine
Society for Nutritional Medicine
PO Box 28
Totton
Southampton
Hampshire SO40 2ZA
Tel. 01703 812124

British Society of Medical and Dental Hypnosis
73 Ware Road
Hertford
Hertfordshire SG13 7ED
Tel. 0181 905 4342

Chartered Society of Physiotherapy
14 Bedford Row
London WC1R 4ED
Tel. 0171 242 1941

The Homoeopathic Trust
2 Powis Place
Great Ormond Street
London WC1N 3HT
Tel. 0171 837 9469

The Institute of Complementary Medicine
PO Box 194
London SE16
Send an SAE for details of practitioners in your area, or for details of support groups.

National Council of Psychotherapists and Hypnotherapy Register
24 Rickmansworth Road
Watford WD1 7HT
Tel. 01483 283592

National Institute of Medical Herbalists
56 Longbrook Street
Exeter
Devon EX4 6AH
Tel. 01392 426022

Osteopathic Information Service
General Osteopathic Council
Premier House
10 Graycoat Place
London SW1P 1SB
e-mail: gosc/uk@dial.pipex.com

Register of Chinese Herbal Medicine
PO Box 400
Wembley
Middlesex HA9 9NZ
Tel. 0171 224 0803

Society for the Promotion of Nutritional Therapy
PO Box 47
Heathfield
East Sussex TN21 8ZX
Tel. 01884 255059

Chapter 16: Well-woman Check

The Health Service Ombudsman for England
11th Floor
Millbank Tower
London SW1P 4QP
Tel. 0171 276 2035

Further Reading

The following is a selection of books which may be of interest to readers who would like to know more about particular subjects.

Beech, Beverly, *Ultrasound, Unsound*, Association for Improvement in Maternity Services, London, 1994

Berryman, Julia, Thorpe, Karen, and Windridge, Kate, *Older Mothers: Conception, Pregnancy and Birth after 35*, Pandora, London, 1995

Blue, Adrianne, *On Kissing*, Indigo, London, 1997

Blythman, Joanna, *The Food We Eat*, Michael Joseph, London, 1996

Bradford, Nikki (Consultant Editor), *The Hamlyn Encyclopaedia of Complementary Health*, Hamlyn, London, 1996

Carper, Jean, *Stop Ageing Now!*, Thorsons, London, 1996

Clarke, Jane, *Body Foods for Women: Eat Your Way to Good Health*, Orion, London, 1997

Cooper, Peter J., *Bulimia Nervosa and Binge Eating: A Guide to Recovery*, Robinson Publishing, London, 1993

Crisp, Professor A.H., *Anorexia Nervosa: The Wish to Change*, Psychology Press, 1996

Davies, Vanessa, *Abortion and Afterwards*, Ashgrove Press, Bath, 1995 (rev.ed.)

Edelman, Hope, *Motherless Daughters*, Hodder and Stoughton, London, 1995

Evennett, Karen, *The PMS Diet Book*, Sheldon Press, London, 1997

Fairburn, Christopher G., *Overcoming Binge Eating*, Guilford Press, New York, 1995 (available through bookshops in UK, and through the Eating Disorders Association, see p.391)

Franklin, Caryn, and Goodman, Georgina, *Breast Health Handbook*, Pandora, London, 1996

Furse, Anna, *The Infertility Companion: A User's Guide to Tests, Technology and Therapies*, Thorsons, London, 1997

Glenville, Marilyn, *Natural Alternatives to HRT*, Kyle Cathie Ltd, London, 1997

Greer, Germaine, *The Change: Women, Age and the Menopause*, Penguin, London, 1992

Guillebaud, John, *The Pill and Other Forms of Hormonal Contraception*, Oxford University Press, 1997 (recommended by the Family Planning Association)

Heiman, Julia R., and LoPiccolo, Joseph, *Becoming Orgasmic: A Sexual and Personal Growth Programme for Women*, Piatkus, London, 1998 (recommended by Relate and the Family Planning Association)

Heyderman, Dr Eadie, *Coping with Breast Cancer*, Sheldon Press, London, 1996

Lacroix, Nitya, *Love, Sex and Intimacy*, Lorenz Books, London, 1996

Lazarides, Linda, *The Nutritional Health Bible*, Thorsons, London, 1997

Love, Dr Susan M. (with Karen Lindsey), *The Hormone Dilemma: Should You Take HRT?*, Thorsons, London, 1997

Mason, Mary-Claire, *Male Infertility: Men Talking*, Routledge, London, 1993

Mears, Jo, *Coping with Endometriosis*, Sheldon Press, London, 1996

Moquette-Magee, E., *Eat Well for a Healthy Menopause: The Low Fat, High Nutrition Guide*, John Wiley & Sons, Chichester, 1996

McConville, Brigid, *Women under the Influence: Alcohol and Its Impact*, Pandora, London, 1995 (rev.ed.)

Regan, Professor Lesley, *Miscarriage: What Every Woman Needs to Know*, Bloomsbury, London, 1997

Richardson, Diane, *Women and the Aids Crisis*, Pandora, London, 1989

Saunders, Peter, *Your Pregnancy Month by Month*, Hodder Headline, London, 1996

Simkin, Sandra, *The Case against Hysterectomy*, Pandora, London, 1996

Stacey, Sarah, and Fairley, Josephine, *The Beauty Bible*, Kyle Cathie Ltd, London, 1997

Stoppard, Dr Miriam, *The Magic of Sex*, Dorling Kindersley, London, 1991

Stoppard, Dr Miriam, *Menopause*, Dorling Kindersley, London, 1994

Thomas, Pat, *Every Woman's Birth Rights*, Thorsons, London, 1996

Wesson, Nicky, *Morning Sickness: A Comprehensive Guide to Causes and Treatments*, Vermilion, London, 1997

Woodham, Anne, and Peters, David, *The Encyclopaedia of Complementary Medicine*, Dorling Kindersley, London, 1997

Index